Hearing Loss in Children

Editors

BRADLEY W. KESSER
MARGARET A. KENNA

OTOLARYNGOLOGIC CLINICS OF NORTH AMERICA

www.oto.theclinics.com

December 2015 • Volume 48 • Number 6

ELSEVIER

1600 John F. Kennedy Boulevard • Suite 1800 • Philadelphia, Pennsylvania, 19103-2899

http://www.oto.theclinics.com

OTOLARYNGOLOGIC CLINICS OF NORTH AMERICA Volume 48, Number 6
December 2015 ISSN 0030-6665, ISBN-13: 978-0-323-41706-8

Editor: Jessica McCool
Developmental Editor: Alison Swety

Otolaryngologic Clinics of North America (ISSN 0030-6665) is published bimonthly by Elsevier, Inc., 360 Park Avenue South, New York, NY 10010-1710. Months of issue are February, April, June, August, October, and December. Business and Editorial Offices: 1600 John F. Kennedy Blvd., Suite 1800, Philadelphia, PA 19103-2899. Customer Service Office: 6277 Sea Harbor Drive, Orlando, FL 32887-4800. Periodicals postage paid at New York, NY and additional mailing offices. Subscription prices is $365.00 per year (US individuals), $692.00 per year (US institutions), $175.00 per year (US student/resident), $485.00 per year (Canadian individuals), $876.00 per year (Canadian institutions), $540.00 per year (international individuals), $876.00 per year (international institutions), $270.00 per year (international & Canadian student/resident). Foreign air speed delivery is included in all *Clinics*' subscription prices. All prices are subject to change without notice. **POSTMASTER:** Send address changes to *Otolaryngologic Clinics of North America*, Elsevier Health Sciences Division, Subscription Customer Service, 3251 Riverport Lane, Maryland Heights, MO 63043. **Telephone: 1-800-654-2452 (U.S. and Canada); 314-447-8871 (outside U.S. and Canada). Fax: 314-447-8029. E-mail: journalscustomerservice-usa@elsevier.com (for print support); journalsonlinesupport-usa@elsevier.com (for online support).**

Reprints. For copies of 100 or more of articles in this publication, please contact the Commercial Reprints Department, Elsevier Inc., 360 Park Avenue South, New York, NY 10010-1710. Tel.: 212-633-3874; Fax: 212-633-3820; E-mail: reprints@elsevier.com.

Otolaryngologic Clinics of North America is also published in Spanish by McGraw-Hill Interamericana Editores S.A., P.O. Box 5-237, 06500 Mexico D.F., Mexico.

Otolaryngologic Clinics of North America is covered in *MEDLINE/PubMed (Index Medicus), Current Contents/Clinical Medicine, Excerpta Medica, BIOSIS, Science Citation Index,* and *ISI/BIOMED.*

PROGRAM OBJECTIVE

The goal of the *Otolaryngologic Clinics of North America* is to provide information on the latest trends in patient management, the newest advances; and provide a sound basis for choosing treatment options in the field of otolaryngology.

LEARNING OBJECTIVES

Upon completion of this activity, participants will be able to:
1. Review the incidence of genetic and acquired hearing loss.
2. Discuss diagnosis, audiometric evaluation, and psychosocial aspects of pediatric hearing loss.
3. Recognize the management of pediatric hearing loss, as well as developing treatments such as cochlear implants and medical therapy for sensorineural hearing loss.

ACCREDITATION

The Elsevier Office of Continuing Medical Education (EOCME) is accredited by the Accreditation Council for Continuing Medical Education (ACCME) to provide continuing medical education for physicians.

The EOCME designates this enduring material for a maximum of 15 *AMA PRA Category 1 Credit*(s)™. Physicians should claim only the credit commensurate with the extent of their participation in the activity. All other health care professionals requesting continuing education credit for this enduring material will be issued a certificate of participation.

DISCLOSURE OF CONFLICTS OF INTEREST

The EOCME assesses conflict of interest with its instructors, faculty, planners, and other individuals who are in a position to control the content of CME activities. All relevant conflicts of interest that are identified are thoroughly vetted by EOCME for fair balance, scientific objectivity, and patient care recommendations. EOCME is committed to providing its learners with CME activities that promote improvements or quality in healthcare and not a specific proprietary business or a commercial interest.

The planning committee, staff, authors and editors listed below have identified no financial relationships or relationships to products or devices they or their spouse/life partner have with commercial interest related to the content of this CME activity:

Karen B. Avraham, PhD; Lori L. Bobsin, PhD, CCC-SLP, LSLS Cert. AVT; Kay W. Chang, MD; Daniel I. Choo, MD, FACS; Aliza P. Cohen, MA; Michael DeMarcantonio, MD; William Dougherty, MD; Anjali Fortna; Patricia Gates-Ulanet, PsyD; John H. Greinwald, MD, FAAP; Samantha Gustafson, AuD; Linda J. Hood, PhD; K. Todd Houston, PhD, CCC-SLP, LSLS Cert. AVT; Claire Iseli, MBBS, MS; Kathleen M. Kelly, MD; Margaret A. Kenna, MD, MPH; Bradley W. Kesser, MD; Tal Koffler, MSc; Anil K. Lalwani, MD; Daniel J. Lee, MD, FACS; Judith E.C. Lieu, MD, MSPH; Jessica McCool; Nancy K. Mellon, MS; Santha Priya; John Drew Prosser, MD; Sidharth V. Puram, MD, PhD; Joseph P. Roche, MD; Alison J. Singleton, AuD; Donna L. Sorkin, MA; Megan Suermann; Alison Swety; Kathy Ushakov, MSc; Susan B. Waltzman, PhD.

The planning committee, staff, authors and editors listed below have identified financial relationships or relationships to products or devices they or their spouse/life partner have with commercial interest related to the content of this CME activity:

Craig A. Buchman, MD is a consultant/advisor for Cochlear Corporation and Advanced Bionics AG.
Sharon L. Cushing, MD, MSc, FRCSC has a patent with The Hospital for Sick Children.
Marlan R. Hansen, MD receives research support from Cochlear Corporation.
Blake C. Papsin, MD, MSc, FRCSC, FACS, FAAP has a patent with The Hospital for Sick Children, and is on the speakers' bureau for Cochlear Ltd.
Anne Marie Tharpe, PhD is on the speakers' bureau for, is a consultant/advisor for, and receives research support from Sonova AG.

UNAPPROVED/OFF-LABEL USE DISCLOSURE

The EOCME requires CME faculty to disclose to the participants:
1. When products or procedures being discussed are off-label, unlabelled, experimental, and/or investigational (not US Food and Drug Administration [FDA] approved); and
2. Any limitations on the information presented, such as data that are preliminary or that represent ongoing research, interim analyses, and/or unsupported opinions. Faculty may discuss information about pharmaceutical agents that is outside of FDA-approved labelling. This information is intended solely for CME and is not intended to promote off-label use of these medications. If you have any questions, contact the medical affairs department of the manufacturer for the most recent prescribing information.

TO ENROLL

To enroll in the *Otolaryngologic Clinics of North America* Continuing Medical Education program, call customer service at 1-800-654-2452 or sign up online at http://www.theclinics.com/home/cme. The CME program is available to subscribers for an additional annual fee of USD 260.

METHOD OF PARTICIPATION

In order to claim credit, participants must complete the following:

1. Complete enrolment as indicated above.
2. Read the activity.
3. Complete the CME Test and Evaluation. Participants must achieve a score of 70% on the test. All CME Tests and Evaluations must be completed online.

CME INQUIRIES/SPECIAL NEEDS

For all CME inquiries or special needs, please contact elsevierCME@elsevier.com.

Contributors

EDITORS

BRADLEY W. KESSER, MD
Director, Otology/Neurotology; Professor, Department of Otolaryngology-Head and Neck Surgery, University of Virginia School of Medicine, Charlottesville, Virginia

MARGARET A. KENNA, MD, MPH
Director of Clinical Research, Department of Otolaryngology and Communication Enhancement, Boston Children's Hospital, Professor of Otology and Laryngology, Harvard Medical School, Boston, Massachusetts

AUTHORS

KAREN B. AVRAHAM, PhD
Department of Human Molecular Genetics and Biochemistry, Sackler Faculty of Medicine and Sagol School of Neuroscience, Tel Aviv University, Tel Aviv, Israel

LORI L. BOBSIN, PhD, CCC-SLP, LSLS Cert. AVT
Coordinator, Aural Habilitation Program, University of Virginia Cochlear Implant Program, University of Virginia Health System, Charlottesville, Virginia

CRAIG A. BUCHMAN, MD
Department of Otolaryngology-Head and Neck Surgery, University of North Carolina at Chapel Hill, Chapel Hill, North Carolina

KAY W. CHANG, MD
Associate Professor, Department of Otolaryngology, Stanford University, Stanford, California

DANIEL I. CHOO, MD, FACS
Professor and Director, Division of Pediatric Otolaryngology, Department of Otolaryngology-Head and Neck Surgery, Cincinnati Children's Hospital Medical Center, University of Cincinnati College of Medicine, Cincinnati, Ohio

ALIZA P. COHEN, MA
Division of Pediatric Otolaryngology-Head and Neck Surgery, Cincinnati Children's Hospital Medical Center, Cincinnati, Ohio

SHARON L. CUSHING, MD, MSc, FRCSC
Archie's Cochlear Implant Laboratory, Department of Otolaryngology-Head and Neck Surgery, The Hospital for Sick Children, University of Toronto, Toronto, Ontario, Canada

MICHAEL DeMARCANTONIO, MD
Department of Otolaryngology-Head and Neck Surgery, Cincinnati Children's Hospital Medical Center, University of Cincinnati College of Medicine, Cincinnati, Ohio

WILLIAM DOUGHERTY, MD
Department of Otolaryngology-Head and Neck Surgery, University of Virginia School of Medicine, Charlottesville, Virginia

PATRICIA GATES-ULANET, PsyD
The River School, Washington, DC

JOHN H. GREINWALD, MD, FAAP
Division of Pediatric Otolaryngology-Head and Neck Surgery, Ear and Hearing Center, Cincinnati Children's Hospital Medical Center; Department of Otolaryngology-Head and Neck Surgery, University of Cincinnati College of Medicine, Cincinnati, Ohio

SAMANTHA GUSTAFSON, AuD
Project Coordinator, Listening and Learning Lab, Department of Hearing and Speech Sciences, Vanderbilt Bill Wilkerson Center, Vanderbilt University School of Medicine, Nashville, Tennessee

MARLAN R. HANSEN, MD
Professor, Departments of Otolaryngology-Head and Surgery and Neurosurgery, The University of Iowa Carver College of Medicine, Iowa City, Iowa

LINDA J. HOOD, PhD
Professor, Department of Hearing and Speech Sciences, Vanderbilt University, Nashville, Tennessee; Honorary Professor, School of Rehabilitation Sciences, University of Queensland, Brisbane, Queensland, Australia

K. TODD HOUSTON, PhD, CCC-SLP, LSLS Cert. AVT
Professor of Speech-Language Pathology, Director, Telepractice and eLearning Laboratory (TeLL) School of Speech-Language Pathology and Audiology, College of Health Professions, The University of Akron, Akron, Ohio

CLAIRE ISELI, MBBS, MS
Department of Otolaryngology-Head and Neck Surgery, University of North Carolina at Chapel Hill, Chapel Hill, North Carolina; North Melbourne, Victoria, Australia

KATHLEEN M. KELLY, MD
Resident, Department of Otolaryngology-Head and Neck Surgery, University of Texas Southwestern Medical Center, Dallas, Texas

MARGARET A. KENNA, MD, MPH
Director of Clinical Research, Department of Otolaryngology and Communication Enhancement, Boston Children's Hospital, Professor of Otology and Laryngology, Harvard Medical School, Boston, Massachusetts

BRADLEY W. KESSER, MD
Director, Otology/Neurotology; Professor, Department of Otolaryngology-Head and Neck Surgery, University of Virginia School of Medicine, Charlottesville, Virginia

TAL KOFFLER, MSc
Department of Human Molecular Genetics and Biochemistry, Sackler Faculty of Medicine and Sagol School of Neuroscience, Tel Aviv University, Tel Aviv, Israel

ANIL K. LALWANI, MD
Professor and Vice Chair for Research Otolaryngology-Head and Neck Surgery; Chief, Division of Otology, Neurology and Skull Base Surgery; Director, Columbia Cochlear

Implant Program, Department of Otolaryngology-Head and Neck Surgery, Medical Director, Perioperative Services, New York Presbyterian – Columbia University Medical Center, Columbia University College of Physicians and Surgeons, New York, New York

DANIEL J. LEE, MD, FACS
Department of Otolaryngology, Massachusetts Eye and Ear Infirmary; Department of Otology and Laryngology, Harvard Medical School, Boston, Massachusetts

JUDITH E.C. LIEU, MD, MSPH
Associate Professor, Program Director, Vice Chair for Graduate Medical Education, Department of Otolaryngology-Head and Neck Surgery, Washington University School of Medicine, St Louis, Missouri

NANCY K. MELLON, MS
Head of School, The River School, Washington, DC

BLAKE C. PAPSIN, MD, MSc, FRCSC, FACS, FAAP
Archie's Cochlear Implant Laboratory, Department of Otolaryngology-Head and Neck Surgery, The Hospital for Sick Children, University of Toronto, Toronto, Ontario, Canada

JOHN DREW PROSSER, MD
Division of Pediatric Otolaryngology-Head and Neck Surgery, Cincinnati Children's Hospital Medical Center, Cincinnati, Ohio

SIDHARTH V. PURAM, MD, PhD
Department of Otolaryngology, Massachusetts Eye and Ear Infirmary; Department of Otology and Laryngology, Harvard Medical School, Boston, Massachusetts

JOSEPH P. ROCHE, MD
Neurotology Fellow, Department of Otolaryngology-Head and Surgery, The University of Iowa Carver College of Medicine, Iowa City, Iowa

ALISON J. SINGLETON, AuD
Audiologist, Department of Otolaryngology, NYU Cochlear Implant Center, NYU Langone Medical Center, NYU School of Medicine, New York, New York

DONNA L. SORKIN, MA
Executive Director, American Cochlear Implant Alliance, McLean, Virginia

ANNE MARIE THARPE, PhD
Professor and Chair, Department of Hearing and Speech Sciences, Associate Director, Vanderbilt Bill Wilkerson Center, Vanderbilt University School of Medicine, Nashville, Tennessee

KATHY USHAKOV, MSc
Department of Human Molecular Genetics and Biochemistry, Sackler Faculty of Medicine and Sagol School of Neuroscience, Tel Aviv University, Tel Aviv, Israel

SUSAN B. WALTZMAN, PhD
Marcia F. Vilcek Professor of Otolaryngology; Co-Director, Department of Otolaryngology, NYU Cochlear Implant Center, NYU Langone Medical Center, NYU School of Medicine, New York, New York

Contents

bilateral hearing loss. The World Health Organization notes that, worldwide, there are 360 million people with disabling hearing loss, with 50% preventable. Although many hearing losses are acquired, many others are manifestations of preexisting conditions. The purpose of a pediatric hearing evaluation is to identify the degree and type of hearing loss and etiology and to outline a comprehensive strategy that supports language and social development and communication.

approach by a team of health professionals, including audiologists, speech pathologists, otolaryngologists, pediatricians, genetic counselors, and early intervention programs. Early diagnosis and intervention offers the best chance for speech and language acquisition. Although hearing aids can provide some of the needed information, they are often not sufficient for spoken language development and a cochlear implant is needed. This must be combined with a strong audiology and speech therapy rehabilitation program.

autosomal-dominant (AD) inheritance. Although AR nonsyndromic SNHL is most commonly caused by GJB2 and SLC26A4, there is no single gene that accounts for any significant proportion of AD SNHL. High-throughput sequencing techniques, also called next-generation sequencing (NGS) or massively parallel sequencing (MPS), may allow for routine definitive diagnosis of all possible genetic causes for hearing loss in the not-too-distant future.

Videos of typical operating room setup for pediatric ABI surgery and key steps in pediatric ABI surgery accompany this article

Auditory brainstem implants (ABIs) provide auditory perception in patients with profound hearing loss who are not candidates for the cochlear implant (CI) because of anatomic constraints or failed CI surgery. Herein, the authors discuss (1) preoperative evaluation of pediatric ABI candidates, (2) surgical approaches, and (3) contemporary ABI devices and their use in the pediatric population. The authors also review the surgical and audiologic outcomes following pediatric ABI surgery. The authors' institutional experience and the nearly 200 cases performed in Europe and the United States indicate that ABI surgery in children can be safe and effective.

Hearing loss is the most common sensory deficit in developed societies. Hearing impairment in children, particularly of prelingual onset, has been shown to negatively affect educational achievement, future employment and earnings, and even life expectancy. Sensorineural hearing loss (SNHL), which refers to defects within the cochlea or auditory nerve itself, far outweighs conductive causes for permanent hearing loss in both children and adults. The causes of SNHL in children are heterogeneous, including both congenital and acquired causes. This article identifies potential mechanisms of intervention both at the level of the hair cell and the spiral ganglion neurons.

OTOLARYNGOLOGIC CLINICS
OF NORTH AMERICA

THE CLINICS ARE AVAILABLE ONLINE!
Access your subscription at:
www.theclinics.com

Preface

The Child with Hearing Loss

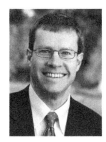 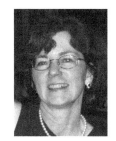

Bradley W. Kesser, MD   Margaret A. Kenna, MD, MPH
Editors

Perhaps no other field in otolaryngology has expanded as rapidly as the evaluation and management of hearing loss in children. From safer and higher-resolution imaging techniques to more focused genetic analyses, the old ratio of congenital sensorineural hearing loss, 25-25-50, idiopathic-acquired-genetic, is rapidly changing as many idiopathic causes for hearing loss are being elucidated, and many specific causes of genetic hearing loss have been discovered. With the widespread mandate of newborn hearing screening in every state, children with hearing loss are being identified earlier and, ideally, diagnosed by 3 months of age with intervention by 6 months of age. However, diagnosing the cause of hearing loss in the young child remains challenging, and clinicians are left to ponder who should be tested, when, and what tests to order. Genotype-phenotype correlations and techniques from linkage algorithms to whole genome screening have mapped deafness and other associated traits to specific chromosomes in the human genome, allowing researchers and clinicians to identify many of the causes of both syndromic and nonsyndromic pediatric sensorineural hearing loss. Interestingly, the genetic analysis of hearing loss has shed light on the structure, physiology, function, and development of the cochlea and other inner ear structures. With over 100 specific genes identified whose mutation causes hearing loss (with likely more by the time this is published!), keeping up with the science is quite challenging for clinicians (see the Hereditary Hearing Loss homepage at hereditaryhearingloss.org).

Whether to order computed tomography (CT) or magnetic resonance imaging (MRI) is often a question asked at otolaryngology meetings in the evaluation of children with hearing loss. The answer, of course, depends on the clinical question being asked and the nature of the hearing loss. One article in this issue comprehensively discusses imaging for pediatric hearing loss, the ideal study, when to pursue it, and what to look for.

Cytomegalovirus (CMV) is now recognized as the most common viral cause of congenital hearing loss and a likely cause of progressive hearing loss. Although the optimal diagnostic test as well as management of CMV remains in flux, this common

Otolaryngol Clin N Am 48 (2015) xv–xvi
http://dx.doi.org/10.1016/j.otc.2015.09.018
0030-6665/15/$ – see front matter © 2015 Published by Elsevier Inc.

oto.theclinics.com

virus needs to be recognized as an important part of the newborn hearing loss diagnostic effort.

Management options for children with hearing loss include any number of interventions from individualized education programs to surgery to hearing aids (conventional and bone conducting), cochlear implantation, and even brain stem implants. Several articles address these options for children with both conductive and sensorineural hearing loss, including an entire article addressing the child with unilateral hearing loss, an often difficult clinical scenario to assess and manage.

In summary, we asked the world's leading pediatric otologic clinicians and scientists to present the most up-to-date, evidence-based recommendations to guide clinicians—otolaryngologists, pediatricians, audiologists, speech-language therapists, and other hearing health care professionals—in the workup and habilitation of these children. And what is coming down the road? Better cochlear implant technology and coding strategies, auditory brainstem implant technology, and finally, gene therapy or stem cell therapy for sensorineural hearing loss are all exciting prospects for the near and distant future.

We also cannot thank enough the authors who have generously donated their time and expertise to make this issue of *Otolaryngologic Clinics of North America* a practical, informative, exciting, and relevant addition to the ever-expanding literature on hearing loss in children, and who provide outstanding care for these children every day.

Bradley W. Kesser, MD
Department of Otolaryngology-Head
and Neck Surgery
University of Virginia School of Medicine
Box 800713
Charlottesville, VA 22908-0713, USA

Margaret A. Kenna, MD, MPH
Department of Otolaryngology
and Communication Enhancement
Boston Children's Hospital
300 Longwood Avenue, BCH 3129
Boston, MA 02115, USA

E-mail addresses:
Bwk2n@virginia.edu (B.W. Kesser)
margaret.kenna@childrens.harvard.edu (M.A. Kenna)

Audiometric Evaluation of Children with Hearing Loss

Alison J. Singleton, AuD, Susan B. Waltzman, PhD*

KEYWORDS

- Pediatric hearing loss • Evaluation • Diagnosis • Measures

KEY POINTS

- Early diagnosis of pediatric hearing loss is possible and desirable.
- Measurement tools are available to diagnosis all types of hearing loss in children of all ages.
- Medical and surgical intervention and rehabilitation can begin at a very young age because of the ability to measure hearing loss effectively.

INTRODUCTION

The goal of pediatric audiologic assessment is to determine if a hearing loss exists and to diagnose the type, degree, and specific nature of the hearing loss. The types of hearing loss include conductive, sensorineural, and mixed; the degree is defined in **Table 1**.

The accuracy of the results is crucial because the treatment plan depends on the outcome of the diagnosis. To choose appropriate techniques, consideration must be given to the child's age, developmental status, physical status, and functional age level. Best practices involve using a test battery approach and not relying solely on one measure to avoid the possibility of error by using the cross-check principle.[1]

SCREENING FOR HEARING LOSS

Early detection of any amount and type of hearing loss leads to earlier intervention increasing the possibility that a child can reach his or her developmental potential in all areas. Mandatory newborn hearing screening has significantly reduced the age

The authors have nothing to disclose.
Department of Otolaryngology, NYU Cochlear Implant Center, NYU Langone Medical Center, NYU School of Medicine, 660 First Avenue, 7th Floor, New York, NY 10016, USA
* Corresponding author.
E-mail address: susan.waltzman@nyumc.org

Otolaryngol Clin N Am **48** (2015) 891–901
http://dx.doi.org/10.1016/j.otc.2015.06.002
0030-6665/15/$ – see front matter © 2015 Elsevier Inc. All rights reserved.
oto.theclinics.com

Abbreviations	
ABR	Auditory brainstem response
BOA	Behavioral observation audiometry
CAPD	Central auditory processing disorder
CPA	Conditioned play audiometry
OAE	Otoacoustic emissions
SRT	Speech reception threshold

at which hearing loss is identified, from approximately 14 months of age for significant hearing loss and from 2.5 years of age for less severe degrees of hearing loss to ideally 3 months of age. Late identification of hearing loss causes a lag in the needed medical and audiologic treatment and increases the possibility of delayed linguistic and overall development. Because approximately 2 to 3 per 1000 babies in the United States are born with some amount of hearing loss in one or both ears, the value of newborn hearing screening programs is evident. Currently in the United States, 95% of newborn babies are screened before hospital discharge, although follow-up of all children has been more difficult to achieve.[2,3] Screening is most frequently accomplished using either auditory brainstem response (ABR) testing and/or otoacoustic emissions (OAEs) testing and is performed ideally before the newborn leaves the hospital.

Otoacoustic Emissions

OAEs are sounds given off by outer hair cells when the cochlea is stimulated by sound. The movement of outer hair cells produces an inaudible sound that echoes back into the middle ear, which can be measured with a small microphone inserted into the ear canal. The status of the middle ear affects OAEs and can prevent their detection while assisting in the diagnosis of middle ear effusion or other middle ear conditions that cause conductive hearing loss.

Auditory Brainstem Response

ABR measures the auditory nerve and brain's response to sound. It uses surface electrodes placed on the head to measure the coordinated electrical activity of the auditory nerve and brainstem relay pathways when the ear is stimulated by sound. Measuring the threshold (minimum sound intensity to elicit the electrical response) greatly assists in the diagnosis of sensorineural hearing loss.

Table 1
Classification of degree of hearing loss

Hearing Level (dB)	Classification of Hearing Loss
≤0–15	Normal hearing
16–25	Slight hearing loss
26–40	Mild hearing loss
41–55	Moderate hearing loss
56–70	Moderately severe hearing loss
71–90	Severe hearing loss
91+	Profound hearing loss

From Clark JG. Puretone evaluation. In: Katz J, editor. Handbook of clinical audiology. 5th edition. Baltimore (MD): Lippincott Williams & Wilkins; 2002. p. 82; with permission.

These two screening techniques can lead to the diagnosis of mild to profound hearing loss be they conductive or sensorineural in nature (and are covered in greater depth later in the article). A definitive diagnosis requires follow-up after hospital discharge. According to the Joint Committee on Infant Hearing 2007 Position Statement, all infants should have access to hearing screening by 1 month of age. If the infant did not pass the hearing screening and subsequent rescreenings, a diagnostic audiologic evaluation and medical evaluation should be performed to confirm the presence of hearing loss by 3 months of age. All infants with confirmed hearing loss should receive intervention by 6 months of age.[3]

BEHAVIORAL AUDIOMETRY

Although these objective electrophysiologic measures provide an estimate of hearing levels, they are not a substitute for behavioral testing. The diagnosis of hearing loss requires at least ear-specific pure tone air and bone testing, which can be accomplished using age-dependent measures. Because behavioral testing is not a viable approach in infants, behavioral observation audiometry (BOA) is often used as an adjunct to electrophysiologic methods when the infant is younger than the age of 6 months. Although BOA does not provide ear-specific information or information regarding absolute thresholds, it does assess the infant's reflexive response to auditory stimuli including warbled pure tones, narrow-band noise, and speech signals presented through speakers in a sound field. Reflexive responses include full body startle, head/limb reflex, and eye blink. Attentive responses include motion cessation; eye widening; and in older infants smiling, laughing, pointing, and the cessation/initiation of crying or babbling. In general, the responses should be seen within a few seconds of the stimulus presentation (**Table 2**).[4]

From the age of approximately 6 months to 2 years, visual reinforcement audiometry is used to estimate auditory thresholds based on responses that have been shown to be closely aligned with pure tone thresholds obtained with the standard hand raising technique used in older children and adults. The goal is to obtain ear- and frequency-specific information before the child loses interest. The method requires that a child turn her or his head toward the sound source that is coupled with conditioned reinforcement, such as a lighted toy. In an ideal situation, two audiologists are used: one to initiate the stimulus and the second to observe the child's response. The response should be time-locked to within a few seconds of the stimulus presentation

Table 2	
Auditory maturation of normal hearing infants	
Age	**Auditory Maturation**
0–4 mo	Newborn behavioral responses to auditory stimulus are limited to reflexive actions
4–7 mo	Response to sound is a horizontal head turn toward the side of the sound source 4-mo head turn is slow 6-mo head turn is definite and brisk
7 mo	Localize sound source in lower plane (looking downward)
9 mo	Locate sound source when presented above head height
12 mo	Locate sound source in any plane on either side of the body easily and briskly

Knowledge of the auditory maturation can provide useful and predictive information in the difficult-to-evaluate child with developmental delays.

Data from Northern JL, Downs MP. Behavioral hearing tests with children. In: Northern JL, Downs MP, editors. Hearing in children. 6th edition. San Diego (CA): Plural Publishing, Inc; 2014. p. 247–307.

for it to be considered a true response. The paradigm is stimulus-response-reinforcement: a stimulus (either a pure tone or speech) is presented and the child learns that a response (turning head toward stimulus source) will result in reinforcement, usually an animated toy enclosed in smoked plexiglass.[4] Note that some children are frightened by some animations so alternatives should be available. To obtain ear-specific information insert earphones or standard headphones should be used. Either is acceptable depending on the will of the child. It is also possible that some children will not accept any form of earphone and sound field testing will have to be substituted. In this case, the results are a reflection of the better hearing ear only. Results should be combined with OAEs, tympanometry, and reflexes to obtain a total picture regarding hearing status.

Conditioned Play Audiometry

Conditioned play audiometry (CPA) is the next level of behavioral testing and can often be used with children 2 years of age through 4 to 5 years of age. The primary goal of CPA is to obtain ear- and frequency-specific thresholds via air and bone conduction allowing for the diagnosis of conductive, sensorineural, or mixed hearing loss. For air conduction testing, insert earphones should be used, whereas a bone oscillator is placed for bone conduction testing. The test used a form of operant conditioning where the child is taught to wait, listen for a tone or speech signal, and then perform an activity as a response.[4] Most popular tasks include putting a block in a box, pegs in a board, or doing a simple puzzle. In some situations with the consent of the parent or guardian, the child can be offered a tangible item (ie, food or candy) as a reward. It is important not only to choose a task that the child can perform with ease but also to switch tasks often to avoid boredom. As with all the evaluation procedures, CPA needs to be combined with OAEs, tympanometry, and reflexes to obtain a complete picture. There can also be situations where the child because of the existence of multiple disabilities and/or delays cannot respond adequately. In these cases, ABR testing is recommended to obtain a clearer picture of hearing status.

By 5 years of age in a child with average cognitive abilities and some extra encouragement, children should be able to be tested using standard pure tone testing techniques, such as hand-raising or button pushing, and ear-specific air and bone conduction thresholds should be obtained with relative ease.

SPEECH AUDIOMETRY

Although pure tone thresholds provide the information regarding type and degree of hearing loss, speech perception measures provide insight into the extent the hearing loss affects the child's ability to hear, recognize, and understand simple and complex speech stimuli. Testing can be performed using headphones for individual ear information and/or sound field, if necessary. The most basic speech testing is the speech detection threshold, which is defined as the lowest level (intensity) that a child is aware that a speech signal is being delivered. The next, and more informative, level of testing is the measurement of the speech reception threshold (SRT), which provides a quick estimate of hearing levels in each ear and is obtained using two-syllable spondee words specifically designed for children. SRT is the minimum intensity (measured in decibels hearing level) at which the child can repeat 50% of a spondee word list. The SRT correlates well to pure tone averages (within 6 dB) providing an excellent validation of degree of hearing loss. There are numerous methods to obtain an accurate SRT including picture cards, spondee toys (ie, toothbrush, airplane, hot dog), and the

Children's Spondee Word list.[5] The method used depends on the age and cognitive level of the child as determined by the clinician.

Speech Perception Testing

The next level of speech testing involves determining the ability of the child to understand speech at suprathreshold levels (ie, conversational speech). The speech perception test provides particular insight into the extent to which a hearing loss affects everyday understanding of speech and often provides the initial clue to additional cognitive disabilities. There are numerous speech discrimination tests to choose from depending on the age and level of the child and the preference of the audiologist. The tests can be administered live voice or recorded depending on the needs of the child and are divided into two categories: closed set and open set tests. In closed set tests, the child has a limited set of test items from which to choose, compared with open-set tests, which are more challenging because the response set is not limited: the child simply repeats what he or she hears.

Table 3 includes some of the standard pediatric speech perception tests available for evaluating children with hearing loss. In recent years perception tests have been developed specifically for those children with moderate-to-severe-to-profound sensorineural hearing loss who are being considered for cochlear implantation and for evaluation following implantation (**Table 4**). There is, however, no reason not to consider these tests for use in children with all levels of hearing loss.

Table 3 Speech perception measures	
Closed-Set Tests	
Auditory Numbers Test (ANT)[6]	Simple auditory test, child must be able to count to 5 Picture pointing response Picture cards have groups of one to five ants on them
Sound Effects Recognition Test (SERT)[7]	An alternative to traditional speech tests to assess children with very limited verbal abilities Test uses familiar environmental sounds instead of speech stimuli (ie, dog barking, toilet flushing, baby crying) Picture pointing response Minimum age 3 y
Pediatric Speech Intelligibility (PSI)[8,9]	20 monosyllabic words and 10 sentences (showing actions) Picture pointing response Minimum age 3 y
Northwestern University Children's Perception of Speech (NU-CHIPS)[10]	Based on receptive vocabulary of 3–5 y olds Picture pointing response Four pictures per card
Word Intelligibility by Picture Identification (WIPI)[11]	Based on receptive vocabulary of children 4–6 y old Picture pointing response Six pictures per card Is more difficult than NU-CHIPS because more test items per card and requires finer auditory skills because the foils are more challenging
Open-Set Tests	
Phonetically Balanced Kindergarten (PB-K)[12]	Based on vocabulary of a typical kindergartener (age 5) 50 monosyllabic words

Note: NU-CHIPS and WIPI can be used without the pictures making them open-set measures.

Table 4
Speech perception measures used with cochlear implants

Closed-Set Tests	
Monosyllabic Trochee Spondee (MTS)[13]	12 words: four monosyllabic, four trochees, four spondees Score is representative of the correct stress pattern and the number of words correctly identified Picture pointing response
Glendonald Auditory Screening Procedure (GASP)[14]	Similar to the MTS 12 words: three monosyllabic, three trochees, three spondees 10 common everyday sentences and phoneme detection task Picture pointing response
Early Speech Perception Test (ESP)[15]	Assesses pattern perception, spondee identification, and monosyllable identification Standard and low verbal versions uses pictures or objects Minimum age 2 y Scoring is based on four categories 　Category 1: no pattern perception 　Category 2: pattern perception 　Category 3: some word identification 　Category 4: consistent word identification
Open-Set Tests	
Multisyllabic Lexical Neighborhood Test (MLNT) and Lexical Neighborhood Test (LNT)[16]	Assesses word recognition and lexical discrimination in children with hearing loss Test vocabulary is that of a profoundly deaf child age 3–5 MLNT: two- and three-syllable words LNT: monosyllabic words
Hearing in Noise Test for Children (HINT-C)[17]	130 sentences divided into 13 lists of 10 sentences each Administered in quiet or speech-shaped noise 5 y of age or older
Pediatric AzBio sentence[18]	320 sentences divided into 16 lists of 20 sentences each Administered in quiet or multitalker babble Sentences have a rather high linguistic complexity

Although these lists are by no means exhaustive, they are representative of the tests available to evaluate the hearing-impaired child. It is up to the clinician to decide the appropriateness of a given measure depending on the age, level of hearing loss, and level of functioning of a particular child.

An additional confounding factor is the presence of a central auditory processing disorder (CAPD), defined as a deficiency in the ability of the brain to fully interpret and process sound. Although children with this disorder by definition have normal peripheral hearing, their failure to respond appropriately to pure tone and speech stimuli particularly in noise can be mistaken for hearing loss. Inconsistencies between subjective and objective testing and behavioral observations, often made by a multidisciplinary team consisting of teachers, psychologists, and speech-language pathologists, can assist with the diagnosis. CAPD is most often accompanied by other disabilities, such as reading and language disorders and attention deficit issues. If CAPD is suspected, a test battery (eg, SCAN-3:C) can be administered (generally to children at least 7 or 8 years old). Electrophysiologic measures can also aid in making the diagnosis when behavioral testing is not feasible. Often neuropsychologists and audiologists, when evaluating children for CAPD, do a battery of tests that look at auditory memory and other auditory processing tasks that seem to be reliable and specific indicators of auditory processing deficits (but only in the presence of normal peripheral hearing).

OBJECTIVE MEASURES

Physiologic measures of auditory system function can be obtained without the child's participation (nonbehavioral; ie, does not require any active response from the child). Although behavioral measures are the "gold standard" for obtaining definitive thresholds, objective measures are a valuable part of the pediatric test battery in that they provide useful information and serve as a cross-check to behavioral methods.[1] The tests can be performed while the child is awake, asleep, in a resting state, or under sedation, and thus are effective in very young children, multiply disabled children, and others who cannot complete the tasks necessary for behavioral testing.

Acoustic Immittance Measures

Acoustic immittance measures help to assess middle ear transfer function and auditory pathway integrity and confirm conductive hearing loss caused by middle ear effusion or other abnormality. Because the middle ear system transfers vibrational energy in air to fluid waves in the cochlea, measures of immittance provide information regarding the integrity of the middle ear sound conducting system and its ability to transfer the mechanical energy of sound to the fluid in the cochlea.[19]

Tympanometry

Tympanometry is the dynamic measure of acoustic immittance of the middle ear as a function of ear canal pressure. A probe placed in the ear canal forms an air-tight seal, delivers a tone, varies the air pressure, and measures the acoustic energy in the canal. A classification system is used to describe the shape of the curve that reflects middle ear admittance and its concomitant middle ear pathology (**Table 5**).

Acoustic Reflex Threshold

The acoustic reflex threshold is a measurement of the suprathreshold sound intensity needed to cause a change in middle ear immittance (increased resistance or stiffness) because of the contraction of the stapedius muscle. Absent or elevated reflex thresholds can indicate either middle ear or cochlear pathology. The amplitude, latency, and decay are quantified to reflect various pathologies. A normal-hearing ear requires a sound of approximately 60 dB sensation level (above threshold) to elicit the reflex. Reflexes may be present at reduced sensation levels for children with sensory loss (ie, cochlear pathology) and may be absent for children with neural loss (ie, retrocochlear pathology/eighth nerve lesion) or a conductive hearing loss.[19] Reflex measurements are still used as part of a test battery particularly when behavioral measures of acoustic thresholds cannot be obtained. Their usefulness as a tool to diagnose eighth nerve lesions, rare in children, is less valuable because of a high number of false positives and the advent of MRI.

Otoacoustic Emissions

OAEs are signals generated by the outer hair cells of the cochlea that travel outward into the middle ear space and ear canal. They are elicited by a stimulus delivered via a probe placed in the ear canal, which then measures the sound reflected back. Currently there are two types of evoked OAEs used for clinical assessment: transient-evoked OAEs, which stimulate the cochlea using a transient signal (ie, click); and distortion product OAEs, which stimulate the cochlea using two different pure

Table 5
Jerger's classification system of tympanograms

Type	Description	Indicative of
Type A	Normal static admittance, normal height of peak Normal ME pressure	Normal ME function
Type A$_s$	Abnormally low static admittance, "shallow" or reduced peak height Normal ME pressure	Reduced TM mobility Ossicular abnormalities or fixation (otosclerosis) Thick or scarred tympanic membrane Severe tympanosclerosis
Type A$_d$	Abnormally high static admittance, "deep" or increased peak height Normal ME pressure	Increased TM mobility Ossicular disarticulation Extremely flaccid eardrum
Type B	No change in static admittance as air pressure in external ear is varied, no peak	"Flat" tympanogram ME effusion (normal ear canal volume) TM perforation (large ear canal volume) Patent ventilation tubes (large ear canal volume) Occluding cerumen (small ear canal volume)
Type C	Near-normal static admittance ME pressure of -200 daPa or worse[a]	"Negative" pressure tympanogram Eustachian tube dysfunction

Abbreviations: ME, middle ear; TM, tympanic membrane.
[a] Limits of normal/abnormal ME pressure may vary and clinics may have their own norms.
Data from Jerger J. Clinical experience with impedance audiometry. Arch Otolaryngol 1970;92:311–24.

tones simultaneously.[19] Because OAEs are usually absent if a hearing loss is greater than 30 dB, they can be helpful in the diagnosis of hearing loss and the monitoring of cochlear function in children too young or not able to complete behavioral testing. It is important to obtain tympanometric measures in conjunction with OAEs to rule out the presence of a conductive hearing loss and middle ear pathology so as not to misdiagnose. Because OAEs are quick to administer, they are often used as a neonatal hearing screening tool and for monitoring cochlear function in children receiving potentially ototoxic medication. OAEs can also be valuable in the diagnosis of auditory neuropathy in children. Present OAEs in the absence of responses on ABR have been associated with a diagnosis of auditory neuropathy and are often the first indication of the pathology (discussed in more detail elsewhere in this issue).

Auditory Brainstem Response

ABR is the electrical potential recorded from a signal, generated by a sound, as it travels along the auditory pathway. It can be performed on children, either under sedation or sleeping, who are too young or incapable of performing behavioral audiometry. The results are used to estimate thresholds using both air and bone conduction transducers. Although the most common stimulus used is a click, tone-bursts can be used to obtain frequency-specific information, and correction factors are applied to convert the results to estimate hearing thresholds. It is common to begin testing at high intensity levels where all waveforms can be seen and systematically reduce the presentation level to where only a wave V is seen when nearing threshold, defined as the minimum intensity of sound needed to generate a reliable wave V repsonse.[19] Screening ABRs are often used for neonatal screening in conjunction with OAEs.

Table 6 Commonly used functional assessment measures		
Measure	**Age Range**	**Description**
Infant Toddler Meaningful Auditory Integration Scale (IT-MAIS)[20]	Birth–3 y	Parent questionnaire 10 questions that evaluate the extent to which a child makes meaningful use of sound in everyday life
Meaningful Auditory Integration Scale (MAIS)[21,22]	3 y+	Parent questionnaire Same purpose as IT-MAIS just designed for older children
Little Ears: Auditory Questionnaire[23]	Birth+	Parent questionnaire 35 questions to address auditory development at various ages
Children's Home Inventory for Listening Difficulties (CHILD)[24]	3–12 y	Questionnaire designed for child and parent Rate how well the child understands speech in 15 situations
Auditory Behavior in Everyday Life (ABEL)[25]	2–12 y	Evaluates auditory behavior in everyday life via a 24-item questionnaire

It is important to emphasize that electrophysiologic methods and behavioral testing are not mutually exclusive and are best used in conjunction with one another. The information obtained from each form of testing is synchronous and provides a total picture of the type and degree of the hearing loss.

FUNCTIONAL AUDITORY ASSESSMENT TOOLS

No discussion of pediatric assessment is complete without a mention of functional assessment tools. In addition to obtaining absolute information regarding the hearing status of a child, it is important to know how the child responds to sound and functions in daily life and the day-to-day effects of hearing impairment. There are numerous questionnaires designed for parents, caregivers, teachers, and so forth that help provide needed information regarding the child so that a total picture is obtained and an accurate treatment plan is developed. **Table 6** provides a list, hardly exhaustive, of some of the more commonly used tools.

SUMMARY

This article provides the reader with basic knowledge regarding the measurement tools needed to assess pediatric hearing loss. It is meant to be a starting point in the evaluation process and designed to be integrated into areas covered elsewhere in this issue. Although it has not specifically addressed the testing of those children with multiple and pervasive disabilities, the test battery described here is adaptable and interchangeable to meet the needs of the entire pediatric population no matter what the age or developmental stage. It is meant to provide the team of professionals involved in the treatment of pediatric hearing disorders with a framework from which the process of diagnosis, treatment, and rehabilitation can begin.

REFERENCES

1. Jerger J, Hayes D. The cross-check principle in pediatric audiometry. Arch Otolaryngol 1976;102:614–20.

2. Centers for Disease Control and Prevention (CDC). Identifying infants with hearing loss—United States, 1999–2007. MMWR Morb Mortal Wkly Rep 2010;59(8):220–3.
3. Joint Committee on Infant Hearing. Year 2007 position statement: principles and guidelines for early hearing detection and intervention programs. Pediatrics 2007;120(4):898–921.
4. Diefendorf A. Detection and assessment of hearing loss in infants and children. In: Katz J, editor. Handbook of clinical audiology. 5th edition. Baltimore (MD): Lippincott Williams & Wilkins; 2002. p. 469–80.
5. Northern JL, Downs MP. Behavioral hearing tests with children. In: Northern JL, Downs MP, editors. Hearing in children. 6th edition. San Diego (CA): Plural Publishing, Inc; 2014. p. 247–307.
6. Erber NP. Use of the auditory numbers test to evaluate speech perception abilities of hearing impaired children. J Speech Hear Disord 1980;45:527–32.
7. Finitzo-Hieber T, Gerling IJ, Matkin ND, et al. A sound effects recognition test for the pediatric audiologic evaluation. Ear Hear 1980;1:271.
8. Jerger S, Lewis S, Hawkins J, et al. Pediatric Speech Intelligibility Test: I. Generation of test materials. Int J Pediatr Otorhinolaryngol 1980;2:217–30.
9. Jerger S, Jerger J, Lewis S. Pediatric Speech Intelligibility Test: II. Effect of receptive language age and chronological age. Int J Pediatr Otorhinolaryngol 1981;3:101–18.
10. Elliott LL, Katz D. Development of a new children's test of speech discrimination [technical manual]. St Louis (MO): Auditec; 1980.
11. Ross M, Lerman J. A picture identification test for hearing-impaired children. J Speech Hear Res 1970;13:44–53.
12. Haskins H. A phonetically balanced test of speech discrimination for children. Evanston (IL): Northwestern University; 1949 [Unpublished master's thesis].
13. Erber NP, Alencewicz CM. Audiologic evaluation of deaf children. J Speech Hear Disord 1972;41:256–67.
14. Erber NP. Auditory training. Washington, DC: Alexander Graham Bell Association for the Deaf; 1982.
15. Moog JS, Geers AE. Early speech perception test for profoundly hearing-impaired children. St Louis (MO): Central Institute for the Deaf; 1990.
16. Kirk KI, Pisoni DB, Osberger MJ. Lexical effects on spoken word recognition by pediatric cochlear implant users. Ear Hear 1995;16:470–81.
17. Nilsson MJ, Soli SD, Gelnett DJ. Development of the sharing in noise test for children (HINT-C). Los Angeles (CA): House Ear Institute; 1996.
18. Spahr AJ, Dorman MF, Litvak LM, et al. Development and validation of the pediatric AzBio sentence lists. Ear Hear 2014;35(4):418–22.
19. Northern JL, Downs MP. Physiologic hearing tests. In: Northern JL, Downs MP, editors. Hearing in children. 6th edition. San Diego (CA): Plural Publishing, Inc; 2014. p. 309–71.
20. Zimmerman-Phillips S, Osberger MF, Robbins AM. Infant-toddler: meaningful auditory integration scale (IT-MAIS). Sylmar (CA): Advanced Bionics Corp; 1997.
21. Robbins AM, Renshaw JJ, Berry SW. Evaluating meaningful integration in profoundly hearing impaired children. Am J Otol 1991;12(Suppl):144–50.
22. Robbins AM, Renshaw JJ, Berry SW. Meaningful auditory integration scale. In: Estabrooks W, editor. Cochlear implants for kids. Washington, DC: AG Bell Assoc. for the Deaf, Inc; 1998. p. 373–86.
23. Kuehn-Inacker H, Weichbold V, Tsiakpini L, et al. Questionnaire for the parent with 35 age-dependent questions that assesses auditory development. Little ears: auditory questionnaire. Innsbruck (Austria): MED-EL; 2003.

24. Anderson KL, Smaldino JJ. Children's Home Inventory for Listening Difficulties (CHILD). 2000.
25. Purdy S, Farrington DR, Moran CA, et al. A parental questionnaire to evaluate children's auditory behavior in everyday life (ABEL). Am J Audiol 2002;11:72–82.

Taking the History and Performing the Physical Examination in a Child with Hearing Loss

Sharon L. Cushing, MD, MSc, FRCSC*, Blake C. Papsin, MD, MSc, FRCSC

KEYWORDS

- Sensorineural hearing loss • Children • Physical examination • History
- Vestibular function • Conductive hearing loss

KEY POINTS

- Hearing loss is one of the most common disorders of childhood and has far reaching impact on communication.
- A working knowledge of the physical features associated with syndromic causes of hearing loss is essential.
- Findings on history and physical examination may help tailor the use of diagnostic and ancillary testing yielding a cost-effective approach.
- Early rehabilitation is essential and should not be delayed while determining the underlying cause.
- Vestibular and balance function should be assessed in all children presenting with hearing loss.

INTRODUCTION

Don't tell me the sky is the limit when there are footprints on the moon
—Paul Brandt (1972), Canadian songwriter from the song,
There's a World Out There, 1999

The limits of the evaluative, diagnostic, and treatment algorithms for pediatric hearing loss are ever changing. What has driven the expansion in these domains

---

Disclosures: No disclosures (S.L. Cushing). B.C. Papsin is a member of the speaker's bureau with Cochlear Americas.
Archie's Cochlear Implant Laboratory, Department of Otolaryngology Head and Neck Surgery, The Hospital for Sick Children, University of Toronto, 555 University Avenue, Toronto, Ontario M5G 1X8, Canada
* Corresponding author. Department of Otolaryngology Head and Neck Surgery, The Hospital for Sick Children, 555 University Avenue, Room 6103C Burton Wing, Toronto, Ontario M5G 1X8, Canada.
E-mail address: sharon.cushing@sickkids.ca

Otolaryngol Clin N Am 48 (2015) 903–912
http://dx.doi.org/10.1016/j.otc.2015.07.010
0030-6665/15/$ – see front matter © 2015 Elsevier Inc. All rights reserved.

oto.theclinics.com

Abbreviations

ANSD	Auditory Neuropathy Spectrum Disorder
BOR	Branchio-oto-renal syndrome
CI	Cochlear implantation
CMV	Cytomegalovirus
CT	Computed tomography
SNHL	Sensorineural hearing loss
USH1	Usher syndrome type 1
VEMP	Vestibular evoked myogenic potentials
WS	Waardenburg syndrome

---

beyond previous limits has been the development and evolution of a variety of diagnostic, surgical, and rehabilitative technologies. The relationship between hearing loss and technology extends back to the industrial revolution when exposure to loud machinery hastened the acquisition of deafness in workers. The technologies of war, and specifically, societies' attempt to accurately document and compensate for damage from hearing loss after the First World War led Fletcher and Munson (1933)[1] to carefully document normal hearing thresholds for the first time. This ability to identify and measure hearing loss was, and remains, essential to its treatment. In the past, noise exposure, and the hearing loss that ensued, was primarily the concern of soldiers, laborers, hunters, and musicians, and safety measures have been put in place to reduce these exposures, minimizing their impact on hearing. However, in this modern day, the evolution of technology continues to put us at risk. In fact, when measured, both the level and the constant nature of noise within our environment are truly remarkable.[2] Consider the daily commute for example, which brings with it the noise associated with traffic and construction. Our days are filled with noise, over which we have little control, as well as considerable noise we volitionally introduce ourselves to, most frequently in the name of entertainment. We do this knowingly as consenting adults, but also expose our infants and children, for example, by introducing white noise machines, which promise the elusive goal of improved sleep at the potential expense of our child's hearing.[3] Technology is obviously not responsible for all forms of hearing loss, particularly in children. In fact, the relationship between hearing loss and technology is deeply entwined in that it is also responsible for some of the most significant advances in the treatment of hearing loss, and it is this relationship that provides the perspective for this article.

The most significant introduction of technology in the therapeutic domain for hearing loss has been the advent of cochlear implantation (CI). Before the introduction of CI, the treatment options and therefore outcomes in severe to profound sensorineural hearing loss (SNHL) were limited. Although there were means available for measuring hearing loss, there was however less of an impetus to identify it early. However, the introduction of CI as an effective treatment option, where performance is ultimately tied to early identification and implantation within critical developmental periods, has driven the development and implementation of early identification strategies such as newborn hearing screening. Similar examples can be found in many domains surrounding pediatric hearing loss and are highlighted throughout this article. This article does not provide a laundry list of all possible features detected on history and all findings on physical examination in the child presenting with hearing loss. Rather, this article aims to arm the clinician with an approach to the child with hearing loss that focuses on the information that is relevant to today's limits in the domains of diagnosis, treatment, and the prediction of outcome. It focuses on how this entwined relationship between hearing loss and technology has shaped the field, focusing on the newest additions to the clinical armamentarium, while also acknowledging that tomorrow there may well be footprints on Mars.

PREVALENCE AND IMPACT HEARING LOSS

Hearing loss is one of the most common disorders of childhood. Approximately 14.9% of US children have low-frequency or high-frequency hearing loss of at least 16 dB hearing level in one or both ears.[4] Profound, early-onset deafness is present in 4 to 11 per 10,000 children,[5] with the overall estimates for congenital onset hearing loss ranging from 1 to 6 per 1000 newborns.[5–7]

The challenges of managing hearing loss extend beyond simply hearing and affect many aspects of communication. Specifically, compared with children who have normal hearing, those with hearing loss will face additional challenges with many aspects of verbal communication and socialization (ie, vocabulary, grammar).[8] There can be demonstrable deficits in language quotients in unrehabilitated hearing loss. These deficits can occur as early as 18 months of age when hearing loss is unrehabilitated.[9] It is therefore important to identify and rehabilitate children with hearing loss as early as possible.

SYMPTOM CRITERIA

Hearing loss can be categorized in any number of ways. Typically, distinction is made between SNHL, which relates to deficits in the cochlea or the neural elements supplying or supplied by it, and conductive hearing loss, which relates to a deficit in the mechanical transmission of sound waves from the external auditory canal, through the eardrum and ossicles, to the cochlea. There are a large number of etiologic mechanisms contained within these 2 categories. Beyond this distinction, hearing loss can be characterized by its onset (ie, congenital vs acquired), its time course (ie, progressive vs nonprogressive), its severity (mild to profound), or its associated cause (ie, syndromic vs nonsyndromic; genetic vs nongenetic). For the purpose of this article, the clinical history and physical examination of the child with SNHL are the main focus.

CLINICAL FINDINGS

In most cases, hearing loss is nonsyndromic in nature, and most commonly, there are no outward signs of the disorder. Although some parents may recognize the failure to startle in children with profound SNHL, it can be exceedingly difficult to interpret the very subtle cues that suggest even very significant hearing loss in an infant or child. The reasons for this are that children remain very motivated to connecting with their environment and those around them. Even in the complete absence of hearing, they have a remarkable ability to use social cues associated with vision, and other sensory cues in their environment, to respond in ways that make it difficult for their caregivers to perceive the hearing loss; this can be compounded by caregiver denial that there is a sensory deficit with their child.

As a result, the most common indicator of hearing loss before infant hearing screening was failure to develop language. In the absence of screening, the age of detection for severe to profound SNHL ranged between 2 and 3 years of age. For less severe or unilateral hearing loss, this age was even older, often only being recognized when the child was able to articulate a difficulty with hearing or had failed a school screening. The challenges of reliably detecting hearing loss coupled with the need for early rehabilitation make hearing loss an ideal disorder to subject to a screening protocol. Jurisdictions in which neonatal screening for hearing loss has been instituted have seen a dramatic reduction in the age of detection, the age at which intervention has been instituted, and ultimately, the outcome. Screening, however, is not perfect, nor is it universal, even in developed countries. In addition, in some cases hearing loss may not occur until later in childhood and will therefore not be picked up by a screening protocol. In these instances, a normal hearing screen may provide undue reassurance to both clinicians and parents. Clinicians should not hesitate to re-refer into screening programs for further audiologic evaluation in children with normal screens where either new risk factors arose following the initial screen (ie, hyperbilirubinemia, meningitis) or with any delay in language or parental/clinician concern.

As mentioned above, most pediatric hearing loss is nonsyndromic in nature, and therefore, in many cases, there are no outward signs of the disorder. Not infrequently in such cases, the clinician may not detect a single abnormality on history or physical examination. In addition, unlike other conditions, even when abnormalities are noted on history and physical examination, this information has, in most cases, little relevance in determining a treatment course. As such, medical clearance for hearing aids should be initiated by the clinician who is first aware of the audiologic diagnosis, even if they do not consider themselves a hearing loss expert. One should not delay the initiation of hearing aids while waiting for a consultation with an expert in pediatric hearing loss or while undertaking the diagnostic evaluation. There is a fear of overamplification in children that is largely unfounded, and the authors suggest immediate and reasonable amplification as soon as it can be applied after diagnosis, regardless of cause.

So why, one might ask, do we continue to perform, teach, and advocate for a complete history and physical examination in children with SNHL? The true utility of the clinical history in this population is to guide the diagnostic protocol aimed at identifying the underlying cause of the hearing loss. In some centers, such as the authors' center, the findings on clinical history and physical examination will be used to create an individualized, so-called "à la carte" approach to the use of further diagnostic modalities with the goal of containing cost. This approach is most relevant in a socialized, envelope-funded system but is increasingly becoming more relevant worldwide. Determining the cause, while again rarely essential to initial treatment, is advantageous for many reasons, not the least of which is providing families with the answer to the question: "Why does my child have a hearing loss?". The psychological impact of answering this question should not be underestimated. In addition, determining the cause can indicate if the child is at risk for any other conditions and can also help predict the recurrence risk for hearing loss within the family. Although knowledge of outcome and performance based on cause is useful at the group level, it may be difficult to predict outcome based on cause at the individual level. Consistent with the underlying theme of this article, when it comes to the clinical history in children with hearing loss, questions are only asked based on access to diagnostic means. Finally, the clinical history also provides the opportunity to educate, which is of particular relevance in the setting of noise exposure and immunization.

As with any clinical complaint, in this case hearing loss, inquiry regarding the onset, variability, and associated signs and symptoms of the presenting complaint, is carried out.

Review of Risk Factors for Hearing Loss

Most importantly, the history should contain a review of known risk factors for hearing loss.

Perinatal history

Risk factors for SNHL can be elucidated by eliciting the prenatal and perinatal history. Specifically of relevance is a history of prematurity and the underlying inciting factor if known. In the setting of prematurity, a thorough history of the course and sequelae (ie, hypoxia, sepsis, hyperbilirubinemia) is relevant, particularly as they may support a cause for an audiologic diagnosis of auditory neuropathy spectrum disorder (ANSD). Exposure to antibiotics or diuretics throughout the course of prematurity may point toward an ototoxic exposure. The occurrence of any intrauterine infections and, in particular, a suspicion or confirmation of cytomegalovirus (CMV) even in the asymptomatic child is becoming increasingly relevant.

Family history

Beyond the perinatal history, a review of family history of hearing loss at a young age as well as a history of consanguinity may increase suspicion for an underlying genetic cause. It should be noted however that the most common genetic causes of hearing loss are recessive in nature; therefore, genetic hearing loss frequently presents in families where no other individual is affected. Families are often surprised by this notion that their child might be the index case, and it is an ideal opportunity to educate them on the importance of heightened awareness for the potential of hearing loss in other siblings and cousins within the family.

Delays of motor milestones

A history of delayed motor milestones (**Table 1**) may increase the suspicion of an associated vestibular disorder, more common in children with cochleovestibular anomalies, some syndromic causes of hearing loss (ie, Usher and Pendred syndromes), acquired infectious causes of hearing loss (ie, meningitis and CMV), ototoxicity, or ANSD.

Infection and immunization

A known history of bacterial meningitis is clearly a risk factor for hearing loss; however, not all meningitis is diagnosed. Therefore, a history of a febrile illness, particularly those requiring hospital admission or intravenous antibiotics, should be noted. In keeping with this, a review of immunization status is important for many reasons. First, the nonimmunized child remains at increased risk of acute otitis media and its complications, including meningitis. Although immunization status is relevant for all children regardless of presenting complaint, it is particularly important in children with an underlying cochleovestibular anomaly who are at increased risk of otogenic meningitis. Clinicians may not yet be aware of the presence of a cochleovestibular anomaly when a child presents to the clinic as an infant; however, it is the practice of the authors to make the assumption that the child is at increased risk until such a time as imaging is obtained.

Table 1	
Red flags indicating delay in motor milestones	
Motor Milestone	**Time Frame (mo)**
Absence of head control	4
Unable to sit unsupported	7–9
Unable to crawl/bottom shuffle	12
Not attempting to walk	18

Noise exposure

As mentioned in the introduction, our modern world presents many opportunities for excessive noise exposure. A history of high-risk activities for noise exposure is particularly relevant in the older child and adolescent presenting with new-onset hearing loss. Although, currently, this may make up a minority of the patients presenting to clinics with hearing loss, asking the question about noise exposure provides an ideal opportunity for parents and older children to reflect and consider the ways in which they may be putting their own and their family's hearing at risk. It indeed provides a teachable moment.

PHYSICAL EXAMINATION

Beyond the otoscopic examination, which rarely reveals the cause of a SNHL, a thorough evaluation of the head and neck, as well as a general examination, is warranted in the child presenting with hearing loss. As outlined above, the physical examination will be completely normal (with the exception of the vestibular examination, which is discussed later) in most children presenting with hearing loss. The examination, however, is of upmost importance in identifying children with syndromic hearing loss. Therefore, the physical examination must be accompanied with a working knowledge of the associated features of a variety of both common and uncommon syndromic causes of hearing loss. Even such prominent features, such as the blue irises, white forelock, vitiligo, and dystopia canthorum associated with Waardenburg syndrome (WS), the blue sclera associated with osteogenesis imperfecta, or small preauricular or cervical pits or skin tags associated with branchio-oto-renal (BOR) syndrome, can be easily missed. These same physical examination findings may occur in other family members who may or may not have the hearing loss, but who could actually have, for example, BOR or WS, whereby hearing loss is a variable feature.

Balance and Vestibular Dysfunction

The most common associated feature of hearing loss is vestibular and balance dysfunction, with the literature indicating that as many as 70% of children with profound SNHL have some degree of vestibular dysfunction and with 20% to 40% displaying severe to profound and often bilateral vestibular loss.[10–14]

Given the high frequency of this associated disorder, it is recommended that all children be screened for vestibular and balance impairments. Clinicians, however, rarely examine vestibular or balance function in children with SNHL, likely a reflection of the challenges of doing so, and a potential lack of time and expertise in the clinic setting. Ideally, formal vestibular testing, including tests of horizontal canal function (ie, caloric and rotary chair or video head impulse testing) as well as tests of otolith function (cervical and ocular vestibular evoked myogenic potentials [VEMP]) would be performed.

The availability of vestibular testing for pediatric patients varies by institution. However, without a vestibular laboratory, a clinically useful minimum battery of tests may be obtained. The authors recommend obtaining a history of motor milestones, a test of static balance (ie, standing on one foot eyes open and eyes closed), and ideally, a clinical test of vestibular end-organ function (ie, head thrust test or dynamic visual acuity testing) to identify children at risk of bilateral vestibular impairment. The authors have recently examined the utility of using simple balance tasks to screen for bilateral vestibular impairment in children with SNHL. They have found that any one of the following 3 tasks has excellent sensitivity and specificity in predicting bilateral vestibular dysfunction in children with SNHL over 4 years of age:

1. One foot standing, eyes open (cutoff <8 seconds)
2. One foot standing, eyes closed (cutoff <4 seconds)
3. Tandem stance, eyes closed (cutoff <8 seconds)

Item 2, one foot standing, eyes closed, displays the best properties and should be preferentially used. Any child who is unable to complete these tasks to the cutoff should be considered at risk of having bilateral vestibular loss. Once identified, suspicion can then be confirmed with end-organ testing as outlined above (Sharon L. Cushing, unpublished data, 2015).

The identification of vestibular impairment is relevant to the child with hearing loss for several reasons, including identification of Usher syndrome type 1 (USH1), a genetic recessive disorder characterized by hearing loss, vestibular dysfunction, and progressive vision loss due to retinitis pigmentosa. In the authors' clinic, children with bilateral profound vestibular end-organ dysfunction (areflexia) without cause (ie, no history of meningitis or cochleovestibular anomaly on imaging) are referred for ophthalmologic assessment, which includes electroretinogram as well as genetic evaluation to assess for USH1. The early identification of USH1 allows for simple interventions (ie, minimizing light exposure, vitamin therapy),[15,16] which may delay the onset and progression of the eventual visual impairment. Although the capacity of these interventions to halt disease progression is limited, the ability as clinicians to obtain an early and definitive diagnosis will be exceedingly important, if and when additional therapeutic strategies, experimental or otherwise, become available for the treatment of retinitis pigmentosa. Such a treatment presents another example of where technology and capacity to treat will drive the evolution and necessity for improved diagnostics. In contradiction to the previous statement that the identification of cause in most cases does not alter the course of treatment, this may not be the case in the setting of USH1. The identification of USH1 supports proceeding with bilateral CI and promoting an auditory verbal approach to communication rather than reliance on visual communication.[17,18] In addition, from a physical therapy standpoint, it supports the use of nonvisual strategies to improve the maintenance of balance.

Finally, identifying vestibular dysfunction in children who are deaf is important beyond etiologic considerations. A recent review of the authors' database demonstrated that an absence of bilateral horizontal canal function (areflexia) increased the odds of cochlear implant device failure 7.6 times,[19] whereby failure is defined as mechanical or electrical malfunction of the surgically implanted internal component. Likewise, poor balance, measured on objective tests of function, and saccular dysfunction, measured by absence of a cervical VEMP, were also significantly more common in children with cochlear implant failure. In summary, balance is poor in children with cochlear implant failure due to vestibular impairment, which increases the odds of failure nearly 8-fold. The likely mechanism is an increase in falls leading to device damage. Vestibular dysfunction is therefore the largest patient-related factor contributing to cochlear implant failure identified to date.[19] In addition, vestibular and balance dysfunction is also monitored for in children who present with magnet displacement, which again, often follows from a traumatic event as well as presentation to the emergency room for concussion, fractures, and other traumatic injuries due to poor balance.

DIAGNOSTIC MODALITIES

Beyond the history and physical examination, there are several important diagnostic modalities to be applied in the setting of pediatric hearing loss. This article does not review the available modalities in detail, but rather provides a summary of the main diagnostic modalities which can be divided into imaging techniques, laboratory evaluation, and genetic evaluation. Different centers will adopt a variety of approaches to the application of these diagnostic modalities with some centers using a more "shotgun" approach, others using an algorithmic approach, and others still applying an "à la carte" approach based on risk factors and findings obtained on history and physical examination. Which approach is adopted will be dependent on the financial and litigious environment, the individual preference of the physician, and at times, the family. As with the clinical history and physical examination, the findings of these diagnostic evaluations are commonly not essential to the treatment of the underlying hearing loss. This finding allows, in some cases, the flexibility of optimally rehabilitating the child's hearing loss while delaying the diagnostic evaluation until a more suitable time (ie, until the child is older and therefore does not require an anesthetic to undergo imaging). An exception to this approach would occur in the setting of hearing loss, whose course and progression could be modified through treatment. Although this scenario is currently uncommon, this may change as the approach to hearing loss due to CMV infection evolves. A further discussion of CMV hearing loss follows in later discussion. Each of these main areas of diagnostic modalities also provides examples of where the evaluative paradigm has followed from the needs of the technology used for treatment. For example, initially, computed tomography (CT) was the preferred modality for imaging of the cochlea. However, CT imaging can miss subtle anomalies of the auditory nerve, which may predispose to a poor outcome after cochlear implantation. As a result, MRI began to be used for the specific purpose of identifying the cochlear nerve within the internal auditory canal, and additionally, better defining the status of the intracochlear fluids (ie, in meningitis) and abnormalities in the brain (ie, increased signal intensity within the globus pallidus following hyperbilirubinemia and temporal gyrus plaques in CMV). In addition, laboratory evaluation for CMV is also an area of diagnostic expansion. Given that CMV may be a potentially treatable cause of hearing loss, much focus is being placed on improved diagnostics, even considering neonatal screening in some jurisdictions. Again, this is another example of where the availability of treatment drives the evolution of the diagnostics.

COLLABORATIVE APPROACH

The successful diagnosis, workup, and treatment of hearing loss in children is a blueprint for the collaborative approach in that it ideally involves audiologists, auditory verbal and speech therapists, social workers, teachers of the deaf, otolaryngologists, pediatricians, and researchers, among other clinicians.

SUMMARY

Hearing loss is one of the most common childhood disorders and has a significant impact on all aspects of development, particularly when diagnosis and treatment are delayed. The prevalence of hearing loss is likely only going to increase given the multitude of opportunities for noise exposure in today's modern environment. The understanding and capacity to determine the cause of hearing loss have greatly improved and have been driven by the introduction of more effective treatments such as cochlear implants. Despite this improvement, cause remains elusive in many children with hearing loss, despite a full diagnostic evaluation, which speaks to our incomplete understanding. History-taking and physical examination in the setting of pediatric hearing loss are straightforward and should include an assessment of motor milestones, balance, and vestibular function. A thorough history and physical examination may provide clues that allow us to tailor our diagnostic evaluation and focus the use of ancillary testing, improving the cost-effectiveness of our workup for hearing loss, an increasingly important and universal consideration in today's health care systems. It also provides an opportunity to educate families regarding hearing health. Outcome in a child with hearing loss is tightly linked to age at diagnosis and rehabilitation, and therefore, treatment should be sought at initial detection of the hearing loss and not be delayed awaiting the completion of a full diagnostic evaluation.

REFERENCES

1. Fletcher H, Munson WA. Loudness, its definition, measurement and calculation. Journal of the Acoustic Society of America 1933;5:82–108.
2. Neitzel R, Gershon RR, Zeltser M, et al. Noise levels associated with New York City's mass transit systems. Am J Public Health 2009;99(8):1393–9.
3. Hugh SC, Wolter NE, Propst EJ, et al. Infant sleep machines and hazardous sound pressure levels. Pediatrics 2014;133(4):677–81.
4. Niskar AS, Kieszak SM, Holmes AE, et al. Estimated prevalence of noise-induced hearing threshold shifts among children 6 to 19 years of age: the Third National Health and Nutrition Examination Survey, 1988–1994, United States. Pediatrics 2001;108(1):40–3.
5. Marazita ML, Ploughman LM, Rawlings B, et al. Genetic epidemiological studies of early-onset deafness in the U.S. school-age population. Am J Med Genet 1993; 46(5):486–91.
6. Cunningham M, Cox EO. Hearing assessment in infants and children: recommendations beyond neonatal screening. Pediatrics 2003;111(2):436–40.
7. Kemper AR, Downs SM. A cost-effectiveness analysis of newborn hearing screening strategies. Arch Pediatr Adolesc Med 2000;154(5):484–8.
8. Deafness and hearing loss. National Information Center for Children and Youth with Disabilities. Washington, DC: 2004; Pub. No. FS3.
9. Yoshinaga-Itano C, Coulter D, Thomson V. Developmental outcomes of children with hearing loss born in Colorado hospitals with and without universal newborn hearing screening programs. Semin Neonatol 2001;6(6):521–9.
10. Cushing SL, Gordon KA, Rutka JA, et al. Vestibular end-organ dysfunction in children with sensorineural hearing loss and cochlear implants: an expanded cohort and etiologic assessment. Otol Neurotol 2013;34(3):422–8.
11. Cushing SL, Papsin BC, Rutka JA, et al. Vestibular end-organ and balance deficits after meningitis and cochlear implantation in children correlate poorly with functional outcome. Otol Neurotol 2009;30(4):488–95.
12. Cushing SL, Papsin BC, Rutka JA, et al. Evidence of vestibular and balance dysfunction in children with profound sensorineural hearing loss using cochlear implants. Laryngoscope 2008;118(10):1814–23.
13. Buchman CA, Joy J, Hodges A, et al. Vestibular effects of cochlear implantation. Laryngoscope 2004;114(10 Pt 2 Suppl 103):1–22.
14. Licameli G, Zhou G, Kenna MA. Disturbance of vestibular function attributable to cochlear implantation in children. Laryngoscope 2009;119(4):740–5.
15. Rayapudi S, Schwartz SG, Wang X, et al. Vitamin A and fish oils for retinitis pigmentosa. Cochrane Database Syst Rev 2013;(12):CD008428.

16. Wang M, Lam TT, Tso MO, et al. Expression of a mutant opsin gene increases the susceptibility of the retina to light damage. Vis Neurosci 1997;14(1):55–62.
17. Ahmed ZM, Riazuddin S, Riazuddin S, et al. The molecular genetics of Usher syndrome. Clin Genet 2003;63(6):431–44.
18. Jatana KR, Thomas D, Weber L, et al. Usher syndrome: characteristics and outcomes of pediatric cochlear implant recipients. Otol Neurotol 2013;34(3): 484–9.
19. Wolter NE, Gordon KA, Papsin BC, et al. Vestibular and balance impairment contributes to cochlear implant failure in children. Otol Neurotol 2015;36(6): 1029–34.

Radiographic Evaluation of Children with Hearing Loss

Michael DeMarcantonio, MD[a], Daniel I. Choo, MD[b],*

KEYWORDS

- CT temporal bone • MRI temporal bone • Childhood hearing loss
- Radiographic evaluation • Enlarged vestibular aqueduct • Common cavity deformity
- Mondini deformity

KEY POINTS

- High-resolution CT of the temporal bone offers excellent visualization of the osseous anatomy of the temporal bone, but has some limitations in the evaluation of soft tissue.
- MRI is associated with a higher cost and probable need for sedation, but offers excellent soft tissue detail and superior identification of intracranial pathology compared to CT.
- For children being considered for cochlear implantation, MRI is the recommended imaging study of choice.
- Enlarged vestibular aqueduct is the most common imaging finding. Findings are bilateral in up to 87% of patients and associated with cochlear malformation in 84%.

INTRODUCTION

Hearing loss is a common problem within the pediatric population, with 6 in 1000 children being diagnosed by the age of 18.[1] Over the past several decades, the universal screening of infants has been significantly expanded to evaluate 95% of newborns for hearing loss.[2] Through the implementation of early screening, the age of diagnosis has been reduced from the previous norm of 2 to 3 years of age, to the current level of 2 to 3 months.[3] As early detection has increased, focus has shifted to the diagnostic workup and the role of genetic, laboratory, and imaging studies. With this review, we seek to provide a guide for the use of imaging in pediatric patients with sensorineural, conductive, or mixed hearing losses. As such, we address the choice of

Disclosures: None relevant.
[a] Department of Otolaryngology-Head and Neck Surgery, Cincinnati Children's Hospital Medical Center, University of Cincinnati College of Medicine, 3333 Burnet Ave., Cincinnati, OH 45229, USA; [b] Division of Pediatric Otolaryngology, Department of Otolaryngology-Head and Neck Surgery, Cincinnati Children's Hospital Medical Center, University of Cincinnati College of Medicine, 231 Albert Sabin Way, Cincinnati, OH 45267, USA
* Corresponding author.
E-mail address: Daniel.Choo@cchmc.org

Otolaryngol Clin N Am 48 (2015) 913–932
http://dx.doi.org/10.1016/j.otc.2015.07.003
0030-6665/15/$ – see front matter © 2015 Elsevier Inc. All rights reserved.

oto.theclinics.com

imaging, findings, and clinical implications based on type of hearing loss at presentation. It is our hope that this format will present the most current information in a concise and more useful manner than cataloging imaging findings by Computed tomography (CT) or MRI.

Choice of Imaging

For a majority of the 20th century, temporal bone tomography was the only imaging modality available to clinicians. Using this technique, studies reported temporal bone abnormalities in up to 18% of typical deaf patients.[4] Despite the obvious limitations, plain films were used to identify congenital aplasia of the cochlea, glomus tumors, and temporal bone fractures.[5] Despite some utility, the use of plain films has been supplanted by more advanced (higher resolution) imaging.

The development of high-resolution CT of the temporal bone has allowed clinicians to dramatically augment the clinical history and physical examination and to arrive at more accurate and precise diagnoses. CT offers excellent visualization of the osseous anatomy of the temporal bone, but has limitations in the evaluation of soft tissues. These limitations are best exemplified by the lower sensitivity/specificity for the detection of acoustic neuromas compared with MRI, the inability to distinguish between soft tissue inflammation versus cholesteatoma consistently, and the inability to detect specific soft tissue lesions (eg, facial neuromas).[6] In practical terms, CT offers the advantage of short image acquisition times and the lack of need for contrast in the vast majority of clinical indications. These characteristics are important in the pediatric population, with the short study duration reducing the need for sedation and the associated potential complications.

MRI of the internal auditory canal (IAC) and temporal bone offers excellent soft tissue detail not afforded by CT. In the 1980s, contrast-enhanced MRI became the standard imaging modality for the detection of lesions of the IAC.[7] More recently, noncontrast fast spin-echo T2-weighted MRI and CISS (constructive interference) imaging protocols have been shown to possess adequate sensitivity and specificity to allow for IAC screening purposes.[8,9] As such, children with sensorineural hearing loss (SNHL), without suspicion of neoplastic, infectious or inflammatory processes, do not necessarily require intravenous contrast.[10] Published data suggest that MRI in the setting of pediatric SNHL workup should be extended to capture images that include the entire brain. Up to 20% of patients with SNHL have detectable intracranial findings, including gliosis, cortical dysplasia, brainstem hypoplasia, and cerebellar tumors.[11] As a balancing factor, the time required for MRI represents a relative disadvantage compared with CT. With MR studies requiring approximately 20 minutes to complete, sedation is required frequently in younger patients.[10]

Although the imaging modality used should be dictated primarily by clinical needs, it is important to acknowledge that other factors may influence decision making. Although the cost of MRI has decreased over recent years, it remains significantly more expensive than CT. For example, at our tertiary pediatric institution, a typical CT of the temporal bones (without contrast) incurs a charge of $1952. MRI is associated with a charge of $3178 without contrast and $3577 with contrast. In an increasingly cost-conscience health care environment, it has been suggested that CT may be a better initial choice in certain patient populations. However, patient safety is another highly relevant (if not more important) factor to consider. Recently, there has been a concerted effort to reduce the radiation exposure of children secondary to imaging studies. In a landmark study, Pearce and colleagues[12] followed 178,604 patients who underwent CT scans over a 24-year period in Great Britain. Use of CT in children delivering a dose of 50 mGy tripled the risk of leukemia, whereas CT in children with a dose of 60 mGy tripled the risk of brain cancer. These exposures resulted in 1 additional case of leukemia and 1 additional case of brain cancer per 10,000 CT scans. It should be noted that because these neoplasms are rare entities, the absolute risk remains low. Nevertheless, it must be remembered that the clinical information obtained via temporal bone CT comes with a very small but real risk of inducing neoplasm. As a result of this and other research, The Alliance for Radiation Safety in Pediatric Imaging has introduced the Image Gently campaign to reduce the radiation exposure in pediatric patients (http://www.imagegently.org). Clinicians should consider global and long-term health risks before ordering imaging and should make every attempt to reduce the exposure of their patients to radiation.

SENSORINEURAL HEARING LOSS

SNHL will be diagnosed in 1 to 2 newborns per 1000 births in the United States each year.[13] The presentation of SNHL in children is variable ranging from profound congenital bilateral deafness to mild adolescent unilateral hearing loss. As such, the diagnostic workup and results will be influenced by a myriad of factors including onset, severity, patient characteristics, genetic or syndromic factors, and laterality.

Imaging Protocols

Bilateral sensorineural hearing loss

Before embarking on a discussion of the workup of bilateral SNHL in children, it is necessary to take a slight tangent and mention the impact of molecular genetic testing and the recognition of the significance of genetic hearing loss as it pertains to contemporary imaging diagnostic algorithms. First described in 1997, mutations of the Gap Junction Beta 2 (GJB2) gene result in defects of the connexin 26 protein.[14] This autosomal-recessive form of hearing loss has been implicated as the cause of hearing loss in up to 40% of children with severe to profound congenital SNHL.[15] It is has been argued that the diagnostic workup in patients with confirmed autosomal-recessive hearing loss can, and should, be limited to only truly necessary studies. To support this proposal, Preciado and associates[16] evaluated the relevance of GJB2 screening on diagnostic workup. Overall, 18% of patients with SNHL were found to be positive for biallelic GJB2 mutations. This detection rate increased to 37% in the subset of patients with severe to profound hearing loss. In patients found to be GJB2 positive, only 1 patient was noted to have an enlarged vestibular aqueduct (EVA), representing a rate of less than 4% in this specific population. Given the low diagnostic yield of imaging in GJB2-positive patients, the authors recommended an updated diagnostic algorithm. This algorithm seeks to avoid unnecessary cost and risk to patients by integrating genetic screening with imaging, in an algorithm that reaches the final diagnoses with the least number of tests and the lowest incurred costs. As depicted in **Fig. 1**, patients with bilateral SNHL and screening negative for deafness-causing mutations would proceed to diagnostic imaging (eg, MRI). The diagnostic yield of imaging studies in these patients is significantly influenced by the severity of hearing loss. In 1 study of patients with bilateral SNHL undergoing MRI, an increase in yield was noted from mild to moderate (21.2%) to moderate to severe (24.7%) and to severe to profound (29.9%).[16] Other authors have demonstrated an even more dramatic difference in diagnostic yield between mild to moderate loss (29%) and severe to profound hearing loss (48%).[11] Accordingly, these data may be useful in identifying patients most likely to have relevant imaging findings in the setting of limited resources.

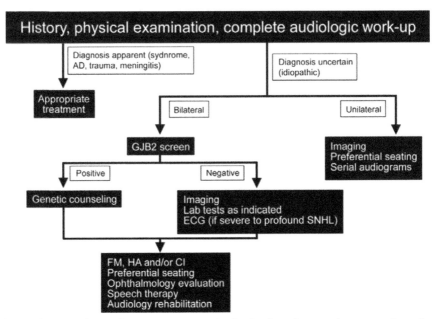

Fig. 1. Algorithm for workup/imaging at our institution based on previous research studies. AD, autosomal dominant; CI, cochlear implant; ECG, electrocardiography; FM, FM amplificaiton system; HA, hearing aid; SNHL, sensorineural hearing loss.

Unilateral sensorineural hearing loss

For patients with unilateral SNHL, temporal bone imaging offers the highest diagnostic yield rate of all available testing. Approximately 35% of studies (MRI or CT imaging[16,17]) will provide a definitive diagnosis as to the etiology of a child's unilateral SNHL. Interestingly, it is not uncommon for patients with unilateral SNHL to have bilateral findings on imaging. Using CT, Song and colleagues[18] demonstrated bilateral findings in 5.6% of patients, with EVA and Mondini malformation representing the most common abnormalities in the otherwise normal hearing ear. This finding is supported by previous audiometric studies showing that 11% of patients with unilateral SNHL will eventually demonstrate bilateral disease.[19] As a result, imaging in unilateral hearing loss is essential to provide diagnoses as well as to evaluate the contralateral ear, and perhaps, provide some prognostic information regarding the child's hearing.

MRI versus computed tomography

The choice of the optimal imaging modality remains a controversial topic. CT is the imaging modality of choice in patients with a conductive hearing loss component, suspected superior semicircular canal dehiscence, or temporal bone trauma. Likewise, MRI is selected when retrocochlear and intracranial pathology must be ruled out. Both MRI and CT can be effective in identifying common inner ear malformations, such as EVA (**Fig. 2**). Unfortunately, few studies have directly compared the two modalities in the same patients. In fact, concurrent CT and MRI have only been evaluated in patients with unilateral SNHL. Concordance between CT and MRI in this setting has been reported as high as 76%.[17] The weaknesses of each modality have been proposed, such as MRI failing to detect EVA, and CT occasionally missing cochlear nerve hypoplasia. Unfortunately, these studies remain limited because fewer than 50% of

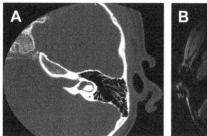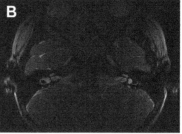

Fig. 2. (*A*) CT and (*B*) MRI imaging in a patient with enlarged vestibular aqueduct.

patients underwent both MRI and CT. This selection bias prevents any meaningful conclusions about the superiority of either modality at this time.

Proposed algorithm

At our institution, patients with SNHL undergo an imaging workup using a structured algorithm (see **Fig. 1**) based on diagnostic yield. Patients presenting with bilateral moderate, severe, or profound congenital SNHL first undergo genetic screening. As discussed, this screening effectively reduces the need for further imaging and laboratory studies, and offers a potential cost savings. Patients with negative genetic testing undergo a noncontrast fast spin-echo T2-weighted MRI to evaluate inner ear and central nervous system structures. In cases of unilateral SNHL, patients proceed directly to MRI regardless of other clinical factors. Despite the need for sedation, MRI has become our imaging modality of choice owing to its superior visualization of the cochlear nerve and central nervous system, its excellent resolution of the inner ear structures, the avoidance of exposure to ionizing radiation, and the ability to perform the study early in the child's life when cochlear implantation is being considered.

For the child with unexplained conductive hearing loss, temporal bone CT imaging is the preferred modality. This imaging, however, can wait until the child is 5 to 6 years old because surgery will not be considered until at least that age, and the larger child receives less total body radiation.

Common Findings

The scope of findings on inner ear imaging in SNHL is exceptionally broad. This review emphasizes the most common findings and their clinical implications.

Enlarged vestibular aqueduct

EVA represents the most common inner ear malformation detected in patients with SNHL.[20] This finding can be bilateral in up to 87% of patients.[21] Although EVA is a congenital condition, hearing loss may not be evident (or even present) immediately from birth, with onset of hearing loss often occurring postlingually.[22] Variability of vestibular aqueduct enlargement and dysmorphology are common in imaging studies (**Fig. 3**). Diagnosis of EVA was initially defined by Valvassori and Clemens[23] as a midpoint vestibular aqueduct greater than 1.5 mm in width. More recently, Vijayasekaran and colleagues[24] have sought to define normative data for vestibular aqueduct size. Using the 95th percentile as a cutoff point, they defined EVAs as having a midpoint and opercular width of 1.0 and 2.0 mm, respectively. The use of these more inclusive criteria is supported by the audiology findings of Madden and colleagues.[21] Their study of EVA patients revealed that borderline EVA (midpoint of

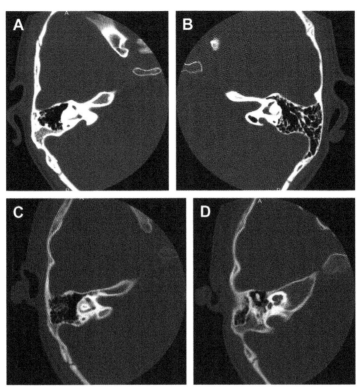

Fig. 3. (*A*) Classic appearance of enlarged vestibular aqueduct (EVA). (*B*) Bulbous appearing EVA. (*C*, *D*) EVA obscured by proximity to a high-riding jugular bulb.

1.0–1.5 mm and operculum of 1.5–2.0) was associated with SNHL that is prone to progression and fluctuation.

EVA is rarely found in isolation, with 84% of patients having an associated cochlear or vestibular anomaly (**Fig. 4**).[25] Associated cochlear anomalies can range from mild asymmetry of the modiolus to classic Mondini malformation.[26] Although progression

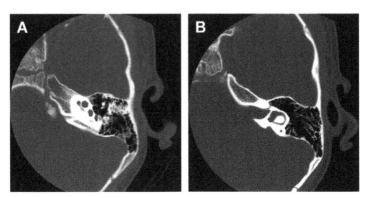

Fig. 4. (*A*) Mondini malformation and (*B*) enlarged vestibular aqueduct are frequently found in combination.

of hearing loss in EVA is variable, profound hearing loss is both possible and common. In particular, head trauma has been linked to progression of hearing loss in up to 4% of patients with EVA.[24] As a result, children are urged to avoid situations where head trauma is a significant possibility or likelihood. The radiographic diagnosis of EVA at an early age allows physicians to offer prognostic information to patients and families, and to counsel those patients at risk for potentially preventable progression of hearing loss.

Congenital cochlear abnormalities

Congenital cochlear malformations represent a common finding on both CT and MRI evaluations. Isolated abnormalities of the cochlea have been detected in 4.1% of patients with SNHL.[20] Mondini malformation, or type II incomplete partition, accounts for 55% of all cochlear deformities (**Fig. 5**). This malformation was first reported by Carlo Mondini in 1791 and was originally described as having an absent interscalar septum and osseous spiral lamina.[27] Imaging classically reveals an absent modiolus and a cochlea limited to 1.5 turns.[28] Mondini malformations are frequently accompanied by other deformities, with 20% of patients having an additional abnormality of the vestibular aqueduct, vestibule, endolymphatic sac/duct, or semicircular canals.[29]

Although less common, other cochlear abnormalities may also be discovered in patients with SNHL on imaging. Complete labyrinthine aplasia (Michel aplasia) represents the most severe and rare malformation of the inner ear. Imaging in these cases reveals a complete absence of inner ear structures that may be unilateral or bilateral.[30] Other findings associated with cochlear anomalies include petrous bone aplasia, narrowed or aplastic IAC, tegmen defects, and middle ear/mastoid hypoplasia.[31] Common cavity deformity occurs with significant frequency, representing 25% of malformations.[29] This deformity is characterized by limited differentiation of the cochlea and vestibule, resulting in a single cavity (**Fig. 6**). Common cavity deformity and complete labyrinthine aplasia can be distinguished by the presence of the IAC in patients with common cavity malformations.[29]

Development of the cochlea can be arrested or perturbed at any point, resulting in deformities ranging from complete aplasia to mild hypoplasia. Cochlear aplasia is characterized by a complete absence of the cochlea in the setting of a normal, dilated, or hypoplastic vestibular system.[32] In cochleovestibular malformation, also known as

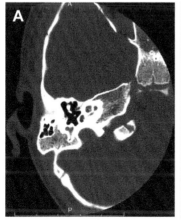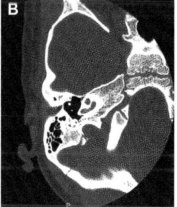

Fig. 5. (*A, B*) Incomplete cochlear partition.

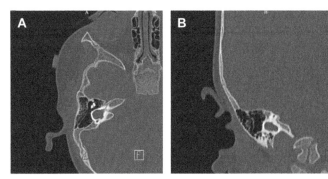

Fig. 6. Axial (A) and coronal (B) CT of common cavity deformity.

type 1 incomplete partition, the modiolus is absent with imaging studies revealing a cystic cochlea and dilated vestibule. In 15% of malformations, the cochlea will be hypoplastic, with imaging demonstrating a small cochlear bud of variable length with only 1 or a partial turn.[27,30]

Recent studies have suggested that, with expanded use of MRI, cochlear abnormalities may be detected with greater frequency than even EVA. In patients with SNHL, McClay and colleagues[11] observed mild cochlear dysplasia in 23% of patients. In this study, the mild dysplasia ranged from isolated deficiency of the modiolus to absence of the cochlear apical turn. The incidence of mild dysplasia in this study is notably greater than both previously reported CT numbers and the accepted frequency of EVA.

Cochleovestibular nerve deficiency

Cochlear nerve deficiency (CND) is defined as an absent or hypoplastic cochlear nerve and is diagnosed in 12% to 18% of patients with SNHL.[10] Using CT, the IAC and cochlear nerve canal are defined as narrow when less than 4 mm and less than 1.8 mm in size, respectively. However, when compared with MRI these criteria have respective sensitivities of only 76% and 68% for the detection of CND.[11] Using IAC size alone is therefore insufficient, because patients with normal caliber IAC may still have detectable CND on MRI.[33] Suspicion for CND should be high in patients with profound congenital SNHL because the cochlear nerve is more likely to be hypoplastic compared to normal controls.[34] In addition, patients may have bilateral nerve deficiency or hypoplasia as well as other associated inner ear abnormalities. Given the propensity for CND, evaluation of the cochlear nerve with MRI is appropriate in the workup of patients with SNHL and may offer useful information, particularly before cochlear implantation (**Fig. 7**).

Special Patient Populations

Syndromic children

Given the accepted prevalence figures, approximately 15% of children with SNHL have an associated syndrome.[35] To date, more than 300 syndromic forms of hearing loss have been described in the literature.[36] Syndromic hearing loss can present in many forms but certain syndromes are more frequently associated with SNHL.

Waardenburg syndrome Waardenburg syndrome is an autosomal-dominant syndrome characterized by heterochomic irides, white forelock, and congenital SNHL.[23] This syndrome represents one of the most common syndromic etiologies

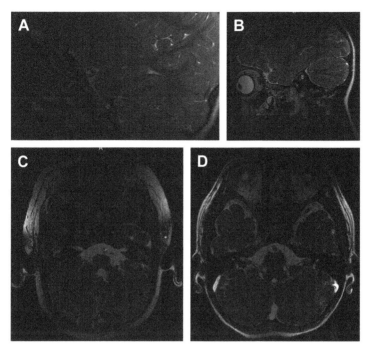

Fig. 7. (*A*) Sagittal and (*C*) axial MRI of cochlear nerve agenesis. (*B*) Sagittal and (*D*) axial MRI of normal cochlear nerve.

of SNHL.[37] Temporal bone abnormalities are common, with approximately 50% of patients having an appreciable deformity on CT.[38] Typical findings include EVA, aplasia of the posterior semicircular canal, and a poorly developed vestibule.[39]

Pendred syndrome Pendred syndrome constitutes up to 7.5% of childhood deafness.[40] Reports commonly describe children presenting with severe to profound SNHL and eventually developing a euthyroid goiter in adolescence.[38] Although the perchlorate discharge test has previously been the standard for diagnosis, advances in molecular diagnostics have now allowed for genetic testing rather than metabolic testing.[41] Goldfeld and colleagues[42] reported bilateral absent modiolus and vestibule enlargement in 100% of the patients studied with definitive Pendred syndrome. In addition, patients were noted to have an absent interscalar septum (75%) and EVA (80%) with high frequency. These findings highlight the triad of goiter, Mondini malformation and EVA classically described in Pendred syndrome. Given the near universality of abnormal inner ear findings in this particular population, imaging is essential in patients with suspected Pendred syndrome.

Branchiootorenal syndrome Branchiootorenal syndrome is an autosomal-dominant syndrome associated with branchial cleft fistulas/cysts, external and inner ear malformations, and renal anomalies[43] Hearing loss occurs in 70% to 93% of patients, and may present as SNHL, conductive hearing loss, or mixed hearing loss with varied severity.[44] Although a wide range of middle and inner ear anomalies are possible, patients with Branchiootorenal syndrome often have a distinctive malformation of the cochlea with a tapered basal turn and hypoplasia of the middle and apical turns (**Fig. 8**). This abnormality bears a resemblance to, but is distinct from, Mondini malformation.[45]

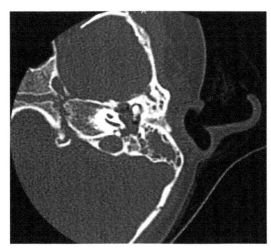

Fig. 8. Patient with branchiootorenal syndrome. The cochlea demonstrates incomplete partition with a classic "unwound" appearance. The mastoid and epitympanum are also opacified incidentally.

CHARGE syndrome CHARGE syndrome is an autosomal-dominant genetic disease characterized by Coloboma, Heart disease, Atresia of the choanae, Retarded growth, Genital hypoplasia, and Ear abnormalities.[46] Patients may present with SNHL, conductive, or mixed hearing loss, with deafness occurring in up to 90% of patients.[47] On CT, the most specific finding for CHARGE syndrome is absence of semicircular canals[48] (**Fig. 9**). The high specificity of this finding has prompted researchers to define the 3 major Cs of CHARGE as coloboma, choanal atresia, and canal hypoplasia.[45] Other findings on MRI and CT include small middle ear clefts, absence of the stapes, aplasia of the round window, hypoplasia of the incus/stapes, ossicular chain fixation, and abnormalities of the facial nerve.[48] Given both soft tissue and bony abnormalities in these children, most patients with CHARGE syndrome eventually undergo both CT and MRI studies for complete evaluation of their ears and hearing.

Infectious etiologies

Reviews of the etiology of hearing loss indicate that prenatal infectious causes have declined with rubella and cytomegalovirus (CMV) accounting for less than 3% of all patients with bilateral SNHL.[37] In the setting of CMV, the role of imaging is limited,

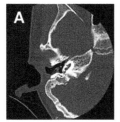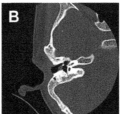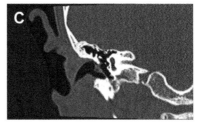

Fig. 9. CHARGE patient. (*A*) An axial view of a hypoplastic cochlea without evidence of lateral or superior semicircular canals. (*B*) Axial and (*C*) coronal view of a remnant rudimentary posterior semicircular canal.

because CMV is not generally associated with inner ear structural abnormalities. Central findings are, however, not uncommon. Abnormalities include intracranial calcifications, ventriculomegaly, white matter abnormalities, neuronal migration abnormalities, and extensive parenchymal destruction.[49] As a result, MRI is a requisite component in the workup of children with suspected or confirmed CMV-related hearing loss.

Meningitis represents the most common cause of postnatal bilateral acquired SNHL.[35] An extensive amount of literature is available on this topic of imaging in the setting of meningitis associated hearing loss. This availability is due to the relevance of postmeningitic scarring and ossifications to cochlear implantation. CT finding vary by stage of disease. During the acute and fibrous stages, imaging may typically seem to be normal. Only during the ossifying stage will osteoplastic bone formation be identified (**Fig. 10**).[38] MRI may play a role in the early evaluation of patients with a history of meningitis and associated SNHL. The use of T2-weighted MRI has proven to be more sensitive in detection of early cochlear ossification, whereas T1-weighted MRI can detect fibrosis and cochlear changes earlier.[50,51] The use of both MRI and CT is recommended in patients with labyrinthine ossification in an attempt to optimize timing of implantation and surgical success.

Sudden sensorineural hearing loss

Sudden SNHL, although extensively studied in adults, remains poorly understood in the pediatric population. The rarity and acute nature of sudden hearing loss makes it a difficult topic for study. Both CT and MRI have been applied in these patients. However, the diagnostic yield remains exceptionally low, with less than 10% of imaging studies providing an etiology.[52] The value of imaging in pediatric patients with sudden SNHL may lie in the potential to identify discrete pathologies such as congenital CMV (via associated intracranial findings, such as brain calcifications) or EVA that may have predisposed the patient to a sudden hearing loss. However, the rarity of this presentation currently offers little objective data to guide its use.

In the setting of SNHL it is important to acknowledge the limitations of imaging in the setting. MRI and CT identify pathology in only a portion of patients. Some common genetic or metabolic defects associated with pediatric SNHL are unlikely to cause structural abnormalities that can be detected on current state of the art clinical imaging (eg, cochlear electrolyte perturbations and hair cell loss in GJB2-related deafness). Even with extensive use of laboratory studies, genetic testing, and imaging, a definitive etiology will remain elusive in as many as 37% of children with bilateral SNHL.[37] Nevertheless, when used appropriately, imaging can yield significant diagnostic and

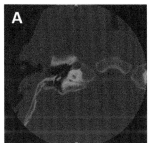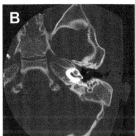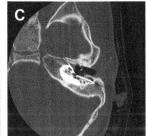

Fig. 10. This patient has a history of meningitis. MRI demonstrates an (A) abnormal cochlea consistent with labyrinthitis ossificans and (B) normal contralateral cochlea (C) labyrinthitis ossificans status post cochlear implant.

prognostic information in pediatric SNHL that can prove invaluable to patients, families, and clinicians.

MIXED HEARING LOSS

Imaging workup in mixed hearing loss is overarchingly guided by practical considerations. Patients are likely to undergo both CT and MRI to adequately assess the middle ear, inner ear, and more central neurologic structures. The possibility of syndromic hearing loss should always be considered in patients with a mixed presentation. As one example, clinicians must be wary of X-linked stapes gusher syndrome. This syndrome, although rare, does represent 50% of all cases of X-linked hearing loss. Patients typically present with mixed hearing loss, but a minority will demonstrate SNHL alone.[53] Given the X-linked transmission, ascertaining an accurate family history is critical. However, it should be remembered that family history can be negative in up to one-third of patients.[54] As a result, this syndrome should be considered in all males with congenital mixed hearing loss. Imaging reveals hypoplasia of the cochleae, absence of bony modioli, enlarged IACs, and abnormal labyrinthine facial nerve canals (**Fig. 11**).[55] It is crucial that patients with X-linked stapes gusher syndrome be

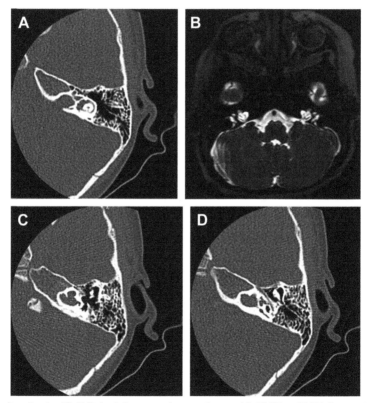

Fig. 11. A patient with X-linked stapes gusher syndrome. (*A, B*) CT and MRI demonstrating a bulbous internal auditory canal. (*C*) CT demonstrating a small oval window and a cochlea with a hypoplastic middle and apical turn. (*D*) CT demonstrating an enlarged fallopian canal of the facial nerve.

identified and imaged before operative intervention to avoid possible significant complications (eg, perilymph or cerebrospinal fluid fistula).

Another syndrome to consider in the setting of mixed hearing loss is Pendred syndrome or EVAS. A fluctuating low frequency conductive hearing loss component is often seen in conjunction with the variable SNHL in patients with EVAS. The mechanism for this mixed hearing loss is believed to be related to a third window effect created by the EVA.[56] The clinical relevance to this conductive hearing loss piece is to avoid the pitfall of unnecessary ventilation tube placement as an attempt to address the low frequency loss (that seems to be very similar to the hearing effect of a chronic fluctuating middle ear effusion).

CONDUCTIVE HEARING LOSS

Conductive hearing loss is very common in the pediatric population. Otitis media is by far the most common cause with 75% of children experiencing at least 1 episode by 6 years of age.[57] The vast majority of patients with conductive hearing loss will not require any imaging workup with their transient conductive hearing losses resolving with infections or effusions. However, CT does play a role in the settings of pediatric chronic, or unexplained congenital conductive hearing losses associated with a history of trauma, cholesteatoma, ossicular malformations and syndromic hearing loss.

Ossicular Malformations

Ossicular malformations are a relatively rare cause of conductive hearing loss in the general pediatric population. Although all of the ossicles are susceptible to deformity and fixation, stapes fixation and incudostapedial discontinuity are the most common anomalies reported in the literature.[58] Stapes fixation alone represents 20% to 35% of all congenital ossicular defects.[59] In patients with congenital conductive hearing loss in the absence of findings on ear examination, imaging is useful to rule out possible stapes gusher (eg, wide IAC orabnormal modiolus) or anomalous/dehiscent facial nerve. These findings on CT predict increased surgical risks and poor hearing outcomes.[60] In comparison, CT imaging in pediatric otosclerosis is more likely to reveal diagnostic findings. In a small study of 7 children, a majority were noted to have poorly calcified foci near the fissula ante fenestram.[61] Given these findings, CT scan will continue to play a role the diagnostic workup of children with conductive hearing loss and normal otoscopic examination.

Temporal Bone Fractures

Temporal bone fractures in children can present along a spectrum of severity involving injury to the skull base, facial nerve, inner ear, and middle ear. Pediatric fractures are typically associated with motor vehicle accidents, falls, biking accidents, and blunt head trauma.[62] Data indicate that hearing loss in pediatric temporal bone fractures is conductive in nature a majority of the time; however, SNHL (17%) and mixed hearing loss (10%) may be encountered as well.[62] Temporal bone fractures have been classically described as longitudinal or transverse in nature, with longitudinal fractures occurring 80% to 90% of the time.[63] In an attempt to further refine the classification system and predict SNHL, fractures have been further categorized as otic capsule violating or otic capsule sparing. Using this system, 90% of temporal bone fractures are described as otic capsule sparing, with the remainder violating the otic capsule. Although both systems are accurate in predicting SNHL, describing fractures in terms of otic capsule involvement increases the accuracy and positive predictive value.[63]

Regardless of the classification system used, CT plays an essential role in the diagnosis and management of pediatric temporal bone fractures. Correlative MR studies may provide additional information about intracranial injury, potential cerebrospinal fluid fistula, brain herniation, and possibly facial nerve integrity. However, as described, the bony detail provided by CT makes it the mainstay in most instances of pediatric temporal bone fractures.

Imaging in Cholesteatoma

In patients with cholesteatoma, preoperative CT imaging has been the modality of choice owing to its high sensitivity and high negative predictive value. However, some limitations of CT imaging in this clinical setting are the low specificity and difficulty differentiating cholesteatoma from granulation tissue, effusion, or other soft tissue lesions (such as chronically inflamed middle ear and mastoid mucosa; **Fig. 12**).[64] As a result, imaging in cholesteatoma has been used primarily for surgery planning and assessment of middle ear, ossicular and mastoid structures. Assessing the labyrinth for fistula or the tegmen for possible defects is also very effectively accomplished by high-resolution CT. However, assessment of the lateral semicircular canal, tegmen, and facial nerve canal may be limited by volume averaging with adjacent soft tissues.[65] Owing to these considerations, it remains common practice for some surgeons to proceed to tympanomastoidectomy without preoperative imaging, with the rationale that the imaging results would not necessarily change the management or decision to proceed with surgery (particularly in the case of confirmed cholesteatoma). Recently, advances in CT and MRI have caused a reexamination of the role of imaging in preoperative evaluation and postoperative surveillance of cholesteatoma. Using fine cut high-resolution CT, Ng and colleagues[65] were able to assess middle and inner ear structures accurately. Correlation of preoperative CT with surgical findings was noted to be particularly strong in cases of tegmen erosion, semicircular canal erosion, and facial canal dehiscence. The authors argue that, in contrast with earlier studies, current generation HRCT offers real value in identifying defects that impact surgical planning. It should be noted that little research has been done in the pediatric population and that any utility of CT must be reconciled with associated radiation exposure considerations.

It has long been hoped that with increased sensitivity and specificity, imaging could be used (instead of second stage surgery) to assess patients for residual or recidivistic disease after primary cholesteatoma surgery. Given the high rates of residual (35%)

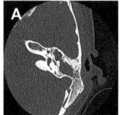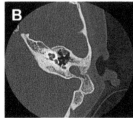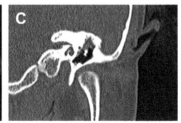

Fig. 12. Postoperative CT scan after canal wall up tympanomastoidectomy for cholesteatoma. (A) CT demonstrates a completely opacified mastoid. (B, C) Axial and coronal views demonstrate opacification of the epitympanic cavity. Differential diagnosis includes cholesteatoma versus granulation tissue. Surgery revealed attic/middle ear cholesteatoma but no evidence of mastoid cholesteatoma.

and recurrent (18%) cholesteatoma, most patients currently undergo planned second look procedures.[66] Previous use of traditional T1- and T2-weighted MRI in this setting has been limited by an inability to differentiate cholesteatoma from surrounding soft tissue. However, the use of postoperative diffusion-weighted MRI has yielded promising results. Diffusion-weighted MRI (DWMRI) applies strong diffusion gradients allowing images to be obtained that depend on the diffusion of water molecules in the section studied. DWMRI has been widely used, with success, in the early detection of acute ischemia.[67] Using DWMRI to detect cholesteatoma, small studies have demonstrated promising rates of sensitivity (77%–100%), specificity (100%), positive predictive value (100%), and negative predictive value (75%–100%).[68,69] The use of DWMRI is not without limitations. In particular, identification of cholesteatoma is limited to disease greater than 5 mm in size[68] and the anatomic precision of the DWMR images is very limited. There also remains a question of whether the use of MRI is warranted given that most patients without disease recurrence on MRI may still require surgery for hearing reconstruction. Although the use of DWMRI in cholesteatoma is promising, further large-scale studies are needed to determine screening application and cost effectiveness.

Syndromic Conductive Hearing Loss

Although many syndromes can present with a conductive component, isolated conductive hearing loss is generally confined to patients with abnormalities in branchial development. In patients with Treacher–Collins syndrome, children typically present with characteristic abnormal development of the face, eyes mandible, and ears. On imaging, these patients have been described as having a unique triad of absent mastoid pneumatization, ossicular disjunction, and a bony cleft in the lateral aspect of the temporal bone.[70] Other findings include atresia or stenosis of the external canal, hypoplasia of the tympanic cavity, a slitlike attic, and abnormal course of the facial nerve.[71] In the setting of hemifacial microsomia, 86% of patients have conductive hearing loss associated with stenosis or atresia of the external auditory canal, ossicular malformation and atresia and hypoplasia of the oval window.[72] Although typically unilateral, up to 30% of patients with hemifacial microsomia have bilateral otologic findings.[73] The Pierre Robin sequence (PRS) is characterized by a triad of glossoptosis, micrognathia and cleft palate.[74] Abnormalities of the middle ear are more variable but not uncommon. Common imaging findings include abnormalities of the ossicles, semicircular canals, and facial nerve canal. A majority of patients with PRS will be noted to have abnormal stapes footplate and dehiscence of the fallopian canal.[75] The possibility of a wide range of varying abnormalities mandates CT imaging before any otologic operative procedures in patients with syndromic conductive hearing loss.

SUMMARY/CLINICAL PEARLS

- Imaging choice
  - Although historically interesting, plain films offer little utility in current practice.
  - CT of the temporal bones offers the advantages of short image acquisition times and excellent visualization of bony anatomy at the cost of a small dose of ionizing radiation.
  - Children with hearing loss (without suspicion of neoplasm, infectious or inflammatory causes), should undergo fast spin-echo T2-weighted MRI or CISS imaging protocols without intravenous contrast.

- CT is the imaging modality of choice in pediatric patients with conductive hearing loss, suspected superior semicircular canal dehiscence, or temporal bone trauma. MRI should be ordered when intracranial pathology must be ruled out.
  - The clinical information obtained via temporal bone CT comes with a very small but real risk of radiation-induced neoplasm.
- SNHL
  - Of pediatric patients with SNHL, 20% will have abnormal intracranial findings. Accordingly, it is reasonable to include brain imaging at the time of temporal bone MRI. The diagnostic yield of imaging in patients with GJB2-related deafness is very low. As a result (and with an eye toward cost effectiveness), it may be reasonable to consider a sequential approach in the diagnostic workup of pediatric SNHL that obtains molecular diagnostic test results before imaging.
  - Five percent of patients with unilateral SNHL have bilateral findings on temporal bone imaging. Bilateral imaging findings are observed even in this population presenting with unilateral hearing loss and provide prognostic information on risks of progressive hearing loss.
  - MRI offers significant benefits (over CT) in patients with bilateral SNHL and should likely be the imaging modality of choice.
  - MRI should be used for patients with severe to profound unilateral SNHL. CT may be used for screening in patients with mild to moderate unilateral SNHL.
- Common findings
  - EVA is the most common imaging finding in patients with SNHL. Findings are bilateral in up to 87% of patients and associated with cochlear malformation in 84%.
  - Mondini, or type II, incomplete partition represents the most common cochlear malformation.
  - Common cavity deformity and complete labyrinthine aplasia can be distinguished by the presence of the IAC in patients with common cavity.
  - The increased use of MRI suggests that mild cochlear dysplasia may occur even more commonly than EVA.
  - CND is diagnosed in 12% to 18% of patients with SNHL. MRI is superior to CT for the detection of CND.
- Syndromic hearing loss
  - Waardenburg syndrome is typically associated with EVA, aplasia of the posterior semicircular canal and poorly developed vestibule.
  - Pendred syndrome is classically associated with the triad of EVA, goiter, and Mondini malformation.
  - Branchiootorenal syndrome is associated with a distinctive malformation of the cochlea with a tapered basal turn and hypoplasia of the middle and apical turns.
  - The 3 major Cs coloboma, choanal atresia, and semicircular canal hypoplasia are highly specific for a diagnosis of CHARGE syndrome
  - X-linked stapes gusher syndrome should be considered in all males with congenital mixed hearing loss. Family history will be negative in one-third of cases.
- Conductive hearing loss
  - Patients with temporal bone fractures typically have conductive hearing loss but SNHL (17%) and mixed loss (10%) are possible.
  - Diffusion-weighted MRI has good sensitivity, specificity, positive predictive value, and negative predictive value for cholesteatoma. However, only cholesteatomas greater than 5 mm are detected effectively.

REFERENCES

1. Billings KR, Kenna MA. Causes of pediatric sensorineural hearing loss: yesterday and today. Arch Otolaryngol Head Neck Surg 1999;125(5):517–21.
2. Russ SA, Hanna D, DesGeorges J, et al. Improving follow-up to newborn hearing screening: a learning-collaborative experience. Pediatrics 2010;126(Suppl 1): S59–69.
3. Harrison M, Roush J, Wallace J. Trends in age of identification and intervention in infants with hearing loss. Ear Hear 2003;24(1):89–95.
4. Unger JM, Shaffer KA. The abnormal temporal bone in the "normal" deaf. Head Neck Surg 1981;3(3):185–92.
5. Carr R. Radiological aspects of recurrent meningitis. Proc R Soc Med 1974; 67(11):1147–50.
6. Parker SW, Davis KR. Limitations of computed tomography in the investigation of acoustic neuromas. Ann Otol Rhinol Laryngol 1977;86(4 Pt 1):436–40.
7. Stack JP, Ramsden RT, Antoun NM, et al. Magnetic resonance imaging of acoustic neuromas: the role of gadolinium-DTPA. Br J Radiol 1988;61(729):800–5.
8. Fukui MB, Weissman JL, Curtin HD, et al. T2-weighted MR characteristics of internal auditory canal masses. AJNR Am J Neuroradiol 1996;17(7):1211–8.
9. Hermans R, Van der Goten A, De Foer B, et al. MRI screening for acoustic neuroma without gadolinium: value of 3DFT-CISS sequence. Neuroradiology 1997; 39(8):593–8.
10. Huang BY, Zdanski C, Castillo M. Pediatric sensorineural hearing loss, part 1: practical aspects for neuroradiologists. AJNR Am J Neuroradiol 2012;33(2):211–7.
11. McClay JE, Booth TN, Parry DA, et al. Evaluation of pediatric sensorineural hearing loss with magnetic resonance imaging. Arch Otolaryngol Head Neck Surg 2008;134(9):945–52.
12. Pearce MS, Salotti JA, Little MP, et al. Radiation exposure from CT scans in childhood and subsequent risk of leukaemia and brain tumours: a retrospective cohort study. Lancet 2012;380(9840):499–505.
13. Brookhouser PE. Sensorineural hearing loss in children. Pediatr Clin North Am 1996;43(6):1195–216.
14. Kelsell DP, Dunlop J, Stevens HP, et al. Connexin 26 mutations in hereditary non-syndromic sensorineural deafness. Nature 1997;387(6628):80–3.
15. Green GE, Scott DA, McDonald JM, et al. Carrier rates in the midwestern United States for GJB2 mutations causing inherited deafness. JAMA 1999;281(23): 2211–6.
16. Preciado DA, Lim LH, Cohen AP, et al. A diagnostic paradigm for childhood idiopathic sensorineural hearing loss. Otolaryngol Head Neck Surg 2004;131(6): 804–9.
17. Simons JP, Mandell DL, Arjmand EM. Computed tomography and magnetic resonance imaging in pediatric unilateral and asymmetric sensorineural hearing loss. Arch Otolaryngol Head Neck Surg 2006;132(2):186–92.
18. Song JJ1, Choi HG, Oh SH, et al. Unilateral sensorineural hearing loss in children: the importance of temporal bone computed tomography and audiometric follow-up. Otol Neurotol 2009;30(5):604–8.
19. Haffey T, Fowler N, Anne S. Evaluation of unilateral sensorineural hearing loss in the pediatric patient. Int J Pediatr Otorhinolaryngol 2013;77(6):955–8.
20. Mafong DD, Shin EJ, Lalwani AK. Use of laboratory evaluation and radiologic imaging in the diagnostic evaluation of children with sensorineural hearing loss. Laryngoscope 2002;112(1):1–7.

21. Madden C, Halsted M, Benton C, et al. Enlarged vestibular aqueduct syndrome in the pediatric population. Otol Neurotol 2003;24(4):625–32.
22. Au G, Gibson W. Cochlear implantation in children with large vestibular aqueduct syndrome. Am J Otol 1999;20(2):183–6.
23. Valvassori GE, Clemis JD. The large vestibular aqueduct syndrome. Laryngoscope 1978;88(5):723–8.
24. Vijayasekaran S, Halsted MJ, Boston M, et al. When is the vestibular aqueduct enlarged? A statistical analysis of the normative distribution of vestibular aqueduct size. AJNR Am J Neuroradiol 2007;28(6):1133–8.
25. Davidson HC, Harnsberger HR, Lemmerling MM, et al. MR evaluation of vestibulocochlear anomalies associated with large endolymphatic duct and sac. AJNR Am J Neuroradiol 1999;20(8):1435–41.
26. Lemmerling MM, Mancuso AA, Antonelli PJ, et al. Normal modiolus: CT appearance in patients with a large vestibular aqueduct. Radiology 1997;204(1):213–9.
27. Jackler RK, Luxford WM, House WF. Congenital malformations of the inner ear: a classification based on embryogenesis. Laryngoscope 1987;97(3 Pt 2 Suppl 40):2–14.
28. Yiin RS, Tang PH, Tan TY. Review of congenital inner ear abnormalities on CT temporal bone. Br J Radiol 2011;84(1005):859–63.
29. Casselman JW, Offeciers EF, De Foer B, et al. CT and MR imaging of congenital abnormalities of the inner ear and internal auditory canal. Eur J Radiol 2001;40(2):94–104.
30. Joshi VM, Navlekar SK, Kishore GR, et al. CT and MR imaging of the inner ear and brain in children with congenital sensorineural hearing loss. Radiographics 2012;32(3):683–98.
31. Ozgen B, Oguz KK, Atas A, et al. Complete labyrinthine aplasia: clinical and radiologic findings with review of the literature. AJNR Am J Neuroradiol 2009;30(4):774–80.
32. Papsin BC. Cochlear implantation in children with anomalous cochleovestibular anatomy. Laryngoscope 2005;115(1 Pt 2 Suppl 106):1–26.
33. Huang BY, Roche JP, Buchman CA, et al. Brain stem and inner ear abnormalities in children with auditory neuropathy spectrum disorder and cochlear nerve deficiency. AJNR Am J Neuroradiol 2010;31(10):1972–9.
34. Russo EE, Manolidis S, Morriss MC. Cochlear nerve size evaluation in children with sensorineural hearing loss by high-resolution magnetic resonance imaging. Am J Otolaryngol 2006;27(3):166–72.
35. Lalwani AK, Castelein CM. Cracking the auditory genetic code: nonsyndromic hereditary hearing impairment. Am J Otol 1999;20(1):115–32.
36. Morton CC, Nance WE. Newborn hearing screening–a silent revolution. N Engl J Med 2006;354(20):2151–64.
37. Morzaria S, Westerberg BD, Kozak FK. Systematic review of the etiology of bilateral sensorineural hearing loss in children. Int J Pediatr Otorhinolaryngol 2004;68(9):1193–8.
38. Huang BY, Zdanski C, Castillo M. Pediatric sensorineural hearing loss, part 2: syndromic and acquired causes. AJNR Am J Neuroradiol 2012;33(3):399–406.
39. Madden C, Halsted MJ, Hopkin RJ, et al. Temporal bone abnormalities associated with hearing loss in Waardenburg syndrome. Laryngoscope 2003;113(11):2035–41.
40. Coyle B, Coffey R, Armour JA, et al. Pendred syndrome (goitre and sensorineural hearing loss) maps to chromosome 7 in the region containing the nonsyndromic deafness gene DFNB4. Nat Genet 1996;12(4):421–3.
41. Reardon W, Trembath RC. Pendred syndrome. J Med Genet 1996;33(12):1037–40.

42. Goldfeld M, Glaser B, Nassir E, et al. CT of the ear in Pendred syndrome. Radiology 2005;235(2):537–40.
43. Melnick M, Bixler D, Nance WE, et al. Familial branchio-oto-renal dysplasia: a new addition to the branchial arch syndromes. Clin Genet 1976;9(1):25–34.
44. Kochhar A, Hildebrand MS, Smith RJ. Clinical aspects of hereditary hearing loss. Genet Med 2007;9(7):393–408.
45. Robson CD. Congenital hearing impairment. Pediatr Radiol 2006;36(4):309–24.
46. Pagon RA, Graham JM Jr, Zonana J, et al. Coloboma, congenital heart disease, and choanal atresia with multiple anomalies: CHARGE association. J Pediatr 1981;99(2):223–7.
47. Sanlaville D, Verloes A. CHARGE syndrome: an update. Eur J Hum Genet 2007; 15(4):389–99.
48. Lemmerling M, Dhooge I, Mollet P, et al. CT of the temporal bone in the CHARGE association. Neuroradiology 1998;40(7):462–5.
49. Boppana SB, Fowler KB, Vaid Y, et al. Neuroradiographic findings in the newborn period and long-term outcome in children with symptomatic congenital cytomegalovirus infection. Pediatrics 1997;99(3):409–14.
50. Coehlo DH, Roland JT Jr. Implanting obstructed and malformed cochlea. Otolaryngol Clin North Am 2012;45(1):91–110.
51. Isaacson B, Booth T, Kutz JW Jr, et al. Labyrinthitis ossificans: how accurate is MRI in predicting cochlear obstruction? Otolaryngol Head Neck Surg 2009; 140(5):692–6.
52. Tarshish Y, Leschinski A, Kenna M. Pediatric sudden sensorineural hearing loss: diagnosed causes and response to intervention. Int J Pediatr Otorhinolaryngol 2013;77(4):553–9.
53. Petersen MB, Wang Q, Willems PJ. Sex-linked deafness. Clin Genet 2008;73(1): 14–23.
54. Phelps PD, Reardon W, Pembrey M, et al. X-linked deafness, stapes gushers and a distinctive defect of the inner ear. Neuroradiology 1991;33(4):326–30.
55. Talbot JM, Wilson DF. Computed tomographic diagnosis of X-linked congenital mixed deafness, fixation of the stapedial footplate, and perilymphatic gusher. Am J Otol 1994;15(2):177–82.
56. Merchant SN, Rosowski JJ. Conductive hearing loss caused by third-window lesions of the inner ear. Otol Neurotol 2008;29(3):282–9.
57. Teele DW, Klein JO, Rosner B. Epidemiology of otitis media during the first seven years of life in children in greater Boston: a prospective, cohort study. J Infect Dis 1989;160(1):83–94.
58. Yuen HY, Ahuja AT, Wong KT, et al. Computed tomography of common congenital lesions of the temporal bone. Clin Radiol 2003;58(9):687–93.
59. Albert S, Roger G, Rouillon I, et al. Congenital stapes ankylosis: study of 28 cases and surgical results. Laryngoscope 2006;116(7):1153–7.
60. De la Cruz A, Angeli S, Slattery WH. Stapedectomy in children. Otolaryngol Head Neck Surg 1999;120(4):487–92.
61. Lescanne E, Bakhos D, Metais JP, et al. Otosclerosis in children and adolescents: a clinical and CT-scan survey with review of the literature. Int J Pediatr Otorhinolaryngol 2008;72(2):147–52.
62. Lee D, Honrado C, Har-El G, et al. Pediatric temporal bone fractures. Laryngoscope 1998;108(6):816–21.
63. Dunklebarger J, Branstetter B 4th, Lincoln A, et al. Pediatric temporal bone fractures: current trends and comparison of classification schemes. Laryngoscope 2014;124(3):781–4.

64. Barath K, Huber AM, Stämpfli P, et al. Neuroradiology of cholesteatomas. AJNR Am J Neuroradiol 2011;32(2):221–9.

65. Ng JH, Zhang EZ, Soon SR, et al. Pre-operative high resolution computed tomography scans for cholesteatoma: has anything changed? Am J Otolaryngol 2014; 35(4):508–13.

66. Migirov L, Tal S, Eyal A, et al. MRI, not CT, to rule out recurrent cholesteatoma and avoid unnecessary second-look mastoidectomy. Isr Med Assoc J 2009;11(3): 144–6.

67. Sugahara T, Korogi Y, Kochi M, et al. Usefulness of diffusion-weighted MRI with echo-planar technique in the evaluation of cellularity in gliomas. J Magn Reson Imaging 1999;9(1):53–60.

68. Dhepnorrarat RC, Wood B, Rajan GP. Postoperative non-echo-planar diffusion-weighted magnetic resonance imaging changes after cholesteatoma surgery: implications for cholesteatoma screening. Otol Neurotol 2009;30(1):54–8.

69. Aikele P, Kittner T, Offergeld C, et al. Diffusion-weighted MR imaging of cholesteatoma in pediatric and adult patients who have undergone middle ear surgery. AJR Am J Roentgenol 2003;181(1):261–5.

70. Jahrsdoerfer RA, Aguilar EA, Yeakley JW, et al. Treacher Collins syndrome: an otologic challenge. Ann Otol Rhinol Laryngol 1989;98(10):807–12.

71. van Vierzen PB, Joosten FB, Marres HA, et al. Mandibulofacial dysostosis: CT findings of the temporal bones. Eur J Radiol 1995;21(1):53–7.

72. Rahbar R, Robson CD, Mulliken JB, et al. Craniofacial, temporal bone, and audiologic abnormalities in the spectrum of hemifacial microsomia. Arch Otolaryngol Head Neck Surg 2001;127(3):265–71.

73. Carvalho GJ, Song CS, Vargervik K, et al. Auditory and facial nerve dysfunction in patients with hemifacial microsomia. Arch Otolaryngol Head Neck Surg 1999; 125(2):209–12.

74. Cohen MM Jr. Robin sequences and complexes: causal heterogeneity and pathogenetic/phenotypic variability. Am J Med Genet 1999;84(4):311–5.

75. Gruen PM, Carranza A, Karmody CS, et al. Anomalies of the ear in the Pierre Robin triad. Ann Otol Rhinol Laryngol 2005;114(8):605–13.

Acquired Hearing Loss in Children

Margaret A. Kenna, MD, MPH

KEYWORDS

- Cytomegalovirus (CMV) • Toxoplasmosis • Meningitis • Rubella • Syphilis • Noise
- Enlarged vestibular aqueduct • Sudden sensorineural hearing loss

KEY POINTS

- Hearing loss is the most common congenital sensory impairment, with an incidence of 4/1000 live births. This number rises to approximately 20% after the age of 12 years for all degrees and laterality of hearing loss.
- The World Health Organization (WHO) notes that 50% of hearing loss is due to preventable causes. These include preventable viruses, such as rubella and cytomegalovirus (CMV); low birth weight and other prenatal, perinatal, and postnatal complications; head injury; ototoxicity; and noise.
- Congenital CMV is the most common viral cause of congenital hearing loss. Early postnatal identification of CMV can identify those who may benefit from medical treatment.
- Hearing loss due to noise is increasingly common but preventable.
- Head injuries, including concussion, can lead to both hearing loss and vestibular dysfunction.

INTRODUCTION

Hearing loss is the most common congenital sensory impairment. Bilateral severe to profound hearing loss is present in 1 to 2/1000 live births, and if unilateral and mild to moderate hearing losses are included, the number rises to 4/1000. According to National Health and Nutrition Examination Survey data from 2001 to 2008, 20.3% of all subjects aged greater than to equal to 12 had a unilateral or bilateral hearing loss, with many of these hearing losses acquired and of later onset.[1] Furthermore, the prevalence of hearing loss increased with every decade, was less prevalent in women compared with men, and in white individuals versus black across nearly all decades. The WHO notes that, worldwide, there are 360 million people with disabling hearing loss and that 50% is preventable.[2] The purpose of pediatric hearing evaluation is to

Disclosures: None relevant.
Otolaryngology and Communication Enhancement, Boston Children's Hospital, Harvard Medical School, 300 Longwood Avenue, BCH3129, Boston, MA 02115, USA
E-mail address: Margaret.kenna@childrens.harvard.edu

Otolaryngol Clin N Am 48 (2015) 933–953
http://dx.doi.org/10.1016/j.otc.2015.07.011
0030-6665/15/$ – see front matter © 2015 Elsevier Inc. All rights reserved.

oto.theclinics.com

Abbreviations	
AIED	Autoimmune inner ear disease
BOR	Branchio-oto-renal syndrome
CDC	Centers for Disease Control and Prevention
CHARGE	Coloboma, heart defect, atresia choanae (ie, choanal atresia), retarded growth and development, genital abnormality, and ear abnormality
CMV	Cytomegalovirus
CRS	Congenital rubella syndrome
CS	Congenital syphilis
ECMO	Extracorporeal membrane oxygenation
EVA	Enlarged vestibular aqueduct
FTA	Fluorescent treponemal antibody absorption test for syphilis
HSV	Herpes simplex virus
HZO	Herpes zoster oticus
NICU	Neonatal intensive care unit
OAE	Otoacoustic emission
OM	Otitis media
PCR	Polymerase chain reaction
PDS	Pendred syndrome
SNHL	Sensorineural hearing loss
TORCHES	Toxoplasmosis, other infections, rubella, cytomegalovirus, herpesvirus, and syphilis
VLBW	Very low birth weight
WHO	World Health Organization

identify the degree and type of hearing loss and the etiology and to outline a comprehensive strategy that supports language and social development and communication. This article reviews the causes and evaluation of acquired and later-onset hearing loss.

NEWBORN HEARING SCREENING

Most newborn hearing screening uses either automated auditory brainstem response testing and/or otoacoustic emissions (OAEs) in the 30-dB to 35-dB range. It is, therefore, entirely possible to pass a newborn hearing screen and have a mild degree of hearing loss. Many infants who pass a newborn hearing screen may subsequently fail a hearing screen in preschool or in the early elementary grades. Although these children may have a progressive or acquired hearing loss, the hearing loss may also just be a more accurate evaluation of a preexisting congenital hearing loss. In addition, newborn hearing screening programs using only OAEs may miss auditory dyssynchrony.[3] Therefore, even if an infant or young child has passed a newborn hearing screen, if hearing loss is suspected, and/or speech and language are delayed, a more complete diagnostic audiometric examination is always warranted.

OVERVIEW OF CAUSES OF HEARING LOSS IN INFANTS AND CHILDREN

Identifying the cause of the hearing loss can provide prognostic and educational information to the family and help support a plan for (re)habilitation. Careful evaluation can now pinpoint a definite or probable cause of the hearing loss 50% to 60% of the time. The etiologies of hearing loss have often been divided into congenital and acquired. Many of the causes that are congenital, however, were "acquired" in utero and may only present at a later time (eg, delayed onset of sensorineural hearing loss [SNHL] from CMV); this is in contrast to those truly acquired after birth (eg, secondary to extracorporeal membrane oxygenation [ECMO], meningitis, or trauma). Although it is important to know if the hearing loss is prelingual or postlingual in onset for management purposes, a more useful way to look at hearing loss etiology is to divide the causes into infectious, anatomic, genetic, traumatic, ototoxic, and other. Many causes of hearing loss present with a similar degree and laterality of the hearing loss, with potential overlap between some of these causes, making the identification of a definite cause more challenging. Some examples of this include children with enlarged vestibular aqueducts (EVAs) and mutations in the SLC26A4 gene (a genetic cause with an anatomic presentation); neonatal intensive care unit (NICU) stays involving possible combinations of ototoxicity, ECMO, prolonged ventilation, and hyperbilirubinemia; and more than 1 statistically common cause presenting in the same child, for example, congenital CMV and mutations in the *GJB2* (connexin 26) gene.

Genetic Causes of Hearing Loss

Genetic hearing loss is primarily discussed elsewhere in this issue.[4,5] Genetic causes of hearing loss, however, may present later in childhood, seemingly as an acquired hearing loss, so genetic causes should always be considered, especially if other causes are not readily identified. For example, hearing loss associated with GJB2 (connexin 26) may present as very mild, or even normal, in the newborn period, then go on to progressively worsen.[6,7] Hearing loss associated with mutations in SLC26A4, usually associated with the presence of EVA, may present as mild, mixed, or even initially conductive and is often progressive and fluctuating.[8] Genetic susceptibility is well documented for hearing loss related to aminoglycosides and may also be a factor in patients with noise-related hearing loss and ototoxicity related to other medications.[9] Although much of congenital or childhood-onset hearing loss is genetic, recessive, and nonsyndromic, audiometric evaluation of biological parents and siblings may document previously unsuspected hearing loss as well, making a genetic cause of what seems an acquired hearing loss more likely.

Infectious Causes

Infectious causes of hearing loss can occur both before and after birth. Historically, the toxoplasmosis, other infections, rubella, CMV, herpesvirus, and syphilis (TORCHES) organisms are described as common causes of congenital hearing loss due to prenatal exposure. As the epidemiology of these organisms has changed, however, only one, CMV, is currently a substantial cause of congenital hearing loss in many countries.

Toxoplasmosis

Toxoplasmosis is caused by the protozoan parasite *Toxoplasma gondii* and, if acquired prenatally, can cause SNHL. *T gondii* is the second leading cause of death from foodborne illness in the United States and has recently been named by the Centers for Disease Control and Prevention (CDC) as 1 of the 5 "neglected parasitic infections."[10] Humans acquire toxoplasmosis by ingesting the oocysts of the parasite. This can occur by eating contaminated undercooked meat or by handling and then accidentally ingesting oocysts from cat feces, soil, or water containing the parasite. (Members of the family Felidae [domestic cats] are the only known definitive hosts for *T gondii*.) Rarely, transmission may be from a contaminated blood transfusion or an organ transplant. The overall prevalence and incidence of congenital toxoplasmosis varies by region and country. In the United States, it is estimated that 22.5% of the population 12 years and older have been infected with *T gondii*, whereas in some parts of the world up to 95% of the population has been infected. Reporting is hampered by the fact that primary infection in most adults (including pregnant mothers) is asymptomatic. The incidence of congenital toxoplasmosis is estimated to be 1/1000 to 1/10,000. In 2000, the CDC reported that there were an estimated 400 to 4000 cases of congenital toxoplasmosis in the United States, based on the seroconversion rate of pregnant mothers.[11] Massachusetts began screening newborns for toxoplasmosis in 1986, and in 1994 a study from the New England Regional Newborn Screening Program found the incidence of toxoplasmosis in newborns to be 1/10,000.[12] The incidence of congenital toxoplasmosis varies outside the United States, with an estimate of 6/1000 births in France, 2/1000 births in Poland, 7 to 10/1000 births in Colombia, and 2/1000 births in Slovenia. Although recently the incidence of congenital toxoplasmosis has been reported to be decreasing, the rates of positive antibody titers remain high among pregnant women, especially outside the United States. Mothers who become primarily infected with T gondii have approximately a 30% to 50% chance of transmitting the infection to their fetus. Although the most severe disease is experienced by fetuses becoming infected during the first trimester, transmission of infection (transplacental) is much more common later in pregnancy, especially during the third trimester, or during delivery. Eighty-five percent of infants with congenital toxoplasmosis are asymptomatic at birth, with those infected later in pregnancy most likely to be asymptomatic. Although vertical transmission of infection is most likely to occur with primary maternal infection, immunocompromised women with chronic infection may also pass on the disease. If new infection is detected in the mother in early pregnancy, treatment with oral spiramycin, which does not cross the placenta, can prevent transmission to the fetus. If infection occurs later in pregnancy, and/or if the fetus is also infected, treatment with pyrimethamine, sulfadiazine, and folinic acid (pyrimethamine is a folic acid antagonist) may prevent transmission to the infant by treating the mother and may also treat the fetus.[13]

The classic symptoms of congenital toxoplasmosis are chorioretinitis, hydrocephalus, and intracranial calcifications. Other symptoms can be seen in other congenital infections, including CMV, rubella, and herpes, and may include hepatosplenomegaly, jaundice, anemia, microcephaly, and lymphadenopathy. Although a 2009 systematic review by Brown and colleagues[14] did not find any cases of hearing loss in infants with appropriately treated congenital toxoplasmosis, others have reported an incidence of hearing loss from 0% to 20%. Earlier studies with a higher incidence of SNHL often included untreated infants, whereas most infants in recent studies had been treated, suggesting that adequate treatment decreases the occurrence of SNHL. Treatment of congenitally infected infants with pyrimethamine and sulfadiazine is generally effective, although infants who present without neurologic disease have somewhat better outcomes than those who present with neurologic impairment. In addition, babies asymptomatic at birth may develop signs later in life, including chorioretinitis.[15]

Toxoplasmosis is diagnosed using serologic testing. Measuring toxoplasma-specific IgG antibodies can determine if a person has been infected, whereas IgM is used to estimate when infection occurred. The lack of specificity of the IgG and IgM antibody test can make testing somewhat difficult to interpret. If the mother is both IgG and IgM positive, then further IgG avidity testing should be performed at a reference laboratory experienced in toxoplasmosis testing. Newborns suspected of having congenital toxoplasmosis should be tested for both IgM- and IgA-capture enzyme immunoassay. Diagnosis can also be made by direct observation of the parasite in stained tissue sections or cerebrospinal fluid. Polymerase chain reaction (PCR) can also be used to detect parasite genetic material and is especially useful if in utero infection is suspected.

Rubella

Rubella is caused by a togavirus of the genus *Rubivirus*. Until the introduction of the rubella vaccine, rubella was the most common viral cause of congenital SNHL. The rate of congenital rubella syndrome (CRS) for infants born to women infected during their first 11 weeks of pregnancy is 90%; if infected during the first 20 weeks of pregnancy it is 20%. The most common features of CRS are cataracts, heart defects, hearing impairment, and developmental delay. After the licensure of live attenuated rubella vaccines in the United States in 1969, the number of reported cases of CRS declined 99%, from 77 cases in 1970 to 4 total cases from 2005 to 2011. Although no longer endemic in the United States, rubella continues to be endemic in many other countries, where vaccination rates may also not be uniformly high in postpubertal girls. Therefore, babies with congenital hearing loss born outside the United States in areas where rubella remains endemic, or born to mothers who may not have been vaccinated, may be more likely to have CRS as a cause of their hearing loss. According to the WHO, the number of countries that have incorporated rubella vaccine into their immunization programs increased from 83 countries (12% of the birth cohort) in 1996 to 134 countries (44% of birth cohort) in 2012.[16] In addition, the development of CRS is a theoretic risk in infants of mothers vaccinated during pregnancy.[17]

Rubella virus can be cultured from nasal, throat, urine, blood, and cerebrospinal fluid specimens in infants with CRS. The serologic tests for rubella in babies with suspected CRS include IgG and IgM antibodies to rubella, with the enzyme immunoassays the most widely used and available. Infants with CRS may have detectable IgM antibody for 6 to 12 months after birth, and IgM can also be detected in cord blood or serum. Reverse transcription–PCR for detection of rubella virus RNA can also be used to detect the virus in clinical specimens, including blood, serum, and tissues.

Cytomegalovirus

Prenatal exposure CMV, a β-herpesvirus, is the most common congenital viral infection and currently the most common viral cause of congenital SNHL. The prevalence of congenital CMV infection is approximately 0.4% to 2.3% of all newborns. A 2008 study in Dallas, Texas, by Stehel and colleagues[18] documented a 6% incidence of congenital CMV in babies with confirmed hearing loss. If the mother has a primary CMV infection during pregnancy, there is a 40% chance that the infant will become infected; and if she has a reactivation infection, there is an approximately 2% chance. The possibility of transmission of primary infection from mother to child is 25% in the first trimester, 50% in the second, and 75% in the third. Infants exposed to the virus during the first trimester, however, are the most likely to develop serious neurologic sequelae. Although 90% of infants with congenital CMV are asymptomatic at birth, 10% to 15% develop hearing loss, whereas 65% to 70% of infants with symptomatic CMV infection at birth also develop hearing loss. In the study by Stehel and colleagues,[18] 75% of the infants with congenital CMV were only diagnosed because they had hearing loss. Because CMV-related hearing loss may not develop until later in infancy/childhood, however, the diagnosis can easily be missed.[19] Infants with symptomatic CMV may present at birth with microcephaly, intrauterine growth restriction, developmental delay, hepatosplenomegaly, chorioretinitis, jaundice, petechiae, thrombocytopenia, hyperbilirubinemia, anemia, and hearing loss. The diagnosis of congenital CMV is made in the first 2 to 3 weeks of life by viral culture or PCR of saliva, urine, blood, or other bodily tissues.[20] Positive PCR using dried blood spots can confirm a diagnosis of congenital CMV outside the newborn period when viral culture or CMV IgG cannot differentiate between congenital and postnatally acquired infection.[21–25] In addition, PCR technology may become a basis for large-scale screening.

In the United States, Utah (2013) and Connecticut (2015) have passed laws mandating the testing of newborns who fail their newborn hearing screen for CMV.

Initially, treatment of symptomatic congenital CMV involved 6 weeks of intravenous ganciclovir; more recently, oral valganciclovir, a prodrug of ganciclovir, has been used.[26] Although the optimal duration of therapy remains unclear, a recent study looking at 6 weeks versus 6 months of valganciclovir showed modestly improved hearing and developmental outcomes at 24 months in babies with symptomatic congenital CMV in the infants who received 6 months of valganciclovir.[23] Although several studies support improved hearing in infants receiving antiviral therapy, the numbers of treated patients remain small, the follow-up is variable, and progression of the hearing loss may occur after the drugs are stopped. Side effects of ganciclovir and valganciclovir include bone marrow suppression (neutropenia, thrombocytopenia, and anemia), and kidney and liver toxicity. Teratogenesis, mutagenesis, inhibition of spermatogenesis, and impaired fertility have been reported, primarily in animal studies, as a result of exposure to these agents. Once a baby is out of the newborn period, making a definite diagnosis of congenital CMV is difficult. It can be suspected, however, based on findings of developmental delay, microcephaly, and hearing loss; some infants have a history of intrauterine growth retardation, prematurity, hepatosplenomegaly, petechiae, and neurologic impairment in the perinatal period. Visual impairment may be present in 10% to 20% of symptomatic babies and includes strabismus, optic atrophy, macular scarring, pigmentary retinitis, and visual loss. Boppana and colleagues[27] have reported late-onset or reactivation chorioretinitis in 7/31 (23%) children after 1 to 10 years of age. Imaging findings can help narrow the diagnosis in older children or confirm the diagnosis in newborns. Intracranial calcifications, migrational abnormalities (eg, polymicrogyria), cerebral and cerebellar volume loss, ventriculomegaly, and white matter disease are commonly seen on a combination of ultrasound, MR imaging, and CT. Characteristic imaging findings in association with neurodevelopmental delay and hearing loss suggest a diagnosis of congenital CMV. Treatment of older children with progressive hearing loss due to congenital CMV has not been studied.

Herpes simplex

Herpes simplex virus types 1 and 2 (HSV-1 and HSV-2) are double-stranded DNA viruses of the Herpesviridae family that commonly infect humans.[28] Neonatal HSV infections occur in approximately 1/3200 births in the United States, with a majority HSV-2.[28] Kimberlin[29] reported that 85% of transmission is peripartum, 10% is postnatal, and 5% is in utero, with primary maternal infection resulting in a higher transmission rate than reactivation disease. Approximately 50% of neonatal HSV infections have CNS involvement. HSV-1 infections have also been associated with hearing loss after infection or reactivation of infection after infancy. Some are associated with HSV meningitis or encephalitis.[30] The incidence of hearing loss in children with neonatal HSV is unclear, with hearing loss secondary to HSV-1 more common than in HSV-2. A recent systematic review of the incidence of SNHL in neonates exposed to HSV found that SNHL occurs rarely in infants with exposure to HSV, and there was no evidence of delayed onset of SNHL in infants with asymptomatic perinatal HSV infection.[31] The few articles that reported audiometric data found a prevalence rate of 0% to 33% for hearing loss associated with intrauterine HSV-2 infection, with all infants also having severe CNS disease; however, all studies were small and audiometric techniques varied. Based on the limited information available, Westerberg and colleagues[31] did not find that routine serologic screening for HSV infection in otherwise asymptomatic neonates with SNHL was justified. If congenital or perinatally acquired HSV infection is suspected, testing using direct viral culture of lesions or blood, or serologic testing, is recommended; if HSV infection is confirmed, audiometric evaluation is recommended.

Syphilis
Transplacental mother-to-child transmission of syphilis has been recognized since the fifteenth century. Congenital syphilis (CS) and syphilis acquired after birth are caused by *Treponema pallidum*, a gram-negative spirochete bacterium. Worldwide, 2 million mothers test positive for *T pallidum* infection during pregnancy, comprising 1.5% of all pregnancies. Prenatal *T pallidum* infection can lead to stillbirths and neonatal death. In the United States, however, CS is uncommon, with the result that hearing loss due to CS may be missed. In a systematic review of CS cases and articles contained in multiple databases published in 2009, Chau and colleagues[32] did not find any reported cases of SNHL in infants with CS born to mothers with syphilis acquired during pregnancy. The number of CS cases reported annually in the United States was 10.6/100,000 live births in 2003, 8.2/100,000 in 2005, 10.1/100,000 in 2008, and 8.7/100,000 in 2013. These rates parallel the primary and secondary syphilis rates among US girls and women from 2005 to 2008 of 1.5/100,000 but with a subsequent decrease in 2013 to 0.9/100,000.[33] Therefore, CS remains uncommon in the United States and, therefore, any associated hearing loss may not be readily recognized or even sought. Although late CS may present as the classic Hutchinson triad of interstitial keratitis, notched incisors, and SNHL, it can present as hearing loss alone. Clutton joint (symmetric hydrarthrosis, especially of the knees) and mulberry molars (malformed first molar resembling a mulberry) were added as additional features of CS by Fiumara and Lessell.[34] Prenatal diagnosis involves testing pregnant mothers, generally at the first prenatal visit and then toward the beginning of the third trimester, with nearly complete elimination of any serious complications in the baby if the mother is treated before 24 weeks' gestation. For babies with CS identified after birth, appropriate treatment with penicillin usually results in a cure. Because syphilis acquired after birth may present as progressive and/or sudden hearing loss or vertigo, the diagnosis should be considered in any sexually active patient who presents with recent-onset hearing loss and/or vertigo.

Other Infectious Diseases Associated with Hearing Loss

Human immunodeficiency virus
Audiologic and vestibular symptoms can occur in children infected with Human immunodeficiency virus (HIV) 1. These include conductive hearing loss (often due to otitis media [OM]), SNHL, tinnitus, vertigo, and ataxia. Hearing loss may occur due to direct infection of the inner ear with HIV or secondary to opportunistic infections (eg, CMV, syphilis, tuberculosis, and cryptococcal meningitis) or ototoxic drug therapy. In several studies, children with perinatally acquired HIV seem to have a higher incidence of hearing loss than normal children, with both SNHL and conductive hearing loss, due mainly to otitis media. A recent study in HIV+ adults compared with HIV− adults showed a higher incidence of both low-frequency and high-frequency hearing loss. In 1 pediatric study, there was a suggestion that lower CD4 counts, longer time with HIV, and higher viral load were associated with an increased prevalence of audiologic or vestibular symptoms.[35] Therefore, children who are HIV+ should have audiometric examinations incorporated into their routine care.[36,37]

Measles (rubeola)
Measles is a paramyxovirus spread via the respiratory route and in the prevaccine era was an identified cause of acquired hearing loss. Although measles was reported to

have been eradicated in the United States in 2000, hundreds of cases have been reported since then, including several large outbreaks in 2008, 2011, 2013, 2014, and 2015[38] These outbreaks occur mainly in unvaccinated children, including those born outside the United States, children too young to vaccinate, and children whose parents have chosen not to vaccinate them. Live attenuated measles virus is included in the standard measles vaccine. Information from the Vaccine Adverse Event Reporting System in the United States estimated the reporting rate of SNHL possibly related to mumps/measles vaccine to be 1 case in 6 to 8 million doses.[39,40] Measles virus has also been possibly implicated in the development of otosclerosis, although whether this is an association or causation remains unclear.[41,42]

Lyme disease

Lyme disease is caused by the bacterium *Borrelia burgdorferi* and is transmitted to humans by the bite of an infected blacklegged tick. It is the most commonly reported vector-borne illness in the United States. In 2013, 95% of cases occurred in 14 states; in the United States, the incidence is highest in the northeast and upper midwest states but has been reported in all 50 states. Although people of any age and both genders are susceptible to tick bites, from 2001 to 2010 Lyme disease was most common among boys aged 5 to 9 years and persons older than 30 years. The CDC reported a 9% incidence of facial palsy among 154,405 patients with Lyme disease between 2001 and 2010. Hearing loss in association with Lyme disease, however, is infrequently reported.[43,44] A 2010 retrospective review by Wilson and colleagues[45] of patients 18 years of age and older presenting with asymmetric SNHL of uncertain etiology showed that of the 88 who were tested for Lyme disease, 3 were positive. Although the endemic nature of Lyme disease in many parts of the country can make confirming a relationship between Lyme disease and hearing loss challenging, Wilson and colleagues[45] thought that of the many tests ordered in their study, Lyme titers and tests for syphilis were potentially the most useful, potentially treatable, and cost-effective.

Mumps

Mumps is a paramyxovirus that results in an acute viral illness characterized by unilateral or bilateral parotitis, and complications, including SNHL, aseptic meningitis, encephalitis, and, in postpubertal age groups, orchitis, oophoritis, and mastitis. Approximately 20% to 40% of infections are asymptomatic, and many symptomatic patients only have respiratory symptoms. Mumps is endemic in most of the world and by the end of 2013 was included in the vaccine programs of 120 countries.[46] Live mumps vaccine was licensed for use in the United States in 1967, with a drop in incidence of mumps cases to 0.1/100,000 persons (314 cases total) in the United States by 2005, a 99% decrease compared with the prevaccine era. There have been several large outbreaks of mumps since then, however, in 2006, 2009, and 2010, often seen on college campuses. The incidence of SNHL after mumps is unclear, but a 2009 study from Japan suggested an incidence of 0.1%, with the hearing loss unilateral and in the moderate to profound range; the CDC states recently the incidence has been less than 1%.[47,48] Hearing loss associated with mumps may occur before or after the parotitis and in otherwise asymptomatic cases. The vaccines against rubella, measles, and mumps contain live attenuated virus, and hearing loss in association with measles, mumps, and rubella vaccination has also been reported, although rarely.[17] A 2008 article using data from the US Vaccine Adverse Event Reporting System for the period 1990 to 2003 estimated the reporting rate of SNHL related to vaccine use to be 1 case in 6 to 8 million doses.[39] Because of the rarity of these reports, a causal relationship between mumps, rubella, and measles vaccination and SNHL requires further study.[48]

Other viruses
Other viral infections have been potentially associated with either congenitally acquired or postnatally acquired hearing loss, including sudden hearing loss. These include lymphocytic choriomeningitis virus, varicella zoster virus, West Nile virus, and human parvovirus B19. Varicella zoster virus causes Ramsay Hunt syndrome, also called herpes zoster oticus (HZO), and involves reactivation of the virus in the geniculate ganglion. In addition to facial paresis, hearing loss and vertigo are 2 of the often multiple presenting symptoms of HZO, which can affect multiple cranial nerves. Up to 5% of patients with HZO will have some degree of permanent hearing loss.[49]

Bacterial meningitis
Hearing loss is a well-documented sequela of bacterial meningitis. A 2010 systematic review and meta-analysis of 132 articles from around the world published between 1980 and 2008 reported a 33.6% incidence of hearing loss due to bacterial meningitis from all causes (Streptococcus *pneumoniae*, Haemophilus *influenzae* type B, Neisseria *meningitidis*, and others).[50] Although *H influenzae* type B meningitis was the most common type of meningitis, hearing loss occurred most often after pneumococcal meningitis. The use of systemic steroids in the management of meningitis remains controversial.[51] A 2013 Cochrane Database review looked at 25 randomized controlled trials of corticosteroid use (4121 subjects) in acute bacterial meningitis. For the group as a whole, they found a significantly reduced rate of hearing loss and neurologic sequelae, although overall mortality was not reduced. The data supported beneficial effects of steroids, including decreased hearing loss and neurologic sequelae, in high-income, but not low-income, countries. Therefore, the benefits of dexamethasone or other steroids in the prevention of hearing loss or other neurologic sequelae due to bacterial meningitis continue to remain unclear.[52,53]

Bacterial meningitis–related hearing loss generally has its onset early in the course of the disease, and the incidence has not been decreased by any specific antibiotic regimen. Although otitis media with direct spread through labyrinthine windows may precede onset of the disease in some cases, a more likely route is penetration of bacteria and bacterial toxins via the cochlear aqueduct or internal auditory canal contents, resulting in perineuritis or neuritis of the cochleovestibular nerve and/or suppurative labyrinthitis. Other pathophysiologic mechanisms operative in producing hearing loss may include serous or toxic labyrinthitis, thrombophlebitis or embolization of labyrinthine vessels, and hypoxia or anoxia of the eighth nerve and central auditory pathways.

If a child with meningitis has normal audiometric studies after the first few days of antibiotic therapy, it is unlikely that significant SNHL will develop later, and some children with initially abnormal hearing may improve, suggesting a resolving serous labyrinthitis. Well-documented late progression of postmeningitic SNHL after years of stability has been reported, however, in a few patients, along with some fluctuation of the hearing for up to a year after the initial episode of meningitis. In addition, Worsøe and colleagues[51] found that many patients who were not suspected of having hearing loss at the time of discharge were later found to have SNHL, supporting the need for close follow-up.

For those children with profound bilateral SNHL after bacterial meningitis, cochlear implantation has been a successful means of auditory rehabilitation. Surgery for cochlear implantation must be expedited, because labyrinthine ossification as a sequela of meningitis may make implantation of the electrode array into the cochlea difficult if not impossible.

Otitis media

Although OM is common, permanent SNHL in the pediatric population as a result of uncomplicated OM is not. SNHL can, however, occur in association with acute suppurative labyrinthitis and with longstanding chronic suppurative otitis media, with or without cholesteatoma. Therefore, the hearing in children with both of these forms of OM must be carefully monitored.[54,55]

HEARING LOSS SECONDARY TO TRAUMA

There are many different categories of trauma that can result in hearing loss in children, including head trauma, exposure to ototoxic medications, chemotherapy and radiation therapy, ECMO, iatrogenic injury due to surgery, and noise. Of all of these, environmental noise is the most common.

Noise-Related Hearing Loss

The outer hair cells in the cochlea, when exposed to loud noise, initially experience transient damage that causes a temporary threshold shift in the hearing; if a person is exposed long enough, the damage becomes permanent. Standard pure tone audiometric tests do not capture these early changes, so by the time the hearing loss can be "seen" in the audiogram, permanent damage has been done. Governmental agencies, including the Occupational Safety and Health Administration and the National Institute for Occupational Safety and Health, have guidelines for occupational and industrial noise exposure and require that individual workers exposed to sound levels greater than 85 A-weighted decibels (dBAs) wear ear protection (dBAs are weighted sound levels and closely match the human perception of sound). These guidelines are based on a calculation of noise "dose," using formulas that include total time of exposure at a specific noise level. These guidelines show how, above 85 dBAs, the potential for permanent hearing loss increases rapidly, with seemingly modest increases in decibel level. Because decibels are measured on a logarithmic scale, for every 3-dB increase in sound pressure the amount of allowable time of exposure to noise above 85 dBAs is cut in half.[56,57]

A 2004 report found that the output levels of common earphones, including insert, supra-aural, vertical, and circumaural, varied across type and manufacturer, but generally the sound pressure level in decibels was highest for the smallest earphones and that insert earphones increased the output level 7 dB to 9 dB.[58] A 2007 article recommends that people using a standard personal music player and headphone combination should limit their listening to no more than 60% volume for 60 minutes (or less) for a CD player and no more than 90 minutes (or less) at 80% volume for an MP3 player during any 24-hour period.[56] Additional recommendations are to use sound-isolating ear phones in the presence of significant background noise. The use of these earphones has been shown to provide as much as 25 dB of sound isolation.[59,60]

In addition, the exposure to noise in the setting of other risk factors for hearing loss, such as systemic aminoglycosides, chemotherapy, and genetic factors (eg, genetic predisposition to noise-induced hearing loss), needs to be studied.

Ototoxicity

Several groups of drugs are well-recognized causes of SNHL, including aminoglycoside antibiotics, systemic chemotherapy (especially cisplatin), macrolides, and loop diuretics. The effects of these drugs on inner ear physiology may be compounded by concurrent medical conditions, including renal failure, the use of ECMO, sepsis, extreme prematurity, diabetes, noise exposure, and genetic factors, all of which are independently related to an increased incidence of hearing loss. Hearing loss related to these drugs may occur both during and long after administration, especially for cisplatin. Radiation therapy involving the temporal bones and cisplatin given within the same time frame have been reported to have an increased incidence of SNHL over either one alone, with the hearing loss often presenting years after the therapy is completed. Although the ototoxicity of the aminoglycosides is strongly related to drug levels (peaks and troughs) and cumulative dosage, genetic susceptibility to ototoxicity, including mutations in mitochondrial genes, especially the homoplasmic 1555A>G and 1494C>T mutations in the mitochondrial 12S ribosomal RNA, is well described, with hearing loss occurring after even 1 dose in some patients who have these mutations. Hearing loss after exposure to macrolides is often reversible when the drugs are discontinued.[61–67] Pharmacologic means to prevent or reverse hearing loss are also being investigated.[68] Identification of particular genetic mutations in certain subpopulations, such as children with cystic fibrosis who often receive aminoglycosides, could guide the use of alternative medications or the institution of preventative interventions.

Head Trauma

It is well known that temporal bone fractures are associated with SNHL. Much less well recognized is the incidence of hearing loss due to closed head trauma, such as concussion and traumatic brain injury, in the absence of obvious temporal bone fractures. A cochlear concussion is classically a notch at 2000 to 4000 Hz in the absence of temporal bone fracture or other organic pathology from head trauma. In a recent study of soldiers returning from Iraq and Afghanistan, more than half the subjects with traumatic brain injury had hearing impairment, and many had both visual impairment and hearing loss.[69] These subjects exhibit both peripheral hearing loss and more subtle central auditory findings, potentially making rehabilitation more challenging. With an increasing recognition of the prevalence of cognitive, behavioral, and vestibular effects of sports-related concussion as well as traumatic brain injury, an auditory and vestibular evaluation should be added to the clinical care of these patients.[70,71]

Sudden Sensorineural Hearing Loss

Sudden SNHL is a well-reported occurrence in adults but little studied in children. Although the definition of idiopathic sudden SNHL includes unilateral onset, many subjects with sudden onset of SNHL actually have bilateral findings. The causes of sudden-onset SNHL are often difficult to identify but include viral, immunologic, traumatic, neoplastic, vascular, toxic, neurologic, and metabolic potential etiologic factors. Unwitnessed head trauma, barotrauma, noise, sudden auditory manifestations of preexisting temporal bone abnormalities, eighth nerve tumors, Meniere disease, progression of unrecognized congenital infections (such as CMV, toxoplasmosis, and syphilis), Lyme disease, or an underappreciated manifestation of a previously existing disease, such as the hereditary periodic fever syndromes, also need to be considered. Ioannis and colleagues[72] studied the records of 48 children with sudden hearing loss presenting to their department between 2002 and 2007. Twenty-six (54%) were found to have pseudohypacusis. Of the 22 patients (46%) with true organic hearing loss, 2 had EVA, 1 had multiple sclerosis, 1 had herpesvirus infection, 2 had acoustic trauma, and the remainder were considered idiopathic. Tarshish and colleagues[73] retrospectively studied 20 children with sudden SNHL. Hearing loss was bilateral in 9/

20 patients and hearing loss ranged from mild to profound. Additional symptoms included tinnitus (n = 9), vertigo (n = 9), sensation of a blocked ear (n = 6), and otalgia (n = 4). Probable causes were viral of unknown type (n = 12), late presentation of congenital CMV (n = 1), noise related (n = 1), nonorganic (n = 1), EVA (n = 1), both acute Epstein-Barr virus and significant ototoxic exposure (n = 1), ototoxic exposure and an inflammatory cerebrovascular incident (n = 1), and unknown (n = 2). Positive diagnostic studies included 1 MR image consistent with congenital CMV and 1 CT scan that showed an EVA; 15/20 patients received systemic steroids, 3 received antivirals, and 4 received antibiotics. Response to steroids varied from complete resolution of SSNHL to worsening.

Suggested treatments for sudden SNHL (without an obvious cause) include systemic steroids, intratympanic steroids, and antivirals, although nearly all treatment series include only patients over 18 years of age.[72] Systemic steroids have been studied the most, with generally modest to mild benefit reported if they are started soon after the SNHL is identified. With regard to antivirals, Tucci and colleagues[74] looked at hearing improvement in patients over 18 years of age with idiopathic SNHL treated with systemic prednisone with or without valacyclovir (antiviral) therapy. No additional benefit over steroids alone was noted in the valacyclovir patients in this trial or in 2 other trials using antivirals.[74,75] Intratympanic steroids, as first or salvage treatment, have also recently been studied. Most studies have small numbers, are retrospective, are limited to case series, do not include a natural history group, and do not include large numbers of (or any) children. The efficacy of intratympanic steroids, therefore, remains unclear.[76–78] Other therapies mentioned in the literature, including hyperbaric oxygen, volume expanders, vasodilators, herbal remedies, anticoagulants, and zinc, have not been studied in a rigorous fashion in any age group for sudden SNHL. Huang and Sataloff[79] reported on 7 children with autoimmune inner ear disease (AIED), with both systemic steroids and cytotoxic medications having some efficacy. Most treatment studies of AIED are small and have not included children, so the long-term efficacy of steroids, as well as diagnostic accuracy, of AIED in children remains unclear.

Hearing loss in babies who require newborn intensive care unit management

It is well recognized that NICU infants, especially those with very low birth weight (VLBW), below 1500 g, have a higher incidence of hearing loss than term infants in the well-baby nursery. The incidence of SNHL in VLBW babies varies between studies, but overall the incidence seems to be decreasing, with a recent study documenting an incidence of 4.1%.[80] Risk factors associated with permanent congenital, delayed-onset or progressive hearing losses are listed in the 2007 Joint Committee on Infant Hearing guidelines[81] and include a NICU stay of more than 5 days or the presence of any of the following: ECMO, assisted ventilation, ototoxic drug exposure, loop diuretics (furosemide), and hyperbilirubinemia requiring exchange transfusion. Robertson and colleagues[82] identified several additional potential markers for hearing loss, including the need for gastrointestinal surgery (colonostomy, ileostomy, or resection associated with necrotizing enterocolitis), patent ductus arteriosus ligation, and lower socioeconomic status (**Box 1**). Additional studies have shown a statistical association between hearing loss and severe hypoxic/ischemic encephalopathy, prolonged mechanical ventilation, persistent pulmonary hypertension, higher serum bilirubin, intraventricular hemorrhage and meningitis, and high-frequency ventilation. Whether some of these are related directly to the hearing loss or occur as a result of factors that may also lead to hearing loss remains unclear.[82–85] Aminoglycoside use, long suspected of being a major risk factor for NICU-related hearing loss, is found only slightly

---

Box 1
Risk indicators associated with permanent congenital, delayed-onset, or progressive hearing loss in infants and children

1. Caregiver concern regarding hearing, speech, language, or developmental delay

2. Family history of permanent childhood-onset hearing loss

3. NICU of more than 5 days or any of the following, regardless of length of stay:

   a. ECMO

   b. Assisted ventilation

   c. Persistent pulmonary hypertension

   d. Exposure to ototoxic medications, including aminoglycosides and loop diuretics

   e. Hyperbilirubinemia requiring exchange transfusion

   f. In utero infections, such as CMV, toxoplasmosis, rubella, and syphilis

4. Craniofacial anomalies, including those that involve the pinna, ear canal, ear tags, ear pits, and temporal bones anomalies

5. Physical findings associated with known syndromes that include a permanent conductive or SNHL

6. Syndromes associated with hearing loss, including congenital, progressive, or late onset. Examples include Usher, Waardenburg, CHARGE, BOR, neurofibromatosis, PDS, Alport, and Jervell and Lange-Nielsen

7. Neurodegenerative disorders, such as the mucopolysaccharidoses, and sensory motor neuropathies, such as Friedreich ataxia or Charcot-Marie-Tooth

8. Culture-positive postnatal infections associated with SNHL, including bacterial meningitis, and some causes of viral meningitis, including herpesvirus and varicella

9. Head trauma, including temporal bone fractures, basilar skull fractures, and severe concussion

10. Chemotherapy

From American Academy of Pediatrics, Joint Committee on Infant Hearing. Year 2007 position statement: principles and guidelines for early hearing detection and intervention programs. Pediatrics 2007;120(4):898–921; with permission.

---

statistically associated.[86] This could be due to better monitoring of peak and trough levels or better management of NICU babies with decreased need for prolonged aminoglycoside courses. Of particular concern is that use of furosemide or other loop diuretics may either be related to hearing loss alone, or they may potentiate the rate of aminoglycoside-induced hearing loss and also be more likely to cause hearing loss in the presence of sepsis. Finally, noise in the NICU, generated by the presence of life support equipment, has been shown to be a contributing factor to hearing loss in NICU infants. This requires further study.[87,88]

Hyperbilirubinemia is a well-recognized cause of hearing loss in newborns, and more recently it has been associated with auditory dyssynchrony.[3] The 2007 Joint Committee on Infant Hearing guidelines[81] list hyperbilirubinemia that requires exchange transfusion as a risk factor for the development of hearing loss. A study by Oh and colleagues[89] suggested that in VLBW infants even a moderate elevation of bilirubin may be related to poorer neurodevelopmental outcomes and hearing loss.[89] A subsequent study by Morris and colleagues[90] assessing aggressive versus conservative phototherapy in VLBW infants showed that infants with even modestly elevated levels of bilirubin had less hearing loss when aggressive phototherapy was used, and the aggressively managed group had better overall neurodevelopmental outcome.[90]

A recent study by Saluja and colleagues,[91] however, found auditory dyssynchrony the only manifestation of acute bilirubin-induced neurotoxicity in late preterm and term infants. The level of hyperbilirubinemia and the optimal management, however, especially in VLBW babies with complicated clinical pictures, remain uncertain.[91]

Middle and inner ear structural anomalies

Congenital anomalies of the middle and/or inner ear may present with progressive and/or fluctuating hearing loss. Although an extensive discussion of these anomalies is beyond the scope of this article,[92,93] these need to be considered in the potential list of causes of "acquired" hearing losses. Structural anomalies resulting in hearing loss can occur at any stage in the embryogenesis of these structures, with a resulting hearing loss that is conductive, mixed, or sensorineural.

In addition, hundreds of syndromes have hearing loss associated with middle and/or inner ear anomalies as one of the features. Many of the patients present with mixed, or occasionally purely conductive, hearing loss. Mutations in the X-linked POU3F4 gene are associated with dilatation of the internal auditory canal and a range of temporal bone anomalies that include stapes fixation and dysplasia of the cochlea and semicircular canals. These patients, who are otherwise nonsyndromic, present with a congenital and subsequently progressive mixed hearing loss. The surgeon may encounter a fixed stapes and perilymphatic gusher at the time of cochlear implant or other middle ear surgery.[94]

Three other syndromes for which the hearing loss is a defining feature include Pendred syndrome (PDS); coloboma, heart defect, atresia choanae (ie, choanal atresia), retarded growth and development, genital abnormality, and ear abnormality (CHARGE) syndrome; and branchio-oto-renal (BOR) syndrome. Patients with PDS present with hearing loss that can be mild to profound, thyroid dysfunction often leading to goiter, and in some cases vestibular dysfunction. Inner ear abnormalities include enlarged bony vestibular aqueducts, enlarged endolymphatic sacs, and cochlear partition defects—50% of PDS patients have mutations in the SLC26A4 gene; up to 10% of patients with hereditary hearing loss have PDS[95]; 70% of CHARGE patients have mutations in the CHD7 gene, with a much smaller number having mutations in the SEMA3E gene; and approximately 40% of BOR patients have mutations in the EYA1 gene, with 5% carrying mutations in the SIX5 gene. Both CHARGE and BOR have characteristic middle and inner ear anomalies and may present with conductive, sensorineural, or mixed hearing losses that can fluctuate or progress. Findings in BOR include a hypoplastic apical turn of the cochlea, facial nerve canal deviated to the medial side of the cochlea, a funnel-shaped internal auditory canal, a patulous eustachian tube, hypoplasia of the horizontal, superior, and posterior semicircular canals and hypoplasia/dysplasia of the malleus and incus.[96,97] Findings in those with CHARGE include cochlear aperture atresia, lack of a cochlear nerve on MR imaging, cochlear dysplasia, round window aplasia or hypoplasia, oval window atresia or aplasia, hypoplastic or dysplastic vestibules, enlarged or anomalous vestibular aqueducts, absent semicircular canals, and facial nerve canals with an anomalous course.[98,99]

In patients with unilateral or bilateral sensorineural or mixed hearing loss, inner ear anomalies are demonstrated by either CT and/or MR imaging of the temporal bones up to 40% of the time.[100] Histopathologically, the hearing losses can involve the membranous and/or bony components of the labyrinth. Although both CT and MR imaging are increasingly effective at demonstrating structural anomalies of the middle and inner ear, subtle bony anomalies, membranous anomalies, or anomalies below the level of resolution of CT or MR imaging still are not appreciated.[92]

The overall evaluation of acquired neonatal and childhood-onset hearing loss
The diagnostic evaluation of acquired hearing loss in newborns and young children is in rapid evolution. In the immediate neonatal period, testing for CMV, even if other potential causes of hearing loss may be present, offers an opportunity to potentially improve or stabilize the hearing loss. Most of the other TORCHES infections are now uncommon in the United States; however, there is established therapy for congenital toxoplasmosis and syphilis, so testing for these should be considered if appropriate. Lin and colleagues[101] recently reported the diagnostic yield of several studies in 270 children with severe to profound SNHL evaluated between 2002 and 2009. They reviewed temporal bone MR imaging and CT, renal ultrasound, ECG, fluorescent treponemal antibody absorption test for syphilis (FTA), GJB2 (connexin 26) sequencing, genetic consultation, and ophthalmologic evaluation. MR imaging revealed structural abnormalities in 24% of the children, abnormalities on CT in 18%, and biallelic GJB2 mutations in 15%. The yield of the other tests was renal ultrasound (4%), ECG (long QT in 1%), FTA (0.5%), genetics evaluation (25%), and ophthalmologic consultation (8%). Nearly all the children with biallelic GJB2 mutations had nonsyndromic SNHL, and several had passed a newborn hearing screen. Although the percentage yield for CT and MR imaging was similar, they did not always find the same abnormalities; EVA was occasionally picked up by MR imaging and not by CT and vice versa. MR imaging of the brain found brain malformations and indications of congenital infections (eg, CMV), which CT of the temporal bones did not. Ophthalmology evaluations revealed myopia and coloboma (in children with CHARGE association) and 2 with retinitis pigmentosa eventually were found to have Usher syndrome. All children with hearing loss are visual learners, so even discovering that they need eyeglasses is useful information, and if they have less common but other important findings that may yield an additional diagnosis that benefits the patient. In addition, this study looked at children with bilateral severe to profound SNHL; the yield of these same tests in children with milder or unilateral hearing loss may be different. The diagnostic yield for specific tests in the Lin and colleagues[101] study is in good agreement with others, including Preciado and colleagues.[102] Testing for diagnoses that are treatable, such as congenital CMV, or dangerous if missed, such as long QT in children with bilateral severe to profound SNHL, should always be considered. Many studies commonly performed in the past to diagnose syndromes associated with hearing loss may now be better evaluated using actual genetic testing. An example of this concept is mutation in the SLC26A4 (PDS gene) associated with bilateral EVA (nonsyndromic EVA, DFNB4) and, in some cases, thyroid dysfunction (the full PDS). A second is Usher syndrome, where genetic testing may be positive in the presence of a normal routine eye examination, especially in young children.[103,104] CMV was not routinely tested in the Lin and colleagues'[101] or most other studies. Because congenital CMV and toxoplasmosis are treatable, however, testing for CMV in infants would be a reasonable place to start in neonates and very young infants. In addition, although CS is uncommon, it is another treatable cause, so testing would be justified if clinically suspected. In addition, patients with biallelic GJB2 mutations seldom have anatomic inner ear abnormalities, so if initial imaging is normal, then mutations in GJB2 are a stronger consideration, whereas if the imaging is abnormal, GJB2 is less likely. For some of the more common causes, occasionally there may be overlap in the same patient. For example, babies with congenital CMV may also have EVA or GJB2 mutations. Therefore, if the presentation does not completely fit the initial

diagnosis, especially as a patient is followed over time, further evaluation for additional causes of hearing loss should be considered. The overall diagnostic yield for these studies taken together (especially imaging, genetics, and CMV) is 50% to 60% and is likely to improve with better genetic testing, higher-resolution imaging, and increased awareness of the incidence of congenital CMV.

SUMMARY

Pediatric hearing loss is common and, with the advent of newborn hearing screening, diagnosed at increasingly younger ages. The identification of a definite cause can aid in prognosis and management. Although many hearing losses are truly acquired, many others are manifestations of preexisting conditions. The yield of diagnostic studies has increased given accurate testing for, and awareness of the frequency of, congenital CMV, anatomic abnormalities of the inner ear, and genetic causes. A methodical approach to diagnostic studies based on laterality and degree of hearing loss, history and physical examination, family history, and overall clinical presentation, frequently yields a cause.

REFERENCES

1. Lin FR, Niparko JK, Ferrucci L. Hearing loss prevalence in the United States. Arch Intern Med 2011;171(20):1851–2.
2. Available at: http://www.who.int/mediacentre/factsheets/fs300/en/. Accessed July 4, 2015.
3. Hood LJ. Auditory Neuropathy/Dys-Synchrony Disorder: Diagnosis and Management. Otolaryngol Clin N Am 2015, in press.
4. Koffler T, Ushakov K, Avraham KB. Genetics of Hearing Loss: Syndromic. Otolaryngol Clin N Am 2015, in press.
5. Chang KW. Genetics of Hearing Loss—Nonsyndromic. Otolaryngol Clin N Am 2015, in press.
6. Chan DK, Chang KW. GJB2-associated hearing loss: systematic review of worldwide prevalence, genotype, and auditory phenotype. Laryngoscope 2014;124(2):E34–53.
7. Kenna MA, Feldman HA, Neault MW, et al. Audiologic phenotype and progression in GJB2 (Connexin 26) hearing loss. Arch Otolaryngol Head Neck Surg 2010;136(1):81–7.
8. Van Camp G, Smith RJH. Hereditary hearing loss homepage. Available at: http://hereditaryhearingloss.org. Accessed July 4, 2015.
9. Lavinsky J, Crow AL, Pan C, et al. Genome-wide association study identifies nox3 as a critical gene for susceptibility to noise-induced hearing loss. PLoS Genet 2015;11(4):e1005094.
10. Available at: http://www.cdc.gov/dpdx/toxoplasmosis/index.html. Accessed July 4, 2015.
11. Lopez A, Dietz VJ, Wilson M, et al. Preventing congenital toxoplasmosis. National Center for Health Statistics. Recommendations Rep 2000;49(rr02): 57–75.
12. Guerina NG, Hsu HW, Meissner HC, et al. Neonatal serologic screening and early treatment for congenital Toxoplasma gondii infection. The New England Regional Toxoplasma Working Group. N Engl J Med 1994;330(26):1858–63.
13. Available at: http://www.cdc.gov/parasites/toxoplasmosis/. Accessed July 4, 2015.

14. Brown ED, Chau JK, Atashband S, et al. A systematic review of neonatal toxoplasmosis exposure and sensorineural hearing loss. Int J Pediatr Otorhinolaryngol 2009;73:707–11.
15. McLeod R, Boyer K, Karrison T, et al, Toxoplasmosis Study Group. Outcome of treatment for congenital toxoplasmosis, 1981-2004: the National Collaborative chicago-based, congenital toxoplasmosis Study. Clin Infect Dis 2006;42(10): 1383–94.
16. Available at: http://www.who.int/topics/rubella/en/. Accessed July 4, 2015.
17. Stewart BJ, Prabhu PU. Reports of sensorineural deafness after measles, mumps, and rubella immunization. Arch Dis Child 1993;69:153–4.
18. Stehel EK, Shoup AG, Owen KE, et al. Newborn hearing screening and detection of congenital cytomegalovirus infection. Pediatrics 2008;121: 970–5.
19. Grosse SD, Ross DS, Dollard SC. Congenital cytomegalovirus (CMV) infection as a cause of permanent bilateral hearing loss: a qualitative assessment. J Clin Virol 2008;41:57–62.
20. Available at: http://www.cdc.gov/cmv/index.html. Accessed July 4, 2015.
21. Boppana SB, Ross SA, Shimamura M, et al, National Institute on Deafness and Other Communication Disorders CHIMES Study. Saliva polymerase-chain-reaction assay for cytomegalovirus screening in newborns. N Engl J Med 2011;364(22):2111–8.
22. Ross SA, Ahmed A, Palmer AL, et al, National Institute on Deafness and Other Communication Disorders CHIMES Study. Detection of congenital cytomegalovirus infection by real-time polymerase chain reaction analysis of saliva or urine specimens. J Infect Dis 2014;210(9):1415–8.
23. Kimberlin DW, Jester PM, Sánchez PJ, et al, National Institute of Allergy and Infectious Diseases Collaborative Antiviral Study Group. Congenital cytomegalovirus disease. N Engl J Med 2015;372:933–43.
24. Koontz D, Baecher K, Amin M, et al. Evaluation of DNA extraction methods for the detection of Cytomegalovirus in dried blood spots. J Clin Virol 2015;66:95–9.
25. Ross SA, Ahmed A, Palmer AL, et al. National Institute on Deafness and Other Communication Disorders CHIMES Study. Urine Collection Method for the Diagnosis of Congenital Cytomegalovirus Infection. Pediatr Infect Dis J 2015. [Epub ahead of print].
26. Lombardi G, Garofoli F, Stronati M. Congenital cytomegalovirus Infection: treatment, sequelae and follow-up. J Matern Fetal Neonatal Med 2010;23(Suppl 3): 45–8.
27. Boppana S, Amos C, Britt W, et al. Late onset and reactivation of chorioretinitis in children with congenital cytomegalovirus infection. Pediatr Infect Dis J 1994;13: 1139–42.
28. Brown ZA, Wald A, Morrow A, et al. Effect of serologic status and cesarean delivery on transmission rates of herpes simplex virus from mother to infant. JAMA 2003;289(2):203–9.
29. Kimberlin DW. Herpes simplex virus infections of the newborn. Semin Perinatol 2007;31(1):19–25.
30. Cohen BE, Durstenfeld A, Roehm PC. Viral causes of hearing loss: a review for hearing health professionals. Trends Hearing 2014;18:1–17.
31. Westerberg BD, Atashband S, Kozak FK. A systematic review of the incidence of sensorineural hearing loss in neonates exposed to Herpes simplex virus (HSV). Int J Pediatr Otorhinolaryngol 2008;72(7):931–7.

32. Chau J, Atashband S, Chang E, et al. A systematic review of pediatric sensorineural hearing loss in congenital syphilis. Int J Pediatr Otorhinolaryngol 2009; 73(6):787–92.
33. Available at: http://www.cdc.gov/std/syphilis/default.htm. Accessed July 4, 2015.
34. Fiumara NJ, Lessell S. Manifestations of late congenital syphilis. An analysis of 271 patients. Arch Dermatol 1970;102(1):78–83.
35. Palacios GC, Montalvo MS, Fraire MI, et al. Audiologic and vestibular findings in a sample of Human Immunodeficiency Virus type-1-infected Mexican children under High Active Antiretroviral Therapy. Int J Pediatr Otorhinolaryngol 2008; 71(11):1671–81.
36. Christopher N, Edward T, Sabrina BK, et al. The prevalence of hearing impairment in the 6 months-5 years HIV/AIDS-positive patients attending paediatric infectious disease clinic at Mulago Hospital. Int J Pediatr Otorhinolaryngol 2013; 77(2):262–5.
37. Torre P, Cook A, Elliott H, et al. Hearing assessment data in HIV-infected and uninfected children of Cape Town, South Africa. AIDS Care 2015;27(8): 1037–41.
38. Available at: http://www.cdc.gov/measles/cases-outbreaks.html. Measles Cases and Outbreaks. Accessed January 29, 2015.
39. Asatryan A, Pool V, Chen RT, et al, Immunization Safety Office, Office of the Chief Science Officer, Centers for Disease Control and Prevention, Atlanta, GA, USA, The VAERS Team. Live attenuated measles and mumps viral strain-containing vaccines and hearing loss: Vaccine Adverse Event Reporting System (VAERS), United States, 1990-2003. Vaccine 2008;26(9):1166–72.
40. Hulbert TV, Larsen RA, Davis CL, et al. Bilateral hearing loss after measles vaccination in an adult. N Engl J Med 1991;325:134.
41. Niedermeyer HP, Arnold W. Otosclerosis and measles virus: association or causation? ORL J Otorhinolaryngol Relat Spec 2008;70(1):63–9.
42. Schrauwen I, Van Camp G. The etiology of otosclerosis: a combination of genes and environment. Laryngoscope 2010;120(6):1195–202.
43. Peeters N, van der Kolk BY, Thijsen SF, et al. Lyme disease associated with sudden sensorineural hearing loss: case report and literature review. Otol Neurotol 2013;34(5):832–7.
44. Available at: www.cdc.gov/lyme/. Accessed July 4, 2015.
45. Wilson YL, Gandolfi MM, Ahn IE, et al. Cost analysis of asymmetric sensorineural hearing loss. Laryngoscope 2010;120(9):1832–6.
46. Available at: http://www.who.int/immunization/monitoring_surveillance/en/. Accessed July 4, 2015.
47. Hashimoto H, Fujioka M, Kinumaki H, Kinki Ambulatory Pediatrics Study Group. An office based prospective study of deafness in mumps. Pediatr Infect Dis J 2009;28(3):173–5.
48. Available at: www.cdc.gov/mumps/about/index.html. Accessed July 4, 2015.
49. Worme M, Chada R, Lavallee L. An unexpected case of Ramsay hunt syndrome: case report and literature review. BMC Res Notes 2013;6:337.
50. Edmond K, Clark A, Korczak VS, et al. Global and regional risk of disabling sequelae from bacterial meningitis: a systematic review and meta-analysis. Lancet Infect Dis 2010;10(5):317–28.
51. Worsøe L, Caye-Thomasen P, Thomas Brandt CT, et al. Factors associated with the occurrence of hearing loss after pneumococcal meningitis. Clin Infect Dis 2010;51(8):917–24.

52. Brouwer MC, McIntyre P, Prasad K, et al. Corticosteroids for acute bacterial meningitis. Cochrane Database Syst Rev 2013;(6):CD004405.
53. Peltola H, Roine I, Fernández J, et al. Hearing impairment in childhood bacterial meningitis is little relieved by dexamethasone or glycerol. Pediatrics 2010; 125(1):e1–8.
54. Yehudai N, Most T, Luntz M. Risk factors for sensorineural hearing loss in pediatric chronic otitis media. Int J Pediatr Otorhinolaryngol 2015;79(1):26–30.
55. Yen YC, Lin C, Weng SF, et al. Higher risk of developing sudden sensorineural hearing loss in patients with chronic otitis media. JAMA Otolaryngol Head Neck Surg 2015;141(5):429–35.
56. Available at: http://www.osha.gov/SLTC/noisehearingconservation/index.html#standards. Accessed July 4, 2015.
57. Available at: http://www.cdc.gov/niosh/topics/noise/default.html. Accessed August 22, 2015.
58. Fligor BJ, Cox LC. Output levels of commercially available portable compact disc players and the potential risk to hearing. Ear Hear 2004;25:513–27.
59. Fligor B. Hearing loss and iPods: what happens when you turn them to 11? Hearing J 2007;60(10):10–6.
60. Kumar A, Mathew K, Alexander SA, et al. Output sound pressure levels of personal music systems and their effect on hearing. Noise Health 2009;11: 132–40.
61. Albert RK, Connett J, Bailey WC, et al, COPD Clinical Research Network. Azithromycin for prevention of exacerbations of COPD. N Engl J Med 2011; 365(8):689–98.
62. Grewal S, Merchant T, Reymond R, et al. Auditory late effects of childhood cancer therapy: a report from the Children's Oncology Group. Pediatrics 2010; 125(4):e938–50.
63. Mick P, Westerberg BD. Sensorineural hearing loss as a probable serious adverse drug reaction associated with low-dose oral azithromycin. J Otolaryngol 2007;36(5):257–63.
64. Mukherjea D, Rybak LP, Sheehan KE, et al. The design and screening of drugs to prevent acquired sensorineural hearing loss. Expert Opin Drug Discov 2011; 6(5):491–505. Available at: Informahealthcare.com.
65. Mulrennan SA, Helm J, Thomas RB, et al. Aminoglycoside ototoxicity susceptibility in cystic fibrosis. Thorax 2009;64:271–2.
66. Rybak LP, Mukherjea D, Jajoo S, et al. Cisplatin ototoxicity and protection: clinical and experimental studies. Tohoku J Exp Med 2009;219(3):177–86.
67. Veenstra DL, Harris J, Gibson RL, et al. Pharmacogenomic testing to prevent aminoglycoside-induced hearing loss in cystic fibrosis patients: potential impact on clinical, patient, and economic outcomes. Genet Med 2007;9(10): 695–704.
68. Esterberg R, Coffin AB, Ou H, et al. Fish in a dish: drug discovery for hearing habilitation. Drug Discov Today Dis Models 2013;10(1).
69. Lew HL, Garvert DW, Pogoda TK, et al. Auditory and visual impairments in patients with blast-related traumatic brain injury: effect of dual sensory impairment on functional independence measure. J Rehabil Res Dev 2009;46(6):819–26.
70. Choi MS, Shin SO, Yeon JY, et al. Clinical characteristics of labyrinthine concussion. Korean J Audiol 2013;17(1):13–7.
71. Zhou G, Brodsky JR. Objective vestibular testing of children with dizziness and balance complaints following sports-related concussions. Otolaryngol Head Neck Surg 2015;152(6):1133–9.

72. Ioannis P, Georgios K, Kontrogiannis A, et al. Pseudohypacusis: the most frequent etiology of sudden hearing loss in children. Eur Arch Otorhinolaryngol 2009;266:1857–61.

73. Tarshish Y, Leschinski A, Kenna M. Pediatric sudden sensorineural hearing loss: diagnosed causes and response to intervention. Int J Pediatr Otorhinolaryngol 2013;77(4):553–9.

74. Tucci DL, Farmer JC, Kitch RD, et al. Treatment of sudden sensorineural hearing loss with systemic steroids and valacyclovir. Otol Neurotol 2002;23(3):301–8.

75. Awad Z, Huins C, Pothier DD. Antivirals for idiopathic sudden sensorineural hearing loss. Cochrane Database Syst Rev 2012;(8):CD006987.

76. Ng JH, Ho RC, Cheong CS, et al. Intratympanic steroids as a salvage treatment for sudden sensorineural hearing loss? A meta-analysis. Eur Arch Otorhinolaryngol 2015;272(10):2777–82.

77. Rauch SD, Halpin CF, Antonelli PJ, et al. Oral vs. intratympanic corticosteroid therapy for idiopathic sudden sensorineural hearing loss: a randomized trial. JAMA 2011;305(20):2071–9.

78. Wei BP, Stathopoulos D, O'Leary S. Steroids for idiopathic sudden sensorineural hearing loss. Cochrane Database Syst Rev 2013;(7):CD003998.

79. Huang NC, Sataloff RT. Autoimmune inner ear disease in children. Otol Neurotol 2011;32(2):213–6.

80. Speleman K, Kneepkens K, Vandendriessche K, et al. Prevalence of risk factors for sensorineural hearing loss in NICU newborns. B-ENT 2012;8(1):1–6.

81. American Academy of Pediatrics, Joint Committee on Infant Hearing. Year 2007 position statement: principles and guide-lines for early hearing detection and intervention programs. Pediatrics 2007;120(4):898–921.

82. Robertson CMT, Howarth TM, Bork DL, et al. Permanent bilateral sensory and neural hearing loss of children after neonatal intensive care because of extreme prematurity: a thirty-year study. Pediatrics 2009;123(5):e797–807.

83. Pruszewicz A, Pospiech I. Low birth weight as a risk factor of hearing loss. Scand Audiol Suppl 2001;52:194–6.

84. Roth DA, Hildesheimer M, Maayan-Metzger A, et al. Low prevalence of hearing impairment among very low birthweight infants as detected by universal neonatal hearing screening. Arch Dis Child Fetal Neonatal Ed 2006;91(4):F257–62.

85. Valkama AM, Laitakari KT, Tolonen EU, et al. Prediction of permanent hearing loss in high risk preterm infants at term age. Eur J Pediatr 2000;159:459–64.

86. Kent A, Turner MA, Sharland M, et al. Expert Aminoglycoside toxicity in neonates: something to worry about? Rev Anti Infect Ther 2014;12(3):319–31.

87. Li H, Wang Q, Steyger PS. Acoustic trauma increases cochlear and hair cell uptake of gentamicin. PLoS One 2011;6(4):e19130.

88. Zimmerman E, Lahav A. Ototoxicity in preterm infants: effects of genetics, aminoglycosides, and loud environmental noise. J Perinatol 2013;33(1):3–8.

89. Oh W, Tyson JE, Fanaroff AA, et al. Association between peak serum bilirubin and neurodevelopmental outcomes in extremely low birth weight infants. Pediatrics 2003;112:773–9.

90. Morris BH, Oh W, Tyson JE, et al. Aggressive vs. conservative phototherapy for infants with extremely low birth weight. N Engl J Med 2008;359:1885–96.

91. Saluja S, Agarwal A, Kler N, et al. Auditory neuropathy spectrum disorder in late preterm and term infants with severe jaundice. Int J Pediatr Otorhinolaryngol 2010;74(11):1292–7.

92. DeMarcantonio M, Choo DI. Radiographic Evaluation of Children with Hearing Loss. Otolaryngol Clin N Am 2015, in press.

93. Dougherty W, Kesser BW. Management of Conductive Hearing Loss in Children. Otolaryngol Clin N Am 2015, in press.
94. de Kok YJ, van der Maarel SM, Bitner-Glindzicz M, et al. Association between X-linked mixed deafness and mutations in the POU domain gene POU3F4. Science 1995;267(5198):685–8.
95. Available at: http://ghr.nlm.nih.gov/condition/pendred-syndrome. Accessed July 13, 2015.
96. Senel E, Gulleroglu BN, Senal S. Additional temporal bone findings on computed tomography imaging in branchio-oto-renal syndrome. Laryngoscope 2009;119:832.
97. Propst EJ, Blaser S, Gordon KA, et al. Temporal bone findings on computed tomography imaging in branchio-oto-renal syndrome. Laryngoscope 2005; 115(10):1855–62.
98. Holcomb MA, Rumboldt Z, White DR. Cochlear nerve deficiency in children with CHARGE syndrome. Laryngoscope 2013;123(3):793–6.
99. Morimoto AK, Wiggins RH, Hudgins PA, et al. Absent semicircular canals in CHARGE syndrome: radiologic spectrum of findings. AJNR Am J Neuroradiol 2006;27:1663–71.
100. Mafong D, Shin E, Lalwani A. Use of laboratory evaluation and radiologic imaging in the diagnostic evaluation of children with sensorineural hearing loss. Laryngoscope 2002;112:1–7.
101. Lin JW, Chowdhury N, Mody A, et al. Comprehensive diagnostic battery for evaluating sensorineural hearing loss in children. Otol Neurotol 2011;32(2):259–64.
102. Preciado DA, Lim LHY, Cohen AP, et al. A diagnostic paradigm for childhood idiopathic sensorineural hearing loss. Otolaryngol Head Neck Surg 2004;131: 804–9.
103. Jacobson SG, Cideciyan AV, Gibbs D, et al. Retinal disease course in usher syndrome 1B due to MYO7A mutations. Invest Ophthalmol Vis Sci 2011;52(11): 7924–36.
104. Kenna MA, Fulton A, Hansen R, et al. Diagnosis of usher syndrome and retinal degeneration in infants. Baltimore (MD): Association for Research in Otolaryngology; 2009.

Management of Conductive Hearing Loss in Children

William Dougherty, MD, Bradley W. Kesser, MD*

KEYWORDS

- Congenital aural atresia • Conductive hearing loss • Middle ear anomaly
- Canalplasty • Chronic otitis media in children

KEY POINTS

- Children with conductive hearing loss (CHL) are identified at several possible diagnostic points of care: newborn hearing screening, parental concern for hearing loss, hearing screening in the pediatrician's office, otoscopic examination either in the pediatrician's or in the otolaryngologist's office, or school hearing screening examination.
- The evaluation of any child with hearing loss involves a thorough history with careful otoscopic examination to include pneumatic otoscopy.
- Audiological assessment is a critical part of the evaluation and depends on the child's age and cooperability (see article by Singleton and Waltzman elsewhere in the issue).
- Any child with an unexplained CHL (normal ear canal, tympanic membrane, middle ear space) should undergo radiologic evaluation, usually high-resolution computed tomography (HRCT) of the temporal bone at some point (see later discussion and article by DeMarcantonio and Choo elsewhere in the issue).
- Management of the child with acquired CHL depends on the cause and may range from simple cerumen disimpaction to ventilation tube insertion, to more complex chronic ear surgery for tympanic membrane perforation or cholesteatoma.
- Management of the child with congenital CHL may include observation with monitoring of the hearing, an individual education (Individual Education Plan [IEP]) or 504(c) plan, amplification (conventional or bone conducting), or surgery. Management depends greatly on the diagnosis, degree of hearing loss, relevant anatomy, parental decision making, and educational and psychosocial factors.

Disclosures: none relevant.
Department of Otolaryngology–Head and Neck Surgery, University of Virginia School of Medicine, Box 800713, Charlottesville, VA 22908-0713, USA
* Corresponding author. Department of Otolaryngology–Head and Neck Surgery, University of Virginia School of Medicine, Box 800713, Charlottesville, VA 22908-0713.
E-mail address: Bwk2n@virginia.edu

Otolaryngol Clin N Am 48 (2015) 955–974
http://dx.doi.org/10.1016/j.otc.2015.06.007
0030-6665/15/$ – see front matter © 2015 Elsevier Inc. All rights reserved.

oto.theclinics.com

INTRODUCTION

While sensorineural hearing loss (SNHL) is far more common in adults, CHL accounts for 90% to 95% of all childhood hearing loss, with middle ear effusion (MEE)/otitis media with effusion (OME) far outpacing all other causes. Whether OME causes lasting deficits in speech and language development remains unclear, probably due to the transient, fluctuating nature of the associated hearing loss, involvement of one or both ears, mild degree of associated hearing loss, and medical and surgical options for management. Fixed, moderate, or moderate to severe congenital CHL such as that caused by congenital aural atresia (CAA) or other ossicular abnormality (eg, congenital stapes ankylosis) is rarer but may cause lasting deficits in speech and language development and educational progress, especially if bilateral and not evaluated and managed early and properly.[1]

Prevalence estimates of congenital SNHL range in the 1 to 3 per 1000 range, whereas estimates for congenital CHL are less well reported; however, clearly, this type of hearing loss, caused by some obstruction, dysfunction, or maldevelopment of the ear canal, eardrum, or middle ear impedance system, is also relatively rare. In a study of 234 Australian infants referred for diagnostic testing from a newborn hearing screening program, prevalence of CHL in the newborns was 2.97 per 1000 while the prevalence of middle ear pathology (with or without CHL) was 4.36 per 1000. As one investigator noted, "In the literature pertaining to CHL in children, the emphasis is on cause rather than severity, making prevalence data difficult to compare."[2] The ongoing and lasting effects of both congenital and acquired CHL in children, especially with regard to OME, have been studied exhaustively, yet no clear conclusions have been made.[3–6]

Options for hearing habilitation in children with congenital CHL include observation with monitoring—both hearing and academic progress—and possible individualized education plan (IEP)/504(c); amplification, either conventional or through bone conduction technology; and surgery. In children with bilateral moderate or moderate to severe fixed CHL such as that seen in CAA, amplification and/or surgical intervention is strongly recommended to support normal speech and language development, but controversy remains on the ideal management of the child with unilateral CHL.

This article provides the clinician with guidelines to inform the evaluation and management of childhood CHL—acquired and congenital as well as unilateral and bilateral.

ACQUIRED CONDUCTIVE HEARING LOSS
Otitis Media with Effusion

Prevalence
By far the most common cause of acquired CHL in children, OME is defined as the presence of fluid in the middle ear without the signs or symptoms of acute, active infection. It is estimated that at any given point in time, approximately 20% of young children have a MEE, with nearly all children having at least 1 episode during their childhood.[7] OME commonly follows an upper respiratory tract infection or is a sequela of acute otitis media and is usually self-limited. Certain populations have a higher prevalence of OME than the general population of young children. Children with Down syndrome have poor eustachian tube function because of decreased motor tone, predisposing them to persistent OME. OME also occurs with increased prevalence in children with cleft palate. In fact, it is nearly universal in children with cleft palate because of abnormal insertion of the levator veli palatini and tensor veli palatini muscles on the eustachian tube, resulting in poor active opening.[8–10] Other risk factors

include male gender, immunodeficiency, ciliary dyskinesia, bottle feeding, cigarette smoke in the house, increased number of siblings in the house, and perhaps the most important—day care.[11]

Almost 85% to 100% of ears affected by OME have a type B, or flat, tympanogram.[12] A type B tympanogram can occur without the presence of MEE, as in the case of tympanosclerosis, or after tympanoplasty. Pneumatic otoscopy should be the primary means by which OME is diagnosed.

Effect of otitis media with effusion on speech and language development

OME causes a CHL by limiting mobility of the tympanic membrane and ossicles, which results in decreased sound transmission through the middle ear. The impact of OME on hearing can range from no hearing loss (0 dB HL) to moderate range hearing loss (55 dB HL). The average hearing loss associated with OME has been estimated at 28 dB HL, but in approximately 20% of children, it exceeds 35 dB HL.[13–16] Even mild degrees of SNHL have been shown in children to cause speech and language delay,[17] so one could presume that a CHL secondary to chronic MEE could similarly impact a child's speech and language development. Hearing loss may be suggested by seeming lack of attentiveness, behavioral changes, excessive volumes on television or listening devices, or failure to respond to normal conversational volumes. It has been previously demonstrated that parents cannot reliably detect mild degrees of hearing loss in children.[18]

If OME has persisted in both ears for 3 months or longer (chronic OME), there is a lower chance of spontaneous resolution. In a meta-analysis, Rosenfeld and Kay[19] found that only 26% of patients with chronic OME showed resolution by 6 months with a 33% resolution rate by 1 year.

Despite evidence of hearing loss associated with OME, there is no evidence that untreated children with OME fair worse developmentally, specifically with respect to language, than do children treated with early tympanostomy tube insertion.[20–22] No studies have been performed on children with an established speech, language, or developmental delay comparing outcomes with versus without surgical treatment of OME.

Management of otitis media with effusion—American Academy of Otolaryngology guidelines

The decision to place ventilation tubes depends on multiple factors including the child's speech and language development to date, the presence of craniofacial abnormalities, recurrence of infections, and the presence of other risk factors cited earlier. The American Academy of Otolaryngology Clinical Practice Guidelines on OME and Tympanostomy Tubes in Children were published in 2004 and 2013, respectively (selected, summarized recommendations are given in **Box 1**).[23,24]

Conductive Hearing Loss Associated with Chronic Otitis Media

Chronic otitis media (COM) is defined as any ear with a tympanic membrane perforation—either with or without cholesteatoma. This section provides guidelines for the management of chronic ear disease in children; it is not meant as an exhaustive review, rather a framework on which to base decisions to optimize outcomes for children with this relatively common disease.

Tympanic membrane perforation

In children, tympanic membrane perforation is most often the result of a retained ventilation tube or a sequela of ventilation tube insertion. Perforations are typically anterior-inferior, the site of ventilation tube placement, and as such, do not cause significant CHL. CHL associated with tympanic membrane perforation is generally in the low

---

Box 1
The American Academy of Otolaryngology Clinical Practice Guidelines on OME and tympanostomy tubes in children

1. Clinicians should distinguish the child with OME who is at risk for speech, language, or learning problems from other children with OME and should more promptly evaluate hearing, speech, language, and need for intervention. This procedure includes children with previously documented delay and those with craniofacial abnormalities, as described above.

2. Clinicians should manage the child with OME who is not at risk with watchful waiting for 3 months from the date of effusion onset (if known) or from the date of diagnosis (if onset is unknown). This fact is supported by the evidence that in most cases OME is self-limited.

3. Antihistamines and decongestants are ineffective for OME and are not recommended for treatment. Antimicrobials and corticosteroids do not have long-term efficacy and are not recommended for routine management. Devices that promote autoinsufflation, however, are useful in children who are old enough to participate.[89]

4. Hearing testing is recommended when OME persists for 3 months or longer, or at any time that language delay, learning problems, or a significant hearing loss is suspected in a child with OME. Language testing should be conducted for children with hearing loss.

5. Children with persistent OME who are not at risk should be reexamined at 3- to 6-month intervals until the effusion is no longer present, significant hearing loss is identified, or structural abnormalities of the eardrum or middle ear are suspected. If a child has a moderate hearing loss, greater than 40 dB HL, then treatment is recommended. If the hearing loss is mild (20–35 dB HL) or normal (0–20 dB HL), then repeat testing can be performed in 3 to 6 months.

6. When a child becomes a surgical candidate, tympanostomy tube insertion is the preferred initial procedure; adenoidectomy should not be performed unless a distinct indication exists (nasal obstruction, chronic adenoiditis). Repeat surgery consists of adenoidectomy plus myringotomy, with or without tube insertion. Tonsillectomy alone or myringotomy alone should not be used to treat OME. Tympanostomy tube insertion has been shown to improve hearing by an average of 6 dB at 6 months.[22] Adenoidectomy has a demonstrated benefit as adjuvant treatment in children requiring reinsertion of tympanostomy tubes, with a 37% to 47% reduction in OME and a 50% reduction in need for reoperation.[20,90]

---

frequencies. Larger perforations are associated with larger CHLs, although the location of perforation has not been shown to affect the degree of CHL.[25]

Before surgical repair, children should undergo audiometric evaluation with air and bone conduction thresholds to evaluate the degree of CHL. Success of pediatric tympanoplasty depends on both intrinsic (patient-derived) and extrinsic (surgeon-derived) factors. Intrinsic factors that should be optimized include patient age, presence of otorrhea, ongoing eustachian tube dysfunction, status of the contralateral ear, health of the child, and size and location of the perforation; extrinsic factors include surgical approach, technique, and surgeon experience.[26,27] Perhaps the greatest predictor of success in pediatric tympanoplasty is age; children younger than 4 years have worse outcomes than older children,[28] but the optimal age for successful tympanoplasty remains uncertain. The status of the contralateral ear is another important consideration.[27]

Techniques for pediatric tympanoplasty are wide ranging and include fat graft myringoplasty (with or without hyaluronic acid[29,30]), underlay, and overlay/lateral grafting techniques. The key to successful tympanoplasty involves evaluating extrinsic and intrinsic factors, optimizing those factors, and practicing practice-based learning—examining personal outcomes and making changes based on a surgeon's own outcomes.

A particular technique that has been successful for closure of one perforation may not carry the same success rates for other perforations. In general, small, posterior central perforations can be managed with a myringoplasty (eg, fat plug) or underlay technique. Marginal perforations do better with underlay or lateral surface grafting. Large, total, or subtotal perforations are generally managed with a lateral surface technique. Other perforations can be managed with any of the techniques, depending on surgeon comfort and experience, and on optimizing those intrinsic factors that play into the success of tympanoplasty in children.

Tympanosclerosis

Tympanosclerosis is the result of recurrent or chronic middle ear inflammation resulting in fibrosis, which can lead to fixation of the ossicles and associated CHL. Tympanosclerosis can be seen innocuously in the tympanic membrane (myringosclerosis) and not associated with CHL, or it can be an insidious cause of progressive CHL as it immobilizes the ossicular chain. Any child with a history of recurrent ear infections and/or myringosclerosis with progressive CHL should be suspected of having ossicular hypomobility due to tympanosclerosis.

Management may include observation with monitoring of the hearing, amplification (conventional or bone conducting), or surgical exploration. Although tympanosclerosis generally has multiple loci in the middle ear,[31] hearing results of lateral chain fixation secondary to tympanosclerosis, in which the surgeon used a partial or total ossicular replacement prosthesis, trend better than those of tympanosclerotic stapes fixation, in which mobilization or partial/total stapedectomy has been performed.[32,33] HRCT of temporal bone can be helpful in elucidating the site of ossicular fixation and can give the surgeon and family preoperative and prognostic information on chances of hearing rehabilitation with surgery. Stapedectomy, either partial or total, can be successful in restoring hearing but is not advised in the presence of a tympanic membrane perforation—a staged approach must be undertaken to close the perforation before opening the footplate.[34]

Of course, any operation to remove or address fibrosis or scar tissue risks further fibrosis, so long-term follow-up is required.

Cholesteatoma

Cholesteatoma refers to stratified squamous epithelium (skin) growing in the middle ear and may be congenital or acquired. Cholesteatoma causes CHL either by mass effect on the ossicular chain or by bony erosion of the ossicles. Primary acquired cholesteatoma starts as a tympanic membrane retraction, potentially as a consequence of eustachian tube dysfunction, either in the posterior pars tensa (sinus cholesteatoma, **Fig. 1**) or in the pars flaccida (attic cholesteatoma, **Fig. 2**). The retracted area of the eardrum forms a pocket lined by healthy stratified squamous epithelium that fills with desquamated epithelium (keratin), and the pocket expands as it fills with keratin. Cholesteatoma may also develop from an eardrum perforation as the skin migrates into the middle ear rather than closing the perforation (secondary acquired cholesteatoma).

Congenital cholesteatoma is usually seen as a pearly mass behind the anterosuperior quadrant of an intact tympanic membrane, thought to originate from an epithelial rest in the middle ear (**Fig. 3**). Congenital cholesteatoma may also arise from the mastoid and reach a large size before being diagnosed. Congenital cholesteatomas represent about 4% of all pediatric cholesteatomas.[35] Cholesteatomas are erosive, and acquired cholesteatoma often presents with otorrhea and chronic, recalcitrant infection. Congenital cholesteatoma presents with a CHL and a white retrotympanic mass.

Comprehensive management of pediatric cholesteatoma, often more invasive and more aggressive than in the adult, is surgical and beyond the scope of this article

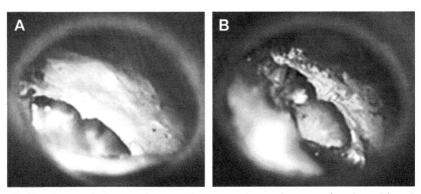

Fig. 1. Otomicroscopic image of a posterior tympanic membrane perforation with a sinus cholesteatoma; (*A*) before cleaning and (*B*) after cleaning with matrix of the cholesteatoma on the promontory, right ear.

(see Weber,[36] Sismanis and colleagues,[37] and Brackmann and colleagues[38]). The primary goal of surgery is a clean, safe, dry ear with no recurrent or residual disease. Recurrence rates are higher in children than in adults possibly related to continued immaturity of the eustachian tube. Secondary goal is rehabilitation of the associated CHL and may involve ossiculoplasty (either at the time of cholesteatoma resection or as a staged procedure), conventional amplification, osseointegrated bone conducting implant, or even preferential seating in class with or without a frequency modulation (FM) system.

Effect of chronic otitis media on hearing and speech/language development

The above-mentioned entities generally affect school-aged children and as a result, are not thought to have a dramatic impact on speech and language development during the critical early years of life. The degree of CHL associated with cholesteatoma, tympanic membrane perforation, and tympanosclerosis varies with the extent of disease. An average pure tone air conduction of 41.3 dB has been reported in a review of 158 cholesteatoma ears.[39] As noted, CHL varies with size but not location of tympanic

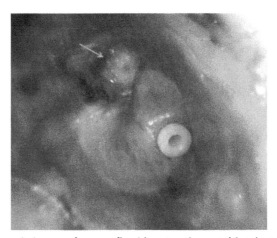

Fig. 2. Otomicroscopic image of a pars flaccida retraction resulting in an attic cholesteatoma; right ear. Arrow points to keratin debris in attic.

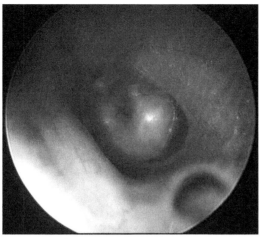

Fig. 3. Otomicroscopic image of a congenital cholesteatoma; left ear.

membrane perforation.[25,40] Cholesteatoma and tympanosclerosis typically affect hearing in only 1 ear, and having a normal contralateral ear, children may cope well with this degree of hearing loss. Careful monitoring of academic progress, preferential seating in class, consideration of an FM system, and amplification are strategies used to rehabilitate children with chronic ear disease. Unilateral CHL in the severe range has been shown to affect academic performance,[41] but the CHL associated with cholesteatoma may not be severe, unless there is complete ossicular discontinuity.

The priority in treating cholesteatoma is to achieve a safe, dry ear; good hearing results are often achievable with ossicular chain reconstruction. Conventional hearing aids and bone conducting hearing aids are also appropriate and successful in hearing rehabilitation.

CONGENITAL CONDUCTIVE HEARING LOSS
Overview

Congenital anomalies of the middle ear are rare causes of CHL in children and are classically divided into major (CAA, defined by absence or stenosis of the external auditory canal [EAC] and some middle ear ossicular underdevelopment) and minor malformations.[42] Minor malformations are characterized by a normal auricle, intact and patent EAC, intact tympanic membrane, and a deformation, fixation, or disruption of ossicular conduction. The hearing loss associated with these minor malformations, including congenital stapes ankylosis, persistent stapedial artery, malleus bar/malleus fixation, and absent oval window can range from mild to severe, can be missed on newborn hearing screening, and may not be diagnosed until the child can sit for behavioral testing. Some of these anomalies include those that are also associated with CAA, such as malleus bar and malleoincudal fixation.

Development and Embryology of the Middle Ear

The eustachian tube develops during the third week of gestation from the endoderm of the first branchial pouch, with the lateral end of the pouch forming the middle ear cleft. Pneumatization of the tympanic cleft begins around week 10. The tympanic membrane forms during the 28th week and is derived from all 3 layers of primitive tissue: ectoderm forming the outer squamous layer, mesoderm forming the middle fibrous layer, and endoderm forming the medial mucosal layer.

The malleus and incus are a single mass at 6 weeks, separating at 8 weeks. The head and neck of the malleus, as well as the body and short process of the incus, are derivatives of Meckel's cartilage (first branchial arch). The manubrium of the malleus, long process of the incus, and the superstructure of the stapes are derivatives of Reichert's cartilage (second branchial arch). Arrest in development of the first branchial arch underlies CAA, which is accompanied by a fused malleus-incus complex, absent manubrium, and often normal stapes bone (second arch derivative), as well as mandibular hypoplasia (hemifacal microsomia).

The stapes begins to form at 4 to 5 weeks from the blastema. Cranial nerve VII divides the blastema into the stapes, interhayle (future stapedius tendon), and laterohayle (future pyramidal eminence).[43] The tympanic portion of the footplate develops from the second branchial arch cartilage, and the vestibular portion of the footplate (lamina stapedalis and annular ligament) originates from the otic capsule. The 2 develop independently and eventually fuse. The interhayle develops into the stapedial muscle and tendon, and the laterohayle becomes the posterior tympanic wall. Ossification begins at week 19 and proceeds from both the stapes superstructure and the otic capsule and, under normal conditions, does not involve the vestibular portion of the footplate, which includes the annular ligament, which should remain cartilaginous throughout life.[44]

An important concept to understand in the embryology of the ear is that the ear canal and middle ear develop from the branchial apparatus; the cochlea, vestibule, labyrinth, and central auditory nervous system structures develop from the otocyst, from the neuropore. The implication is that most patients with congenital CHL have just that—a conductive and not a mixed or sensorineural loss. That said, patients with CAA can have morphologic inner ear abnormalities identified on computed tomographic (CT) scan, but these abnormalities do not necessarily translate into an SNHL.[45] Proper audiometric evaluation with air and bone conduction testing will best characterize the hearing.

Patient Evaluation

Diagnosing CHL in the child with grade II or III microtia and associated CAA (**Fig. 4**) is very straightforward—the disability is easily seen on physical examination and appropriate testing can be performed. After newborn hearing screening, recommended

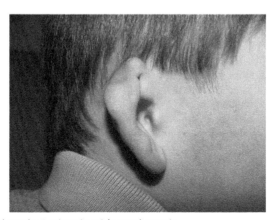

Fig. 4. Congenital grade II microtia with aural atresia.

testing protocols include otoacoustic emissions testing in the normal ear or the ear with a minor malformation, air and bone conduction auditory brainstem response (ABR) testing in the normal ear, and bone conducting testing in the atretic ear if unilateral, and bone conducting ABR if bilateral.[46] The child with a CHL secondary to a minor malformation or the child with a normal auricle and CAA can be deceiving, but the hearing loss is usually identified at newborn hearing screening, or occasionally later in life, at a school screening. Careful binocular microscopic examination either in the office or under anesthesia with air and bone conduction ABR testing can diagnose CAA or minor malformation and CHL.

Although exploratory tympanotomy is the gold standard for diagnosing most minor middle ear anomalies (and offers simultaneous therapeutic intervention), the authors recommend that any child with an unexplained CHL (normal ear canal, eardrum, and middle ear space) be referred for temporal bone HRCT imaging before surgical exploration. Conditions causing a conductive or mixed hearing loss *not* amenable to surgical intervention should be identified and include enlarged vestibular aqueduct or dehiscence of the superior semicircular canal (incidence unknown in children but known to occur[47]). In addition, the surgeon should rule out a possible middle ear neoplasm causing mass effect on the ossicles (eg, paraganglioma, facial nerve hemangioma, middle ear adenoma, or congenital cholesteatoma in the epitympanum not seen on otoscopic examination) as the cause of CHL before embarking on middle ear surgery.

Some middle ear anomalies, such as absence of the oval window (**Fig. 5**), can be detected on HRCT and may offer the surgeon some prognostic information on the outcome of surgery (correction of this anomaly has shown poor long-term hearing

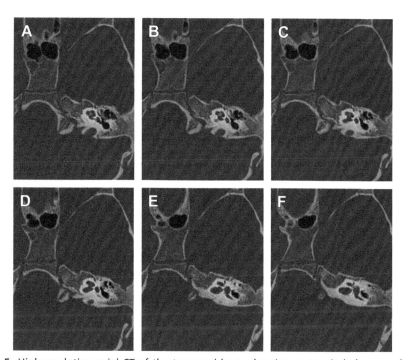

Fig. 5. High-resolution axial CT of the temporal bone showing congenital absence of the oval window (*A–F,* inferior to superior; note inferior displacement of the facial nerve).

outcomes[48]). Persistent stapedial artery may also be identified alerting the surgeon to an anatomic abnormality not amenable to surgical correction. A middle and inner ear predisposed to X-linked stapes gusher may also be identified on CT imaging and possibly preclude surgical exploration in favor of amplification.[49]

Minor Malformations

Teunissen and colleagues[50] classified and reported the observed frequencies of minor congenital malformations in 144 patients (**Table 1**).

These malformations, in general, are not apparent on otoscopic examination, and may not be apparent on imaging. Exploratory tympanotomy can be discussed with the goal of restoring ossicular conduction. Patients with CHL due to minor malformations of the middle ear are generally good candidates for exploration and surgical rehabilitation of hearing, although some minor malformations such as congenital absence of the oval window (CAOW) do not show good long-term hearing outcomes with surgery.

Congenital stapes ankylosis

Isolated congenital stapes ankylosis is a rare disorder, but it has been reported consistently in the literature. Similar, but acquired disease processes include juvenile otosclerosis and stapes fixation due to tympanosclerosis. Division of isolated congenital stapes ankylosis into (1) those with footplate fixation and (2) those with superstructure fixation has been proposed.[43] Footplate fixation is far more commonly reported in the literature. The superstructure fixations are further divided as follows[43]:

1. Elongation of the pyramidal process and ossification of the stapedius tendon
2. Stapes-promontory fixation
3. Stapes-facial canal fixation
4. Stapes-pyramidal fixation with a normal stapedius tendon
5. Double fixation

These investigators postulate that the cause of congenital footplate fixation is abnormal ossification of the annular ligament around the 16th week of gestation, when the otic capsule is undergoing ossification. Previously, it was hypothesized that this represented an arrest in development and differentiation of the ligament, leading to congenital stapes fixation.[51] Regardless, histopathologic evaluation of temporal bones with suspected congenital stapes fixation demonstrated that the annular ligament was partly fibrous, partly cartilaginous, and partly bone,[51] although this finding is not identifiable on temporal bone CT imaging.

Surgical management of congenital stapes fixation is similar to that of otosclerosis. Welling and colleagues[52] reported their experience with pediatric stapedectomy for both juvenile otosclerosis and congenital stapes fixation. The investigators report

Table 1	
Classification of congenital ossicular anomalies	
Class 1	Ankylosis or isolated congenital fixation of the stapes (30.6%)
Class 2	Stapes ankylosis associated with other malformations of the ossicular chain (38.1%)
Class 3	Congenital anomalies of the ossicular chain with a mobile stapes footplate (21.6%)
Class 4	Congenital aplasia or severe dysplasia of the oval and round windows (includes persistent stapedial artery; 9.7%)

Adapted from Teunissen EB, Cremers WR. Classification of congenital middle ear anomalies. report on 144 ears. Ann Otol Rhinol Laryngol 1993;102(8 Pt 1):606–12.

similar results in both cohorts, with good closure of the air-bone gap. Similar reviews exist with successful operations performed in children as young as 8 years of age.[53,54] Stapes mobilization as an alternative to stapedectomy can provide good hearing improvement, but there is a risk of refixation. Surgery is similar to that of stapedectomy in the adult.

Surgery for stapes superstructure fixation is targeted, most often using a laser or microdrill, to address the site of ankylosis. Excellent surgical outcomes can be achieved by analyzing the different sites of fixation and using specific maneuvers to address each.[43,55]

Stapes superstructure malformations may be seen in conjunction with footplate or superstructure fixation, as well as with normal hearing ears. Superstructure abnormalities may coexist with stapes ankylosis up to 30% of the time.[53] The most commonly reported stapes malformation is the collumellar or monopodial type, in which the stapes superstructure is rodlike and attaches to the footplate centrally.[43,56] It is postulated that the malformation may be due to failure of the stapedial artery to develop and canalize the stapes crura. Additional malformations include unicrurate stapes, in which either the anterior or posterior crus is absent, and the dangling crura malformation, in which neither crus attaches to the footplate.

Malleoincudal fixation and malleus bar

After congenital stapes ankylosis, fixation of the malleus or incus in the epitympanum is the second most common isolated congenital middle ear malformation (**Fig. 6**). Fixation can also be seen as an acquired deformity. The incus and malleus can be fused and fixed to the epitympanum producing a maximal CHL.[57] Fixation of the malleus is more common.[58] This malformation can be associated with a normal EAC and auricle, or an atretic ear. The diagnosis may be suspected with pneumatic otoscopy, and imaging can be confirmatory.[59] When present as an isolated anomaly, surgical intervention involves a transcanal approach with an atticotomy to free the complex from fixation.[57,58,60] Alternatively, the incudostapedial joint can be disarticulated and

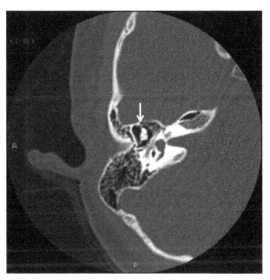

Fig. 6. High-resolution axial CT scan showing fixation of the head of the malleus in the epitympanum, right ear. *Arrow* shows point of fixation between head of malleus and epitympanic wall.

reconstruction can proceed with a partial ossicular replacement prosthesis on top of the mobile stapes bone.

Malleus bar is a rare ossicular malformation that can be seen in isolation or can coincide with CAA.[61] The malleus bar is a bony bar connecting the manubrium or neck of the malleus to the posterior tympanic wall.[62] As opposed to many other ossicular malformations, malleus bar can often be identified on imaging.[63] Excellent hearing recovery is attained with drilling and severing of the bony partition, when it is not coincident with other middle or inner ear malformations. Care must be taken not to transmit the high energy of the drill to a mobile ossicular chain.

Congenital incudostapedial discontinuity

Congenital absence of the long process of the incus is a rare phenomenon. As some have pointed out, in some instances, it is challenging to differentiate whether the discontinuity at the incudostapedial joint is congenital or related to erosion from recurrent otitis media or COM, owing to the tenuous blood supply of the lenticular process.[64] A histopathologic study of 21 cases of suspected congenital absence of the incus long process found 13 of 21 specimens to be associated with an abnormality of the stapes superstructure.[64] This finding supports a developmental origin, as both the long process and stapes superstructure are second arch (Reichert's cartilage) derivatives. Wehrs[65] described a family with 3 successive generations of females with severe bilateral CHL because of absence of the long process of the incus and the capitulum of the stapes, hypothesizing that the congenital anomaly was inherited as an autosomal dominant mutation, or possibly as an X-linked dominantly inherited mutation. Correction is with ossicular chain reconstruction, the extent depending on the presence or absence of a mobile stapes superstructure.

Congenital absence of the oval window

CAOW results from failure of the otic capsule bone to open into the vestibule, from failure of the footplate to develop, or from failure of the stapes to fuse with the vestibule.[66] CAOW results in maximal CHL. As opposed to stapes ankylosis, CAOW can be identified on thin-cut temporal bone CT (see **Fig. 5**). Radiographically, failure of the oval window to develop results in osseous obliteration and concentric narrowing, resulting in a dimplelike depression along the medial tympanic wall, or by a thick bony plate.[67] It is proposed that the origin of CAOW is related to an anteroinferiorly displaced facial nerve during the early weeks of gestation, preventing contact between the developing stapes footplate and the otic capsule, resulting in aplasia of the oval window.[67–70] CAOW is often associated with an absent or rudimentary stapes. As with the other minor malformations, CAOW can be coincident with CAA.

Surgical rehabilitation, an oval window drill-out (OWD), is targeted at restoring ossicular continuity with a neo-oval window. de Alarcon and colleagues[48] reported their experience with 17 OWD procedures: a postauricular approach is used with transection of the posterior canal wall skin with a tympanomeatal flap to enter the middle ear. The new oval window is drilled to the vestibule and ossicular continuity is reestablished using a total ossicular prosthesis over a temporalis fascia graft. In this series, 4 of 17 cases were aborted and the remaining 13 had improvement in hearing at 1 month, and 9 of 13 had continued improved hearing at long-term follow-up. Revision surgery was attempted in 4 patients whose hearing deteriorated and was unsuccessful at improving hearing. It has been similarly reported by others that the initial hearing gain was lost over time, and revision surgery failed to improve outcome.[69] However, a recent large retrospective study reported sustained improvement at 6 months in the vast majority of patients.[71] Bone-anchored hearing aids are an additional appropriate surgical intervention depending on patient and surgeon preference.

Persistent stapedial artery

The stapedial artery develops during the fetal period but normally atrophies at the third fetal month. Persistence of the stapedial artery is a rare finding, first reported by Hyrtl in 1836. Moreano and colleagues[72] reported a 0.48% (5/1045) prevalence of persistent stapedial artery in their histopathologic review of 1045 temporal bones.

The artery develops as the source for the middle meningeal artery before losing that connection. If present, a stapedial artery courses through the floor of the middle ear, superiorly through the obturator foramen of the stapes, and through the fallopian canal into the middle cranial fossa as the middle meningeal artery.[73] If the stapedial artery persists, foramen spinosum will be absent and there will be an aberrant internal carotid artery (**Fig. 7**).

Persistent stapedial artery can cause pulsatile tinnitus and CHL by limiting stapes mobility (can also be associated with stapes ankylosis), and possibly SNHL if there is erosion into the otic capsule. Although there are case reports of successful surgery using a malleus-stapes stapedotomy with Teflon wire prosthesis,[74] most surgeons would exercise caution because of the proximity of the artery to the facial nerve and possible sequela of hemiplegia if cauterized (although this notion has been challenged).[75]

Congenital Aural Atresia

With an estimated incidence of 1 per 10,000 to 20,000, CAA causes a fixed, moderate/moderate to severe CHL; bone conduction thresholds are usually normal. About 70% of microtia/atresia occurs unilaterally, boys are more commonly affected than girls, and the right ear is more commonly involved than the left, all for unknown reasons. Microtia/atresia prevalence rates tend to be higher in Hispanic (especially those from Ecuador) and Asian patients. The cause is unknown, but scientists have speculated that an arrest in the development of the ear canal and middle ear prevents the first branchial arch from completing its full development. Abnormalities of chromosome 18 (and 22[76]) have been implicated in CAA, especially in the absence of microtia, a rare finding.[77] Disruption of blood flow due to the position of the fetus in utero has also been proposed.

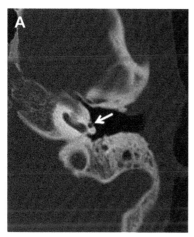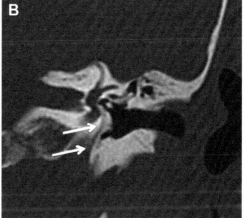

Fig. 7. High-resolution axial (*A*) and coronal (*B*) CT scan of the temporal bone demonstrating a persistent stapedial artery (*arrow on left*) as it courses cranially through the tympanic canaliculus (*arrows on right*). (*Courtesy of* P. Raghavan, MD, Baltimore, MD.)

The diagnosis of CAA is straightforward because of the accompanying microtia. However, CAA can occur in the absence of microtia, so careful otoscopic examination to identify the ear canal is necessary. Search for other associated anomalies including renal, spine, and craniofacial/structural abnormalities should also be considered. Syndromic conditions associated with CAA include hemifacial microsomia/Goldenhar and Treacher Collins syndromes.

Once diagnosed, audiometric evaluation involves air and bone conduction ABR testing (for both normal and atretic ears if unilateral) and bone conduction thresholds for the child with bilateral CAA. Hearing should be monitored at 3- to 6-month intervals for the first 2 years and yearly after that, mostly to ensure that the normal hearing ear continues to hear normally in patients with unilateral CAA. Parental monitoring of speech and language development is also a key adjunct along with speech/language therapy if the child is not progressing. Normal hearing in 1 ear is sufficient for normal speech and language development; however, expressive speech development should be monitored closely, and interventions such as speech therapy or bone conducting amplification can be instituted.[41,78]

To support normal speech and language development, the child with bilateral CAA should wear a properly fitted and programmed bone conducting hearing device. These devices come on a soft band or a hard band. Children with bilateral CAA tolerate these devices well because of the greatly perceived benefit derived. The decision to place a bone conducting hearing device on a child with unilateral CAA is very much a health care professional/family decision. Some children with unilateral CAA take to these devices and wear them willingly, whereas others absolutely refuse to wear them, most likely because of the lack of perceived benefit given their 1 normal hearing ear. No study has demonstrated a clear benefit of these devices in children with unilateral CAA, so it does not have to be a struggle for families to make these children with unilateral CAA wear them. The atretic ear is being stimulated internally when the child talks, babbles, sings, eats, cries, and so on, and is also being given some external stimulation if the sound is loud enough. Owing to the crossed nature of central auditory pathways, both temporal lobes are being stimulated by both ears.

School-aged children encounter more difficult listening situations, locating sound in space and hearing in background noise (noisy classroom, school cafeteria). Some families reintroduce the bone conductor at this stage to assist their child, mostly for school. Bone conducting hearing devices, though, do not help locating a sound source, although they do have some benefit with the head shadow effect.[79,80] Other, potentially useful management strategies for school include preferential seating in class, an individualized education/504(c) plan, and an FM system, where the teacher wears a microphone and the student wears a receiver-speaker at the desk, earbud, or hearing aid in the normal ear to improve the signal-to-noise ratio.

Over a quarter century ago, Bess and Tharpe[81] demonstrated that a subset of patients with unilateral SNHL were at great risk for grade retention. A similar study in 2013 showed that children with unilateral CHL secondary to CAA did not repeat grades at the same rate as children with unilateral SNHL but used resources to a greater degree than did the children in the Bess and Tharpe cohort.[41] Resources used included speech therapy and individualized education programs (IEPs/504(c) plans); only 12% used some type of bone conducting hearing device. Surgery for CAA neither improved nor worsened these results (Kesser, personal communication, 2012).

Surgery for CAA remains a difficult operation[82] with variable hearing outcomes and decline of early hearing gains in a subset of patients undergoing surgery.[83,84] Good long-term (>1 year) hearing outcomes studies are still needed to evaluate atresia surgery as well as more quantitative predictors of surgical success. Although major complications of SNHL and facial paralysis are low because of vastly improved imaging studies, facial nerve monitoring, a deeper understanding of the surgical anatomy, and improvements in surgical technique, minor complications including meatal stenosis, mucosalization with resultant moisture/otorrhea, and loss of early hearing gains remain problematic.[85] Children with unilateral CAA are able to hear better in background noise after surgery, mostly because of the effects of summation and head shadow.[86] Data examining sound localization show improved ability to locate sound in space but still not approaching that of normal binaural listeners (unpublished data).

So what are the best evidence-based management strategies for children with CAA? Certainly for children with binaural CAA, bone conducting hearing technology early in life greatly supports, and is arguably essential for speech and language development. For children with unilateral CAA, the story is not as clear. Although the use of a bone conductor in this setting is never discouraged, one can never be so dogmatic as to say that the child will do poorly or the ear will never respond to sound if a bone conductor is not placed on the child—as mentioned, this is very much a health care professional/family decision. For the school-aged child, preferential seating and an IEP/504(c) plan have been shown to be effective.[41] Other options include the FM system, a trial of a bone conductor, and atresia surgery if the child is a good anatomic candidate.[87,88] Further research into the academic needs of these children with a fixed, congenital CHL due to CAA may also inform decisions regarding children with acquired unilateral CHL because of other causes including OME, ETD, and COM with or without cholesteatoma.

SUMMARY

Acquired CHL due to MEE/eustachian tube dysfunction remains the most common cause of hearing loss in children. Middle ear fluid (OME) is managed through generally established guidelines and recommendations.[24] Cholesteatoma with ossicular erosion is managed surgically with ossicular reconstruction, but ongoing eustachian tube dysfunction and middle ear atelectasis may thwart attempts to restore hearing. Conventional amplification and bone conducting technology are effective means to rehabilitate hearing. Preferential seating in class, IEPs, and FM systems should not be overlooked for this patient population as well.

Congenital CHL may be amenable to surgical intervention, but any child with an unexplained CHL should have an HRCT of the temporal bone to rule out nonsurgical causes of CHL (eg, enlarged vestibular aqueduct, superior semicircular canal dehiscence) and to evaluate for congenital cholesteatoma and neoplastic disease that cannot be seen under binocular microscopy. In addition, the imaging study may identify an anatomic anomaly not amenable to surgical exploration (persistent stapedial artery) or one with mixed postoperative hearing results (absent oval window).

Hearing (re)habilitation may include close monitoring of the hearing with preferential seating in class, IEP, speech therapy, conventional amplification, bone conducting hearing devices, or surgical repair. The choice is best made based on a thorough discussion and common understanding of all risks and benefits shared between hearing health care professional and family.

REFERENCES

1. Downs MP. Relationship of pathology to function in congenital hearing loss. II. The auditory function in congenital hearing loss. Audiology 1972;11(5):330–6.
2. Davidson J, Hyde ML, Alberti PW. Epidemiologic patterns in childhood hearing loss: a review. Int J Pediatr Otorhinolaryngol 1989;17(3):239–66.

3. Gravel JS, Wallace IF. Effects of otitis media with effusion on hearing in the first 3 years of life. J Speech Lang Hear Res 2000;43(3):631–44.
4. Khodaverdi M, Jorgensen G, Lange T, et al. Hearing 25 years after surgical treatment of otitis media with effusion in early childhood. Int J Pediatr Otorhinolaryngol 2013;77(2):241–7.
5. Roberts J, Hunter L, Gravel J, et al. Otitis media, hearing loss, and language learning: controversies and current research. J Dev Behav Pediatr 2004;25(2):110–22.
6. Wallace IF, Gravel JS, McCarton CM, et al. Otitis media and language development at 1 year of age. J Speech Hear Disord 1988;53(3):245–51.
7. Casselbrant ML. Epidemiology of otitis media in infants and preschool children. Pediatr Infect Dis J 1989;8(1 Suppl):S10–1.
8. Broen PA, Moller KT, Carlstrom J, et al. Comparison of the hearing histories of children with and without cleft palate. Cleft Palate Craniofac J 1996;33(2):127–33.
9. Sheahan P, Blayney AW, Sheahan JN, et al. Sequelae of otitis media with effusion among children with cleft lip and/or cleft palate. Clin Otolaryngol Allied Sci 2002; 27(6):494–500.
10. Flynn T, Moller C, Jonsson R, et al. The high prevalence of otitis media with effusion in children with cleft lip and palate as compared to children without clefts. Int J Pediatr Otorhinolaryngol 2009;73(10):1441–6.
11. Friedman RA, Kesser BW, Derebery JM. Surgery of ventilation and mucosal disease. In: Brackman DE, Shelton C, Arriaga MA, editors. Otologic surgery. 3rd edition. Philadelphia: Elsevier; 2010. p. 73–91.
12. Fiellau-Nikolajsen M. Epidemiology of secretory otitis media. A descriptive cohort study. Ann Otol Rhinol Laryngol 1983;92(2 Pt 1):172–7.
13. Bluestone CD, Klein JO, Paradise JL, et al. Workshop on effects of otitis media on the child. Pediatrics 1983;71(4):639–52.
14. Bluestone CD, Fria TJ, Arjona SK, et al. Controversies in screening for middle ear disease and hearing loss in children. Pediatrics 1986;77(1):57–70.
15. Bluestone CD. Studies in otitis media: Children's Hospital of Pittsburgh-University of Pittsburgh progress report–2004. Laryngoscope 2004;114(11 Pt 3 Suppl 105): 1–26.
16. Fria TJ, Cantekin EI, Eichler JA. Hearing acuity of children with otitis media with effusion. Arch Otolaryngol 1985;111(1):10–6.
17. Davis JM, Elfenbein J, Schum R, et al. Effects of mild and moderate hearing impairments on language, educational, and psychosocial behavior of children. J Speech Hear Disord 1986;51(1):53–62.
18. Brody R, Rosenfeld RM, Goldsmith AJ, et al. Parents cannot detect mild hearing loss in children. Otolaryngol Head Neck Surg 1999;121(6):681–6.
19. Rosenfeld RM, Kay D. Natural history of untreated otitis media. Laryngoscope 2003;113(10):1645–57.
20. Paradise JL, Campbell TF, Dollaghan CA, et al. Developmental outcomes after early or delayed insertion of tympanostomy tubes. N Engl J Med 2005;353(6): 576–86.
21. Rovers MM, Straatman H, Ingels K, et al. The effect of ventilation tubes on language development in infants with otitis media with effusion: a randomized trial. Pediatrics 2000;106(3):E42.
22. Rovers MM, Straatman H, Ingels K, et al. The effect of short-term ventilation tubes versus watchful waiting on hearing in young children with persistent otitis media with effusion: a randomized trial. Ear Hear 2001;22(3):191–9.
23. Rosenfeld RM, Culpepper L, Doyle KJ, et al. Clinical practice guideline: otitis media with effusion. Otolaryngol Head Neck Surg 2004;130(5 Suppl):S95–118.

24. Rosenfeld RM, Schwartz SR, Pynnonen MA, et al. Clinical practice guideline: tympanostomy tubes in children. Otolaryngol Head Neck Surg 2013;149(1 Suppl): S1–35.
25. Mehta RP, Rosowski JJ, Voss SE, et al. Determinants of hearing loss in perforations of the tympanic membrane. Otol Neurotol 2006;27(2):136–43.
26. James AL, Papsin BC. Ten top considerations in pediatric tympanoplasty. Otolaryngol Head Neck Surg 2012;147(6):992–8.
27. Hardman J, Muzaffar J, Nankivell P, et al. Tympanoplasty for chronic tympanic membrane perforation in children: systematic review and meta-analysis. Otol Neurotol 2015;36(5):796–804.
28. Duval M, Grimmer JF, Meier J, et al. The effect of age on pediatric tympanoplasty outcomes: a comparison of preschool and older children. Int J Pediatr Otorhinolaryngol 2015;79(3):336–41.
29. Gross CW, Bassila M, Lazar RH, et al. Adipose plug myringoplasty: an alternative to formal myringoplasty techniques in children. Otolaryngol Head Neck Surg 1989;101(6):617–20.
30. Saliba I, Froehlich P. Hyaluronic acid fat graft myringoplasty: an office-based technique adapted to children. Arch Otolaryngol Head Neck Surg 2011; 137(12):1203–9.
31. Ho KY, Tsai SM, Chai CY, et al. Clinical analysis of intratympanic tympanosclerosis: etiology, ossicular chain findings, and hearing results of surgery. Acta Otolaryngol 2010;130(3):370–4.
32. Stankovic MD. Hearing results of surgery for tympanosclerosis. Eur Arch Otorhinolaryngol 2009;266(5):635–40.
33. Aslan H, Katilmis H, Ozturkcan S, et al. Tympanosclerosis and our surgical results. Eur Arch Otorhinolaryngol 2010;267(5):673–7.
34. Celik H, Aslan Felek S, Islam A, et al. Analysis of long-term hearing after tympanosclerosis with total/partial stapedectomy and prosthesis used. Acta Otolaryngol 2008;128(12):1308–13.
35. Potsic WP, Korman SB, Samadi DS, et al. Congenital cholesteatoma: 20 years' experience at the Children's Hospital of Philadelphia. Otolaryngol Head Neck Surg 2002;126(4):409–14.
36. Weber PC. Chronic otitis media. In: Pensak ML, Choo DI, editors. Clinical otology. 4th edition. New York: Thieme; 2015. p. 215–30.
37. Sismanis AA, Poe DS, Haynes DS, et al. Surgery of the ear. In: Gulya AJ, editor. Chapters 28–31. 6th edition. Shelton (CT): People's Medical Publishing House; 2010.
38. Brackmann DE, Shelton C, Arriaga MA. Otologic surgery. 3rd edition. Philadelphia: Saunders Elsevier B.V.; 2010.
39. Martins O, Victor J, Selesnick S. The relationship between individual ossicular status and conductive hearing loss in cholesteatoma. Otol Neurotol 2012;33(3):387–92.
40. Saliba I, Abela A, Arcand P. Tympanic membrane perforation: size, site and hearing evaluation. Int J Pediatr Otorhinolaryngol 2011;75(4):527–31.
41. Kesser BW, Krook K, Gray LC. Impact of unilateral conductive hearing loss due to aural atresia on academic performance in children. Laryngoscope 2013;123(9): 2270–5.
42. Bellucci RJ. Congenital aural malformations: diagnosis and treatment. Otolaryngol Clin North Am 1981;14(1):95–124.
43. Nandapalan V, Tos M. Isolated congenital stapes ankylosis: an embryologic survey and literature review. Am J Otol 2000;21(1):71–80.
44. Rodriguez K, Shah RK, Kenna M. Anomalies of the middle and inner ear. Otolaryngol Clin North Am 2007;40(1):81–96.

45. Vrabec JT, Lin JW. Inner ear anomalies in congenital aural atresia. Otol Neurotol 2010;31(9):1421–6.
46. Singleton AJ, Waltzman SB. Audiometric Evaluation of Children with Hearing Loss. Otolaryngol Clin North Am 2015. in press.
47. Hegemann SC, Carey JP. Is superior canal dehiscence congenital or acquired? A case report and review of the literature. Otolaryngol Clin North Am 2011;44(2): 377–82.
48. de Alarcon A, Jahrsdoerfer RA, Kesser BW. Congenital absence of the oval window: diagnosis, surgery, and audiometric outcomes. Otol Neurotol 2008;29(1): 23–8.
49. Kumar G, Castillo M, Buchman CA. X-linked stapes gusher: CT findings in one patient. AJNR Am J Neuroradiol 2003;24(6):1130–2.
50. Teunissen EB, Cremers WR. Classification of congenital middle ear anomalies. Report on 144 ears. Ann Otol Rhinol Laryngol 1993;102(8 Pt 1):606–12.
51. Lindsay JR, Sanders SH, Nager GT. Histopathologic observations in so-called congenital fixation of the stapedial footplate. Laryngoscope 1960;70(12): 1587–602.
52. Welling DB, Merrell JA, Merz M, et al. Predictive factors in pediatric stapedectomy. Laryngoscope 2003;113(9):1515–9.
53. Albert S, Roger G, Rouillon I, et al. Congenital stapes ankylosis: study of 28 cases and surgical results. Laryngoscope 2006;116(7):1153–7.
54. Teunissen B, Cremers WR, Huygen PL, et al. Isolated congenital stapes ankylosis: surgical results in 32 ears and a review of the literature. Laryngoscope 1990;100(12):1331–6.
55. Kuhn JJ, Lassen LF. Congenital incudostapedial anomalies in adult stapes surgery: a case-series review. Am J Otolaryngol 2011;32(6):477–84.
56. Plester D. Congenital malformation of the middle ear. Acta Otorhinolaryngol Belg 1971;25(6):877–84.
57. Tabb HG. Symposium: congenital anomalies of the middle ear. I. Epitympanic fixation of incus and malleus. Laryngoscope 1976;86(2):243–6.
58. Armstrong BW. Epitympanic malleus fixation: correction without disrupting the ossicular chain. Laryngoscope 1976;86(8):1203–8.
59. Ginat DT, Sedaghat AR, Robson CD, et al. Radiology quiz case 3. Malleus fixation. Arch Otolaryngol Head Neck Surg 2012;138(8):775–6.
60. Seidman MD, Babu S. A new approach for malleus/incus fixation: no prosthesis necessary. Otol Neurotol 2004;25(5):669–73.
61. Carfrae MJ, Jahrsdoerfer RA, Kesser BW. Malleus bar: an unusual ossicular abnormality in the setting of congenital aural atresia. Otol Neurotol 2010;31(3): 415–8.
62. Nomura Y, Nagao Y, Fukaya T. Anomalies of the middle ear. Laryngoscope 1988; 98(4):390–3.
63. Kurosaki Y, Tanaka YO, Itai Y. Malleus bar as a rare cause of congenital malleus fixation: CT demonstration. AJNR Am J Neuroradiol 1998;19(7):1229–30.
64. Park K, Choung YH, Shin YR, et al. Conductive deafness with normal eardrum: absence of the long process of the incus. Acta Otolaryngol 2007;127(8): 816–20.
65. Wehrs RE. Congenital absence of the long process of the incus. Laryngoscope 1999;109(2 Pt 1):192–7.
66. Harada T, Black FO, Sando I, et al. Temporal bone histopathologic findings in congenital anomalies of the oval window. Otolaryngol Head Neck Surg 1980; 88(3):275–87.

67. Zeifer B, Sabini P, Sonne J. Congenital absence of the oval window: radiologic diagnosis and associated anomalies. AJNR Am J Neuroradiol 2000;21(2):322–7.
68. Jahrsdoerfer RA. Embryology of the facial nerve. Am J Otol 1988;9(5):423–6.
69. Lambert PR. Congenital absence of the oval window. Laryngoscope 1990;100(1): 37–40.
70. Gerhardt HJ, Otto HD. The intratemporal course of the facial nerve and its influence on the development of the ossicular chain. Acta Otolaryngol 1981;91(5–6): 567–73.
71. Su Y, Yuan H, Song YS, et al. Congenital middle ear abnormalities with absence of the oval window: diagnosis, surgery, and audiometric outcomes. Otol Neurotol 2014;35(7):1191–5.
72. Moreano EH, Paparella MM, Zelterman D, et al. Prevalence of facial canal dehiscence and of persistent stapedial artery in the human middle ear: a report of 1000 temporal bones. Laryngoscope 1994;104(3 Pt 1):309–20.
73. Tubbs RS, Hansasuta A, Loukas M, et al. Branches of the petrous and cavernous segments of the internal carotid artery. Clin Anat 2007;20(6):596–601.
74. Sugimoto H, Ito M, Hatano M, et al. Persistent stapedial artery with stapes ankylosis. Auris Nasus Larynx 2014;41(6):582–5.
75. Hitier M, Zhang M, Labrousse M, et al. Persistent stapedial arteries in human: from phylogeny to surgical consequences. Surg Radiol Anat 2013;35(10):883–91.
76. Boudewyns A, van den Ende J, Boiy T, et al. 22q11.2 microduplication syndrome with congenital aural atresia: a family report. Otol Neurotol 2012;33(4):674–80.
77. Dostal A, Nemeckova J, Gaillyova R, et al. Identification of 2.3-Mb gene locus for congenital aural atresia in 18q22.3 deletion: a case report analyzed by comparative genomic hybridization. Otol Neurotol 2006;27(3):427–32.
78. Jensen DR, Grames LM, Lieu JE. Effects of aural atresia on speech development and learning: retrospective analysis from a multidisciplinary craniofacial clinic. JAMA Otolaryngol Head Neck Surg 2013;139(8):797–802.
79. Kunst SJ, Leijendeckers JM, Mylanus EA, et al. Bone-anchored hearing aid system application for unilateral congenital conductive hearing impairment: audiometric results. Otol Neurotol 2008;29(1):2–7.
80. Priwin C, Jonsson R, Hultcrantz M, et al. BAHA in children and adolescents with unilateral or bilateral conductive hearing loss: a study of outcome. Int J Pediatr Otorhinolaryngol 2007;71(1):135–45.
81. Bess FH, Tharpe AM. Case history data on unilaterally hearing-impaired children. Ear Hear 1986;7(1):14–9.
82. Kesser BW. Repair of congenital aural atresia. In: McKinnon BJ, editor. Operative techniques in otolaryngology-head and neck surgery, vol. 21, 4th edition. New York: Elsevier, Inc; 2010. p. 278–86.
83. Lambert PR. Congenital aural atresia: stability of surgical results. Laryngoscope 1998;108(12):1801–5.
84. De la Cruz A, Teufert KB. Congenital aural atresia surgery: long-term results. Otolaryngol Head Neck Surg 2003;129(1):121–7.
85. Oliver ER, Hughley BB, Shonka DC, et al. Revision aural atresia surgery: indications and outcomes. Otol Neurotol 2011;32(2):252–8.
86. Gray L, Kesser B, Cole E. Understanding speech in noise after correction of congenital unilateral aural atresia: effects of age in the emergence of binaural squelch but not in use of head-shadow. Int J Pediatr Otorhinolaryngol 2009; 73(9):1281–7.
87. Jahrsdoerfer RA, Yeakley JW, Aguilar EA, et al. Grading system for the selection of patients with congenital aural atresia. Am J Otol 1992;13(1):6–12.

88. Shonka DC Jr, Livingston WJ 3rd, Kesser BW. The Jahrsdoerfer grading scale in surgery to repair congenital aural atresia. Arch Otolaryngol Head Neck Surg 2008;134(8):873–7.

89. Bidarian-Moniri A, Ramos MJ, Ejnell H. Autoinflation for treatment of persistent otitis media with effusion in children: a cross-over study with a 12-month follow-up. Int J Pediatr Otorhinolaryngol 2014;78(8):1298–305.

90. Coyte PC, Croxford R, McIsaac W, et al. The role of adjuvant adenoidectomy and tonsillectomy in the outcome of the insertion of tympanostomy tubes. N Engl J Med 2001;344(16):1188–95.

Diagnostic Evaluation of Children with Sensorineural Hearing Loss

John Drew Prosser, MD[a], Aliza P. Cohen, MA[a],
John H. Greinwald, MD[b,c,]*

KEYWORDS

- Pediatric hearing loss • Sensorineural hearing loss
- Diagnostic evaluation of hearing loss • Genetic • Cytomegalovirus
- Enlarged vestibular aqueduct • Syndromes

KEY POINTS

- Sensorineural hearing loss (SNHL) occurs in approximately 2 to 4 per 1000 live births.
- The cause of pediatric SNHL may be genetic, acquired, or idiopathic.
- Approximately 50% of cases have a genetic cause.
- Of all genetic cases, 15% to 30% occur as part of a syndrome and 80% are transmitted in an autosomal-recessive pattern.
- Approximately 35% of SNHL patients have an acquired cause resulting from intrauterine infections (eg, cytomegalovirus), environmental exposures, meningitis, or prematurity.

INTRODUCTION

Sensorineural hearing loss (SNHL) is the most common sensory deficit in humans, occurring in 2 to 4 per 1000 live births and affecting an estimated 40,000 children in the United States annually.[1,2] This deficit can be unilateral or bilateral and is graded as mild to profound, based on the degree of hearing loss. Although the cause of SNHL can be broadly classified as genetic, acquired, or idiopathic, approximately 50% of children with moderate to profound congenital SNHL have a genetic cause.[3,4]

Disclosures: None.
[a] Division of Pediatric Otolaryngology–Head and Neck Surgery, Cincinnati Children's Hospital Medical Center, 3333 Burnet Avenue, Cincinnati, OH 45229-3039, USA; [b] Division of Pediatric Otolaryngology–Head and Neck Surgery, Ear and Hearing Center, Cincinnati Children's Hospital Medical Center, 3333 Burnet Avenue, MLC 2018, Cincinnati, OH 45229-3039, USA; [c] Department of Otolaryngology–Head and Neck Surgery, University of Cincinnati College of Medicine, 234 Goodman Drive, Cincinnati, OH 45229, USA
* Corresponding author. Division of Pediatric Otolaryngology–Head and Neck Surgery, Cincinnati Children's Hospital Medical Center, 3333 Burnet Avenue, MLC 2018, Cincinnati, OH 45229-3039.
E-mail address: John.Greinwald@cchmc.org

Otolaryngol Clin N Am 48 (2015) 975–982
http://dx.doi.org/10.1016/j.otc.2015.07.004
0030-6665/15/$ – see front matter © 2015 Elsevier Inc. All rights reserved.

Abbreviations	
CMV	Cytomegalovirus
CT	Computed tomography
EKG	Electrocardiogram
PCR	Polymerase chain reaction
PDS	Pendred syndrome
SNHL	Sensorineural hearing loss

Most of these genetic phenotypes are not associated with a named syndrome or other anomaly (nonsyndromic), with only 15% to 30% occurring as part of a recognized syndrome.[5] Of all hereditary hearing loss cases, 80% are transmitted in an autosomal-recessive pattern (designated DFNB_), whereas the remaining are autosomal-dominant (DFNA_), mitochondrial, or sex-linked (DFNX_).[6]

Approximately 35% of children with SNHL have an identifiable acquired cause, which may be attributed to a wide array of causes, including intrauterine infections such as cytomegalovirus (CMV), environmental exposures, meningitis, ototoxic medications, maternal drug or alcohol use, prematurity, or low Apgar scores.[7] Hearing loss without an identified cause is classified as idiopathic.

Widespread adoption of universal newborn hearing screening has improved the ability to identify SNHL; however, the best approach to establishing the cause of the hearing loss has been controversial, and a wide variety of diagnostic tests have been used. Historically, patients underwent a comprehensive simultaneous "shotgun" test battery, which included temporal bone imaging, laboratory tests, and an electrocardiogram (EKG). Patients were also concurrently referred for consultation with specialists. Over the past decade, however, research pertaining to individual test yields and the optimization of genetic testing has shown that a stepwise sequential diagnostic approach is more prudent, because it reduces costs as well as utilization of resources.[8,9] This paradigm is now widely accepted and is discussed in this article.

IDENTIFYING PATIENTS WITH SENSORINEURAL HEARING LOSS

In 2007, the American Academy of Pediatrics Joint Committee on Infant Hearing issued a position statement that outlined recommendations for newborn hearing screening.[10] The report recommended that all infants be screened for hearing loss within the first month of life. More specifically, those at high risk should be screened with auditory brainstem response testing, whereas those at lower risk may be screened with otoacoustic emission testing. Infants who fail the initial screening should have repeat testing, and those who fail this testing should receive a comprehensive audiometric evaluation by 3 months of age. Infants who pass the initial screening should undergo surveillance of communication milestones, starting at the 2-month well-child checkup. If concerns arise, a referral for an audiometric evaluation should be made. Intervention should be initiated by 6 months of age.[10]

The degree or severity of hearing loss must also be documented. A loss between 20 and 40 dB is considered mild, a loss between 41 and 54 dB is moderate, a loss between 55 and 70 dB is moderately severe, and a loss between 71 and 90 dB or greater is considered profound.

CLINICAL HISTORY AND PHYSICAL EXAMINATION

Once the diagnosis of SNHL is established, a thorough medical history should be taken to identify possible risk factors for the hearing loss. The clinician should endeavor to ascertain prenatal, perinatal, and postnatal risk factors for the loss. After a birth history is taken, a thorough review of the family history should be obtained, with construction of a pedigree including at least 3 generations. This information can guide diagnostic evaluations. A comprehensive review of systems should also be carried out and may lead to identification of additional pathology, such as CMV, rubella, toxoplasmosis, or syphilis.

The physical examination should include both an otologic examination and a systemic examination, looking for any dysmorphic features that may indicate the presence of a syndrome associated with SNHL. Although many syndromes involve facial dysmorphism, cardiac, ocular, neck/thyroid, and extremity examinations should not be overlooked. Although a thorough history and physical examination are essential, these assessments alone generally have low diagnostic yield, and additional laboratory and radiologic testing are indicated.

DIAGNOSTIC TESTING
Laboratory Tests

An array of diagnostic laboratory tests that may assist in determining cause is provided in **Table 1**. Given that the diagnostic yield of these tests is low (ranging from 0% to 2%),[7,8,11] they should be ordered only if indicated by medical or family history.

Table 1
Laboratory tests used to evaluate children with sensorineural hearing loss

wTest	Finding	Disease/Syndrome	Approximate Yield (%)
Complete blood count	Abnormalities may signal leukemias associated with hearing loss	Leukemia	<1
Platelet count	Macrothrombocytopenia	Fechtner syndrome	<1
Antinuclear antibody	Elevated	Lupus/other autoimmune disorders associated with hearing loss	<1
Erythrocyte sedimentation rate	Elevated	Lupus/other autoimmune disorders associated with hearing loss	<1
Rheumatoid factor	Elevated	Lupus/other autoimmune disorders associated with hearing loss	<1
Thyroid stimulating hormone	Hypothyroidism	PS	2
Blood urea nitrogen	Elevated	Alport syndrome	<1
Creatinine	Elevated	Alport syndrome	<1
Urinalysis	Proteinuria	Alport syndrome	<1
Blood glucose	Elevated	Alstrom syndrome/diabetes	<1
Fluorescent treponemal antibody-absorbed	Positive	Syphilis	<1
Rapid plasma reagent	Positive	Syphilis	<1
Lipids	Elevated	Hyperlipidemia associated with hearing loss	<1

Genetic Tests

Since the discovery of the role that mutations in the gap-junction β-2 gene (*GJB2*) play in the cause of pediatric SNHL, *GJB2* testing has emerged as an integral part of the overall assessment. *GJB2* codes for the connexin 26 protein, which functions in the intercellular transfer of ions and small molecules. Biallelic mutations segregate in an autosomal-recessive pattern (DFNB1A). Forty percent to 50% of children with severe to profound bilateral SNHL have mutations in this gene, whereas as many as 15% to 20% of children with mild to moderate SNHL have *GJB2* mutations. In addition, large deletion mutations in a neighboring gene (*GJB6*) may work in tandem with single *GJB2* mutations to cause SNHL (DFNB1B). Overall, *GJB2* testing has been shown to have a diagnostic yield of approximately 20%.[8]

Mutations in the *SLC26A4* gene comprise the second most frequent cause of autosomal-recessive nonsyndromic hearing loss.[12] Mutations in this gene produce a phenotypic spectrum of hearing loss disorders encompassing both syndromic (Pendred syndrome [PDS]) and nonsyndromic (DFNB4) phenotypes.[13,14] *SLC26A4* codes for the anion transporter protein pendrin, which plays a key role in maintaining the endocochlear potential.[15] PDS and DFNB4 mutations typically present with congenital bilateral SNHL, which can be progressive. There is considerable variability of audiometric profiles; however, enlargement of the vestibular aqueduct is universally present and vestibular dysfunction may also be present. PDS can be associated with goiter, which may be related to hypothyroidism. A goiter can be present at birth but is more likely to develop in late childhood to early adulthood. DFNB4 is also known as nonsyndromic enlarged vestibular aqueduct and is not associated with abnormalities of the thyroid gland.

Mutations in the 12S ribosomal RNA mitochondrial gene (*MTRNR1*) have been associated with both aminoglycoside antibiotic-induced and nonsyndromic hearing loss.[16] Although mutations in this gene are maternally inherited, phenotypic expression of the associated hearing loss can be variable; hearing loss is worsened by the parenteral administration of aminoglycoside antibiotics.

More than 100 genes have been implicated in the genetic cause of SNHL, and gene-specific testing is available for many of these genes (for an excellent reference, see Hereditary Hearing Loss home page, www.hereditaryhearingloss.org). High throughput genetic testing has led to the ability to screen for a large number of genes involved in hearing loss. **Table 2** provides a list of several of the higher yield genes and their inheritance patterns. Because nearly all hearing loss in young children has a recessive genetic pattern, genetic testing that focuses on these genes is critical. Because many syndromes (eg, Usher, Pendred, Jervell, and Lange-Nielsen) have no outward phenotype in young children, genetic testing is crucial in establishing an early diagnosis. Commercially available genetic screening tests for hearing loss are also now available. The SoundGene panel is one such test (www.pediatrix.com/SoundGene). It is important to understand that these tests are not comprehensive: they are screening tests that can identify some of the more common genetic mutations associated with hearing loss.

Imaging

Both computed tomography (CT) and MRI are an integral part of the overall assessment of children with hearing loss, and both have advantages and disadvantages. High-resolution CT of the temporal bone has the advantage of being more rapid (and hence requiring no sedation in most cases) and less costly than MRI. In addition, CT reveals superior bony detail. However, as compared with MRI, CT is less likely to

Table 2		
Genes related to early childhood sensorineural hearing loss		
Gene	Disorder/Syndrome	Inheritance
CDH23	DFNB12, USH1D	Autosomal recessive
CLRN1	USH3A	Autosomal recessive
EYA1	BOR/BOS1	Autosomal dominant
FOXI1	PS	Autosomal recessive
GJB2	DFNB1A, DFNA3A	Autosomal recessive/dominant
GJB6	DFNB1B, DFNA3B	Autosomal recessive/dominant
GPR98	USH2C	Autosomal recessive
KCNJ10	DFNB4 and Sesame syndrome	Autosomal recessive
MYO6	DFNA22, DFNB37	Autosomal dominant/recessive
MYO7A	DFNB2, DFNA11, USH1B	Autosomal recessive/dominant
OTOF	DFNB9, AUNB1	Autosomal recessive
PCDH15	DFNB23, USH1F	Autosomal recessive
POU3F4	DFNX2 (DFN3)	X-linked recessive
SIX1	BOS3	Autosomal dominant
SIX5	BOR2	Autosomal dominant
SLC26A4	PS/DFNB4	Autosomal recessive
TMC1	DFNB7/11, DFNA36	Autosomal recessive/dominant
TMIE	DFNB6	Autosomal recessive
TMPRSS3	DFNB8/10	Autosomal recessive
USH1C	USH1C, DFNB18	Autosomal recessive
USH1G	USH1G	Autosomal recessive
USH2A	USH2A	Autosomal recessive
WHRN	DFNB31, USH2D	Autosomal recessive

identify cochlear nerve anomalies[17] and is associated with a small dose of ionizing radiation. MRI of the temporal bone has the advantage of revealing superior soft tissue anatomic detail; however, it is more costly, takes longer to carry out, and generally requires sedation or anesthesia in young children. Important to note, a large (n = 270) study of children with severe to profound SNHL found that MRI revealed anomalies explaining the cause of hearing loss in 24% of patients, whereas CT identified the cause in only 18%.[18]

MRI has become the imaging test of choice at the authors' institution. The most common abnormality found on imaging is enlargement of the vestibular aqueduct, with or without incomplete cochlear partitioning. Various degrees of vestibular and cochlear dysplasia can also be found. In addition, absent or deficient cochlear nerves, which may have implication in the decision for cochlear implantation, may be seen, particularly in patients with unilateral hearing loss.

Cytomegalovirus Testing

CMV is a double-stranded DNA virus member of the herpesvirus family and is the leading nongenetic cause of congenital SNHL.[19] SNHL related to CMV can be present at birth or later in childhood. It can be unilateral or bilateral and can vary widely in severity from mild to profound. In 30% to 50% of affected children, the hearing loss fluctuates, and in 50%, the hearing loss is progressive.[19] Laboratory culture has traditionally been the gold standard for diagnosing CMV; however, culture results can take as long as 6 weeks. CMV polymerase chain reaction (PCR) can also be used to diagnose CMV infection, using blood, urine, or saliva tested within the first 3 to 4 weeks of life, or a dried blood spot taken at the time birth. PCR is much more rapid than traditional culture techniques and has good sensitivity and specificity.

PCR in infants older than 3 to 4 weeks of age should be interpreted with caution, because infections can occur during the perinatal or postnatal period that also give a positive result but are not associated with hearing loss. The result may therefore not be conclusively interpreted as evidence of congenital CMV infection—making the timing of testing critically important.[9] In infants, CMV testing should be part of the initial diagnostic evaluation, because if diagnosed, it can be medically treated.

An EKG is warranted in children with severe SNHL and no other identifiable cause of the loss.[8,18] EKG identifies patients with a prolonged QT interval, which is associated with Jervell and Lange-Nielsen syndrome. Although the yield of this test is less than 1%, the consequences of unrecognized prolonged QT can be life-threatening.

CONSULTATION WITH SPECIALISTS

All children with SNHL should be referred for an ophthalmologic evaluation.[18,20–23] The rationale for this is 2-fold. First and more common, in children with SNHL, unrecognized decreased visual acuity can lead to additional communication problems, which may be critical in these children, who are already at risk for speech and language delays.[21–23] The overall yield of a consultation is 20% to 57% for identifying an ophthalmologic abnormality (predominantly unrecognized refractive errors but also strabismus and amblyopia).[18,20,21,24] Second, ophthalmologic findings may be associated with syndromic SNHL, thereby helping to identify a known syndrome (eg, Usher, Stickler). In 2% to 8% of patients, the ophthalmologic finding leads to the identification of the cause of the hearing loss.[18,20,21]

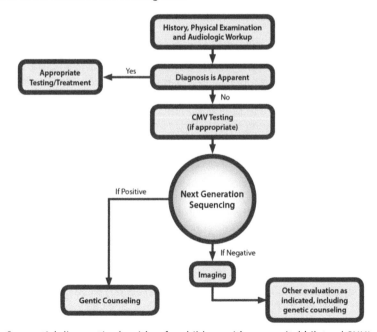

Fig. 1. Sequential diagnostic algorithm for children with congenital bilateral SNHL.

A genetics consultation has been shown to be helpful in identifying a syndrome in 25% to 37% of patients.[18,24] Because the interpretation of complex genetic testing is challenging, all patients should be referred for genetic counseling.

Up to 20% of children with SNHL may also have a developmental disorder or delay[24]; at the authors' institution, they typically refer children older than 1 year of age for consultation with a developmental pediatrician. This consultation may identify a diagnosis such as autism, which has a significant impact on communications skills.

TESTING GUIDELINES

For infants and children with bilateral SNHL who are younger than 5 years of age, CMV and genetic testing using high throughput multigene panels should be at the forefront of the diagnostic evaluation. If genetic testing is negative, imaging studies should be considered and further tests should be ordered if clinically indicated (**Fig. 1**). For patients with unilateral SNHL and older children with bilateral SNHL, imaging studies have the highest diagnostic yield, and the usefulness of genetic testing is uncertain. The exception to this uncertainty is patients with temporal bone anomalies such as enlarged vestibular aqueduct. These patients should have testing for mutations in the *SLC26A4* gene. Testing for CMV is indicated for infants with unilateral SNHL.

REFERENCES

1. Brookhouser P. Sensorineural hearing loss in children. Pediatr Clin North Am 1996;43:1195–216.
2. Mehl AL, Thomson V. Newborn hearing screening: the great omission. Pediatrics 1998;101:E4.
3. Tomaski SM, Grundfast KM. A stepwise approach to the diagnosis and treatment of hereditary hearing loss. Pediatr Clin North Am 1999;46:35–48.
4. Grundfast KM, Lalwani AK. Practical approach to diagnosis and management of hereditary hearing impairment (HHI). Ear Nose Throat J 1992;71:479–84.
5. Cohen M, Gorlin R. Epidemiology, etiology and genetic patterns. In: Gorlin R, Torriello H, Cohen M, editors. Hereditary hearing loss and its syndromes. New York: Oxford University Press; 1995. p. 9–21.
6. Billings KR, Kenna MA. Causes of pediatric sensorineural hearing loss: yesterday and today. Arch Otolaryngol Head Neck Surg 1999;125:517–21.
7. Mafong DD, Shin EJ, Lalwani AK. Use of laboratory evaluation and radiologic imaging in the diagnostic evaluation of children with sensorineural hearing loss. Laryngoscope 2002;112:1–7.
8. Preciado DA, Lawson L, Madden C, et al. Improved diagnostic effectiveness with a sequential diagnostic paradigm in idiopathic pediatric sensorineural hearing loss. Otol Neurotol 2005;26:610–5.
9. Park AH, Duval M, McVicar S, et al. A diagnostic paradigm including cytomegalovirus testing for idiopathic pediatric sensorineural hearing loss. Laryngoscope 2014;124:2624–9.
10. American Academy of Pediatrics, Joint Committee on Infant Hearing. Year 2007 position statement: principles and guidelines for early hearing detection and intervention programs. Pediatrics 2007;120:898–921.
11. Ohlms LA, Chen AY, Stewart MG, et al. Establishing the etiology of childhood hearing loss. Otolaryngol Head Neck Surg 1999;120:159–63.
12. Hilgert N, Smith RJ, Van Camp G. Forty-six genes causing nonsyndromic hearing impairment: which ones should be analyzed in DNA diagnostics? Mutat Res 2009;681:189–96.

13. Everett LA, Glaser B, Beck JC, et al. Pendred syndrome is caused by mutations in a putative sulphate transporter gene (PDS). Nat Genet 1997;17:411–22.

14. Li XC, Everett LA, Lalwani AK, et al. A mutation in PDS causes non-syndromic recessive deafness. Nat Genet 1998;18:215–7.

15. Royaux IE, Belyantseva IA, Wu T, et al. Localization and functional studies of pendrin in the mouse inner ear provide insight about the etiology of deafness in pendred syndrome. J Assoc Res Otolaryngol 1998;4:394–404.

16. Prezant TR, Agapian JV, Bohlman MC, et al. Mitochondrial ribosomal RNA mutation associated with both antibiotic-induced and non-syndromic deafness. Nat Genet 1993;4:289–94.

17. Licameli G, Kenna MA. Is computed tomography (CT) or magnetic resonance imaging (MRI) more useful in the evaluation of pediatric sensorineural hearing loss? Laryngoscope 2010;120:2358–9.

18. Lin JW, Chowdhury N, Mody A, et al. Comprehensive diagnostic battery for evaluating sensorineural hearing loss in children. Otol Neurotol 2011;2:259–64.

19. Fowler KB. Congenital cytomegalovirus infection: audiologic outcome. Clin Infect Dis 2013;57(S4):S182–4.

20. Sharma A, Ruscetta MN, Chi DH. Ophthalmologic findings in children with sensorineural hearing loss. Arch Otolaryngol Head Neck Surg 2009;135:119–23.

21. Mafong DD, Pletcher SD, Hoyt C, et al. Ocular findings in children with congenital sensorineural hearing loss. Arch Otolaryngol Head Neck Surg 2002;128:1303–6.

22. Regenbogen L, Godel V. Ocular deficiencies in deaf children. J Pediatr Ophthalmol Strabismus 1985;22:231–3.

23. Fillman RD, Leguire LE, Rogers GL, et al. Screening for vision problems, including Usher's syndrome, among hearing impaired students. Am Ann Deaf 1987;132:194–8.

24. Wiley S, Arjmand E, Jareenmeinzen-Derr, et al. Findings from multidisciplinary evaluation of children with permanent hearing loss. Int J Pediatr Otorhinolaryngol 2011;75:1040–4.

Management of Children with Mild, Moderate, and Moderately Severe Sensorineural Hearing Loss

Anne Marie Tharpe, PhD*, Samantha Gustafson, AuD

KEYWORDS

- Pediatric hearing loss • Hearing aid use • Progressive hearing loss
- Late-onset hearing loss • Hearing technologies

KEY POINTS

- Management of children with hearing loss requires collaborative, interprofessional teams focused on patient-centered goals and shared problem solving.
- Referrals to otolaryngologists, audiologists, and speech-language pathologists with expertise working with children should be made for diagnosis, treatment, and management of hearing loss.
- The hearing of every child should receive ongoing monitoring throughout childhood to detect late-onset or progressive hearing loss.
- A variety of hearing technologies are appropriate and available for children with mild, moderate, and moderately severe sensorineural hearing losses.

OVERVIEW: NATURE OF THE PROBLEM

Childhood hearing loss impacts almost all areas of child development: speech and language, psychosocial, and psychoeducational development, among others. The earlier management is implemented, the better chance there is to ameliorate the negative impact on development. Although we currently screen the hearing of 97% of newborns in the United States, a significant percentage of infants who fail the screening do

Disclosure Statement: Dr A.M. Tharpe is Chair of the Phonak Research Advisory Board and serves as principal investigator of a research grant from Phonak. Dr S. Gustafson has nothing to disclose.
Department of Hearing and Speech Sciences, Vanderbilt Bill Wilkerson Center, Vanderbilt University School of Medicine, 1215 21st Avenue South, 6308 Medical Center East, Nashville, TN 37232-8718, USA
* Corresponding author.
E-mail address: anne.m.tharpe@Vanderbilt.Edu

not return for follow-up testing. According to the Centers for Disease Control and Prevention, only 70% of infants with hearing loss receive appropriate diagnostic testing by 3 months of age and only 56% receive intervention before 6 months of age.[1] Therefore, it is incumbent on pediatricians and otolaryngologists who treat these children to ensure that families understand the importance of follow-up and management to their children's outcomes.

Effective management of childhood hearing loss requires the collaborative efforts of the child's family and numerous professionals, including audiologists, pediatricians, otolaryngologists, educators, speech-language pathologists, and early interventionists, and others. Exposure to consistent, meaningful sounds during the first few years of life is essential for auditory neural pathways in the brain to develop, leading to spoken language and cognitive growth. Hearing technologies are now available for all types and degrees of hearing loss, and eligibility for these technologies has changed considerably over the past decade. With the rapidly evolving landscape of hearing technologies, communication among professionals becomes more important than ever before to ensure that families receive consistent and accurate counseling about their options.

IDENTIFICATION OF CHILDHOOD HEARING LOSS

Before universal newborn hearing screening, a child born with congenital hearing loss was likely to be identified after the first 2 years of life. The evaluation and diagnosis of children was generally requested and often welcomed by the family, who suspected something was wrong based on their child's lack of language development. For those families, the hearing loss of their child had an obvious impact on their lives, allowing them to accept the diagnosis and to see direct benefit from intervention. This might not be the case for many families of children with hearing loss today. When identified in the newborn period, parents have not yet observed any obvious indications of hearing loss. The "problem" of hearing loss is invisible to them. For these families, acceptance of a diagnosis of hearing loss might be especially difficult and will require a consistent message and reassurance from the family's medical home. Furthermore, we know that infants born to teenage mothers and those born to mothers with less than a high school education are less likely to seek intervention services than older mothers and those with college degrees[1]; thus, these mothers will require additional counseling and encouragement for their infants to receive the hearing services they need.

The Joint Committee on Infant Hearing Guidelines (JCIH[2]) recommends newborn hearing screening that targets permanent, bilateral or unilateral hearing loss averaging 40 dB or greater. This includes those with moderate losses (41–55 dB HL), moderately severe (56–70 dB HL), severe (71–90 dB HL), and profound (91+ dB HL); however, those with minimal or mild loss will likely not be detected. There is now a large body of evidence that suggests children with mild degrees of bilateral and any degree of unilateral permanent hearing loss are at risk of psychoeducational and behavioral difficulties (eg, Refs[3–6]). Minimal or mild bilateral hearing loss can be defined as follows:

- Pure-tone average (500, 1000, 2000 Hz) between 20 and 40 dB HL, OR
- High-frequency hearing loss with pure-tone thresholds greater than 25 dB HL at 2 or more frequencies above 2000 Hz.[3,7]

Fig. 1 illustrates that children with mild degrees of hearing loss are identified and fit with hearing aids later than children with greater degrees of loss. Additionally, because

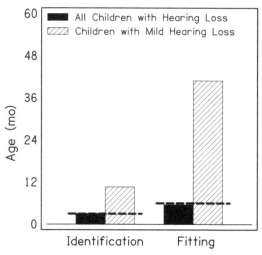

Fig. 1. Median age (months) of hearing loss identification and recommended hearing aid fitting for children with any degree of hearing loss (*filled bars*) and children with mild degrees of hearing loss (*hashed bars*). Horizontal lines represent recommended JCIH guidelines for identification and intervention for children with hearing loss. (*Data from* Refs.[2,8,9])

children with mild degrees of hearing loss can hear and respond to some sounds, there might be less parental concern for the child's hearing behavior and reduced awareness of delayed auditory development, even if the child has been diagnosed with a mild hearing loss.

MANAGEMENT GOALS

Studies have consistently shown that early identification of and intervention for childhood hearing loss results in improved communication abilities, including language, speech perception, and speech production.[10–12] Physicians and other health care providers play a significant role in this process. Although the screening and diagnosis[13] might initially appear as the "main event" in the family's life, the longer journey begins *after* the identification of hearing loss. **Fig. 2** illustrates some of the steps involved in the management of children with hearing loss. Although the management team works together to provide services for the child and family, the frequency of the follow-up visits will be tailored to the individual child and family needs for each aspect of intervention. For example, a young child might receive weekly services from a speech-language pathologist during the first couple of years following identification, but those services will likely be reduced in frequency and eventually cease once the child has achieved age-appropriate speech and language skills. Alternatively, this child's follow-up with an audiologist will continue through adulthood, likely on at least an annual basis.

Medical providers should consider the following management steps for children with newly diagnosed hearing loss:

- State Medicaid programs cover hearing screening, diagnosis, and intervention as part of the Early and Periodic Screening, Diagnostic and Treatment benefit. Children from birth to age 3 years who have been diagnosed with hearing loss

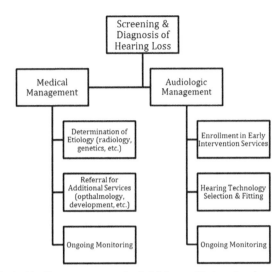

Fig. 2. Steps included in the management of children with hearing loss.

receive free, early intervention services through the Individuals with Disabilities Education Act (IDEA) Part C. School-age children ages 3 to 21 years receive services through IDEA Part B. Ensure that the families of children with hearing loss are aware of their rights for free and appropriate services.
- Refer children to geneticists in cases of suspected genetic hearing loss.
- Incidence of vision impairments is higher in children with hearing loss than in the general population (22% and 14%, respectively[14]). Routine ophthalmologic examinations are recommended by the American Academy of Pediatrics periodicity schedule.[15]
- Refer children to audiologists and speech-language pathologists with expertise in working with children who have hearing loss.[16]

Communication Mode

One of the early decisions a family must make on receiving a diagnosis of hearing loss in their young child is that of communication mode. In 2005, 85% of parents chose listening and spoken language for their child with hearing loss.[17] This is expected because approximately 97% of children with hearing loss are born to normal-hearing parents who use spoken language. However, parents might choose another option based on their experiences, family culture, and communication goals for their child. Other options, especially for those with severe hearing loss or those families who identify with deaf culture, might include some type of visual or manual communication (eg, American Sign Language, Signing Exact English), or a combination of oral and manual communication (eg, Total Communication).

Hearing Assistive Technology

Hearing aids

When a child's family elects to pursue listening and spoken language as the primary mode of communication, the recommended course of treatment includes the fitting of hearing aids. The function of hearing aids is to provide the user with an audible broad frequency range of speech at various input levels (soft, average, and loud), and to ensure that loud inputs to the hearing aid are comfortable for the user. **Fig. 3** shows a schematic of a behind-the-ear (BTE) hearing aid, the most common type of hearing aid used by children. An alternative to the BTE hearing aid is in-the-ear (ITE) technology. In this style of hearing aid, all electronics are housed in the plastic casing that fits in the canal or concha of the pinna. Because of the swallowing risk associated with the small size of ITEs, among other reasons, the American Academy of Audiology[18] does not recommend their use for young children. For children with bilateral hearing loss, regardless of the symmetry of loss between ears, the American Academy of Audiology[18] recommends bilateral hearing aids. Wearing 2 hearing aids provides binaural advantages over a single hearing aid for enhanced auditory localization, signal detection, and speech perception in noise.

The Pediatric Working Group[19] recommends that audiologic appointments following hearing aid fittings be conducted every 3 months during the first 2 years of amplification use. In addition to monitoring auditory status and development, these frequent appointments are important for young children because earmolds must be

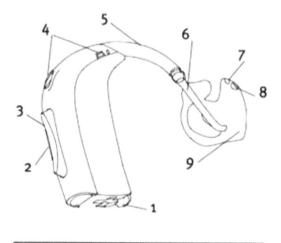

1. Battery compartment

2. Push button

3. Volume control (Optional)

4. Microphone opening

5. Sound hook

6. Earmold tubing

7. Sound outlet

8. Ventilation opening

9. Earmold

Fig. 3. Schematic of a BTE hearing aid. (*Courtesy of* Oticon, Inc, Somerset, NJ; with permission.)

replaced often because of rapid ear canal size growth during early life. Earmolds must fit snugly within the ear to avoid acoustic feedback, and a good fit is also needed for device retention. The timeline of follow-up visits for management will be adjusted based on individual factors such as whether the child has additional handicapping conditions, or is at risk for progressive hearing loss.

The management team should encourage families to aim for full-time use of hearing aids to maximize auditory experiences. Young children (birth to 3 years) and children with mild degrees of hearing loss are at risk for less device use than older children (4–7 years) and children with greater degrees of hearing loss.[20,21] This might be because families see their child with mild hearing loss responding to sound when they are not wearing hearing aids and might feel inclined to discontinue use of the devices. Repeated counseling might be required to remind families that even mild hearing loss can have a negative psychosocial and psychoeducational impact on children.

Remote microphone technology

Children with hearing loss have greater difficulty understanding speech in suboptimal conditions than their normal-hearing counterparts; yet, like all children, children with hearing loss are frequently in noisy conditions, such as day care settings and class-rooms. Although personal hearing aids improve audibility of speech for children with hearing loss, they also improve audibility of the interfering noise. To facilitate optimal learning and communication, the speech signal of interest should be at least 20 dB above the background noise (ie, 20-dB signal-to-noise ratio[22]). Remote microphone technology (eg, frequency-modulation systems) improves the signal-to-noise ratio for listeners. This technology requires a microphone to be placed close to the target speaker's mouth (eg, teacher, therapist, parent), where the decibel level of the speech is well above that of the interfering noise. The high-quality signal from this microphone is then delivered to the listener via a wireless carrier frequency directly to a receiver (personal system) or to a loudspeaker positioned near the listener (audio distribution system). All children who wear hearing aids are candidates for remote microphone technologies. Although all young children with hearing loss can benefit from remote microphone technologies, the utility of this technology increases markedly as they enter the school environment.

Cochlear implants

Hearing aids provide significant benefit to those with mild to severe hearing loss who have good speech perception ability. However, there are some children with severe losses and poor speech perception who derive little if any benefit from hearing aids, but do not meet Food and Drug Administration candidacy criteria for cochlear implantation. Although in years past, only children with severe-to-profound hearing loss were eligible for cochlear implantation, some children with lesser degrees of hearing loss might now be eligible depending on their auditory progress with hearing aids alone. A recent review of 51 children who had more residual hearing than specified by current guidelines, found that all received speech perception benefit following implantation.[23] These investigators called for consideration of cochlear implantation for all children with sensorineural hearing loss who use hearing aids on a full-time basis, and comply with therapy recommendations, but who are not making expected auditory and speech-language progress.

When being considered for implantation, children should maintain full-time hearing aid use, even after their child's auditory progress has been deemed "inadequate" with hearing aids alone. Maintaining device use increases the child's opportunity for continued auditory stimulation before implantation, which might reduce the effects of auditory deprivation. This continued hearing aid use might also help families maintain a routine of device placement and retention, facilitating a smooth transition to full-time use of a cochlear implant following activation.

Interprofessional Collaborative Approach

Advocacy by pediatricians and otolaryngologists is imperative for the success of early hearing detection and intervention programs as well as timely, ongoing monitoring and follow-up services. Pediatricians are typically the first health care providers to whom parents turn when they have concerns about their child's hearing. By virtue of their regular contact with children throughout the first year of life, pediatricians play a central role in directing families through the diagnostic and intervention process. When caring for children with hearing loss and their families, teamwork is required to coordinate the numerous professionals involved, including audiologists, speech-language pathologists, early interventionists, pediatricians, otolaryngologists, and educators. Because a large percentage of children with hearing loss also have additional disabilities (30%–40%), the primary care physician should monitor developmental milestones and initiate referrals for specialty evaluations, as needed. Therefore, other professionals, such as geneticists, social workers, ophthalmologists, neurologists, psychologists, and developmental specialists, also could be part of the professional team. Staying focused on patient-centered goals and shared problem solving will create an effective team and result in optimum care of these families. The knowledge and skills required of providers for effective collaboration are provided in **Box 1**.

Box 1
Knowledge and skills required of providers for effective collaboration

Providers have the knowledge and skills to

1. Recognize roles and responsibilities of families and other individuals with expertise in deafness

2. Support consultation across disciplines and collaborate with families

3. Recognize the roles and the importance of service coordination and medical homes

4. Promote collaboration with community programs and resources to support families and children

5. Recognize intra/interpersonal variables that influence the development of collaborative relationships

6. Apply principles and strategies to support family members and professionals

7. Implement collaborative strategies for communicating, decision-making, and resolving conflict

8. Provide for a continuum of service delivery models to meet the needs of the individual child and family (eg, direct service, collaborative consultation, playgroup based)

9. Assume a leadership role affecting collaboration, including self-evaluating, mentoring, networking, and advocating for families and organizations

From American Academy of Pediatrics. Supplement to the JCIH 2007 position statement: principles and guidelines for early intervention after confirmation that a child is deaf or hard of hearing. Pediatrics 2013;131:e1344; with permission.

Monitoring

Transient conductive hearing loss

At one time, it was estimated that by 3 years of age, 80% of children in the United States would have experienced one or more bouts of otitis media, with more than 40% having 3 or more bouts.[24,25] Since the routine use of the 7-valent pneumococcal conjugate vaccine (PCV-7) in 2000, the incidence and prevalence of otitis media have declined markedly.[26] Moreover, with the advent of the 13-valent vaccine (PCV-13) and recommendations for routine childhood vaccinations,[27] there has been a further reduction of otitis media–related pediatric health care visits, including a reduction in ventilating tube insertion rate by 19% from 2010 to 2011.[28]

The average degree of hearing loss associated with otitis media with effusion (OME) is 25 dB in the speech frequency range.[29] Many typically developing children with these transient losses might experience little difficulty communicating with this added deficit; however, for children with an underlying permanent sensorineural hearing loss who already struggle with auditory and speech-language deficits, the effects of OME can be greater than for those with normal hearing.[30] Therefore, it is of utmost importance that children with permanent hearing loss be monitored to ensure that OME resolves and hearing returns to its typical level.

Progressive and late-onset hearing loss

Although approximately 97% of newborns now receive hearing screening in the United States, it is important for pediatricians and otolaryngologists to remember that approximately 4% to 30% of children have progressive or late-onset hearing loss.[30,31] Hearing loss can occur at any time in a child's life, and these losses can result from trauma, noise exposure, teratogens, or genetic factors. Furthermore, because the JCIH does not target minimal and mild hearing losses, children with these losses might not be identified early. Therefore, it is imperative that the hearing of all children, even those who passed newborn hearing screening, be monitored on a periodic basis consistent with the American Academy of Pediatrics (AAP) periodicity schedule (2014). **Box 2** lists risk indicators associated with permanent congenital, delayed-onset, or progressive hearing loss in childhood.[2]

Ongoing surveillance

The JCIH[2,16] recommends the following surveillance program within the medical home:

- Monitoring for auditory skills, middle-ear status, and developmental milestones at each visit according to the AAP periodicity schedule (2014); a validated global screening tool should be administered to all infants at 9, 18, and 24 to 30 months or at any time if there is health care professional or family concern about hearing or language.
- Children should be referred immediately for further evaluation by an audiologist and a speech-language pathologist for a speech and language evaluation with validated tools if they do not pass the speech-language portion of the global screening in the medical home, or if there is physician or caregiver concern about hearing or spoken-language development.
- Siblings of an infant diagnosed with hearing loss who are at increased risk of having hearing loss should be referred for audiological evaluation.
- All infants with risk indicators for hearing loss,[2] regardless of surveillance findings, should be referred for an audiological assessment at least once by 24 to 30 months of age; children with risk indicators that are highly associated with

---

Box 2
Risk indicators associated with permanent congenital, delayed-onset, or progressive hearing loss in childhood

Risk Indicators

1. Caregiver concerns regarding hearing, speech, language, or developmental delay

2. Family history of permanent childhood hearing loss

3. Neonatal intensive care of more than 5 days or any of the following regardless of length of stay: extracorporeal membrane oxygenation, assisted ventilation, exposure to ototoxic medications, and hyperbilirubinemia that requires exchange transfusion

4. In utero infections, such as cytomegalovirus, herpes, rubella, syphilis, and toxoplasmosis

5. Craniofacial anomalies, including those that involve the pinna, ear canal, ear tags, ear pits, and temporal bone anomalies

6. Physical findings, such as white forelock, that are associated with a syndrome known to include a sensorineural or permanent conductive hearing loss

7. Syndromes associated with hearing loss or progressive or late-onset hearing loss, such as neurofibromatosis, osteopetrosis, and Usher syndrome; other frequently identified syndromes include Waardenburg, Alport, Pendred, and Jervell and Lange-Nielson

8. Neurodegenerative disorders, such as Hunter syndrome, or sensory motor neuropathies, such as Friedreich ataxia and Charcot-Marie-Tooth syndrome

9. Culture-positive postnatal infections associated with sensorineural hearing loss, including confirmed bacterial and viral (especially herpes viruses and varicella) meningitis

10. Head trauma, especially basal skull/temporal bone fracture that requires hospitalization

11. Chemotherapy

From American Academy of Pediatrics. Year 2007 position statement: principles and guidelines for early hearing detection and intervention programs. Pediatrics 2007;120(4):921; with permission.

---

delayed-onset hearing loss should have more frequent audiological assessments.

- All infants for whom the family has significant concerns regarding hearing or communication should be promptly referred for an audiological and speech-language assessment.
- Careful assessment of middle-ear status (using pneumatic otoscopy and/or tympanometry) should be completed at all well-child visits, and children with persistent middle-ear effusion that lasts for 3 months or longer should be referred for otologic evaluation.

Information for the General Otolaryngologist or Pediatrician

Hearing screening beyond the newborn period

Hearing screenings administered to children in physician's offices and in the school system are an important step in identifying children with late-onset and progressive hearing loss. Although these screenings are critical to identifying childhood hearing loss, data suggest that even the most rigorous pure-tone screening protocol (20 dB HL at 1000, 2000, and 4000 Hz) will not identify all children with minimal/mild degrees of loss.[32] Thus, in addition to hearing screenings, physicians should listen for the signs reported by parents listed in **Table 1** and refer children for full audiologic evaluations, even if they have passed a hearing screening, if any of these concerns are expressed.

Table 1
Explanations for parental concerns that may indicate progressive or late-onset hearing loss

Parental Comments	Explanations
"He has been getting into trouble at school lately. His teacher says he's always daydreaming and not paying attention in class."	Children with hearing loss may appear to be off-task at school because they have a hard time following the instruction or conversation.
"My child has recently been listening to the TV and radio at really high volumes."	Children with hearing loss will adjust the volume to meet their listening needs.
"Lately, she doesn't seem to listen to me, but that is, so unlike her."	Children with hearing loss can sometimes appear to be ignoring instruction when it was not heard due to their hearing loss.
"My child complains that she can't understand her teacher."	Children with hearing loss may have difficulty listening to classroom instruction due to classroom noise or distance.
"He has started to ask 'what?' and 'huh?' when we ask him to do something."	Children with hearing loss may not hear portions of speech, resulting in misunderstandings.

SUMMARY

Children with hearing losses in the mild to moderately severe range are a varied group. Although, in general, we expect a positive correlation between degree of hearing loss and its impact on child development, the distinctions across these categories are influenced by many factors, including age of identification and intervention, technology selection and wearing compliance, and quality of intervention. The roles of pediatricians and otolaryngologists in referring children for appropriate assessments and interventions, and encouraging families to comply with hearing technology use and therapeutic intervention are crucial to ensuring the best possible outcomes.

REFERENCES

1. Centers for Disease Control and Prevention. Early hearing detection and intervention among infants–hearing screening and follow-up survey, United States, 2005–2006 and 2009–2010. MMWR Surveill Summ 2014;63(Suppl 2):20–6. Available at: http://www.cdc.gov/mmwr/preview/mmwrhtml/su6302a4.htm.
2. American Academy of Pediatrics. Year 2007 position statement: principles and guidelines for early hearing detection and intervention programs. Pediatrics 2007;120(4):898.
3. Bess FH, Dodd-Murphy J, Parker RA. Children with minimal sensorineural hearing loss: prevalence, educational performance, and functional status. Ear Hear 1998; 19(5):339–54.
4. Bess FH, Tharpe AM. Unilateral hearing impairment in children. Pediatrics 1984; 74(2):206–16.
5. Most T. The effects of degree and type of hearing loss on children's performance in class. Deafness Education Int 2004;6(3):154–66.
6. Wake M, Hughes EK, Collins CM, et al. Parent-reported health-related quality of life in children with congenital hearing loss: a population study. Ambul Pediatr 2004;4(5):411–7.
7. Centers for Disease Control and Prevention. National workshop on mild and unilateral hearing loss: workshop proceedings. Breckenridge (CO): 2005. Available online at: http://www.cdc.gov/ncbddd/ehdi/.

8. Fitzpatrick EM, Durieux-Smith A, Whittingham J. Clinical practice for children with mild bilateral and unilateral hearing loss. Ear Hear 2010;31(3):392–400.
9. Sininger YS, Martinez A, Eisenberg L, et al. Newborn hearing screening speeds diagnosis and access to intervention by 20-25 months. J Am Acad Audiol 2009; 20(1):49–57.
10. Kennedy CR, McCann DC, Campbell MJ, et al. Language ability after early detection of permanent childhood hearing impairment. N Engl J Med 2006; 354(20):2131–41.
11. Moeller MP. Early intervention and language development in children who are deaf and hard of hearing. Pediatrics 2000;106(3):1–9.
12. Yoshinaga-Itano C, Sedey AL, Coutler DK, et al. Language of early-and later-identified children with hearing loss. Pediatrics 1998;5:1161–71.
13. Singleton AJ, Waltzman SB. Audiometric Evaluation of Children with Hearing Loss. Otolaryngol Clin N Am 2015, in press.
14. Sharma A, Ruscella MN, Chi DH. Ophthalmologic findings in children with sensorineural hearing loss. Arch Otolaryngol Head Neck Surg 2009;135(2):119–23.
15. American Academy of Pediatrics. Recommendations for preventive pediatric health care. 2014. Available at: https://www.aap.org/en-us/professional-resources/practice-support/periodicity/periodicity%20schedule_FINAL.pdf. Accessed March 10, 2015.
16. American Academy of Pediatrics. Supplement to the JCIH 2007 position statement: principles and guidelines for early intervention after confirmation that a child is deaf or hard of hearing. Pediatrics 2013;131:e1324–50.
17. Brown C. Early intervention: strategies for public and private sector collaboration. Paper presented at the 2006 Convention of the Alexander Graham Bell Association for the Deaf and Hard of Hearing, Pittsburgh, PA, 2006.
18. American Academy of Audiology. American Academy of Audiology clinical guidelines: pediatric amplification. 2013. Available at: http://audiology-web.s3. amazonaws.com/migrated/PediatricAmplificationGuidelines.pdf_539975b3e7e9f1. 74471798.pdf. Accessed March 17, 2015.
19. The Pediatric Working Group. Amplification for infants and children with hearing loss. Am J Audiol 1996;5(1):53–66.
20. Walker EA, Spratford M, Moeller MP, et al. Predictors of hearing aid use time in children with mild-to-severe hearing loss. Lang Speech Hear Serv Schools 2013;44(1):73–88.
21. Muñoz K, Preston E, Hicken S. Pediatric hearing aid use: how can audiologists support parents to increase consistency? J Am Acad Audiol 2014;25(4):380–7
22. Bistata S, Bradley J. Reverberation time and maximum background-noise level for classrooms from a comparative study of speech intelligibility metrics. J Acoust Soc Am 2000;107:861–75.
23. Carlson ML, Sladen DP, Haynes DS, et al. Evidence for the expansion of pediatric cochlear implant candidacy. Otol Neurotol 2014;36(1):43–50.
24. Teele DW, Klein JO, Chase C, et al. Greater Boston Otitis Media Study Group. Otitis media in infancy and intellectual ability, school achievement, speech, and language at age 7 years. J Infect Dis 1990;162(3):685–94.
25. The Centers for Disease Control and Prevention. 2011 Annual Data Early Hearing Detection and Intervention (EHDI) program. 2013. Available at: http://www.cdc. gov/ncbddd/hearingloss/2011-data/2011_ehdi_hsfs_summary_a.pdf. Accessed March 30, 2015.
26. Zhou F, Shefer A, Kong Y, et al. Trends in acute otitis media-related health care utilization by privately insured young children in the US, 1997-2004. Pediatrics 2008;121:253–60.

27. American Academy of Pediatrics Committee on Infectious Diseases. Recommendations for the prevention of *Streptococcus pneumoniae* infections in infants and children: use of 13-valent pneumococcal conjugate vaccine (PCV13) and pneumococcal polysaccharide vaccine (PPSV23). Pediatrics 2010;126(1):186–90.

28. Marom T, Tan A, Wilkinson GS, et al. Trends in otitis media-related health care use in the United States, 2001-2011. JAMA Pediatr 2014;168(1):68–75.

29. Fria TJ, Cantekin EI, Eichler JA. Hearing acuity of children with otitis media with effusion. Arch Otolaryngol 1985;111(1):10–6.

30. Brookhouser P, Worthington D, Kelly W. Fluctuating and/or progressive sensorineural hearing loss in children. Laryngoscope 1994;104:958–64.

31. Berrettini S, Ravecca F, Sellari-Franceschini S, et al. Progressive sensorineural hearing loss in childhood. Pediatr Neurol 1999;20(2):130–6.

32. Dodd-Murphy JD, Murphy W, Bess FH. Accuracy of school screenings in the identification of minimal sensorineural hearing loss. Am J Audiol 2014;23(4): 365–73.

Management of Children with Severe, Severe-profound, and Profound Sensorineural Hearing Loss

Claire Iseli, MBBS, MS[a,b], Craig A. Buchman, MD[a,]*

KEYWORDS

- Hearing loss • Pediatric • Severe • Profound • Cochlear implant

KEY POINTS

- Early diagnosis of hearing loss with a combination of electrophysiological and behavioral test measures is critical in initiating treatment during a period of maximal neural plasticity.
- Medical assessment involves history, examination, imaging, and other testing to identify a possible cause, allow counseling regarding risk of progression of hearing loss and potentially modifiable factors, and search for anatomic factors that can adversely affect prognosis using a cochlear implant (CI).
- Early fitting with hearing aids (HAs) before 3 months of age and commencement of an early intervention program by 6 months is recommended by the Joint Commission on Infant Hearing.
- If auditory-verbal communication is the aim, HAs are rarely sufficient in this population. Therefore, CIs are the mainstay of care. Implanting should ideally occur at or before 12 months of age to maximize speech and language outcomes.
- When expected outcomes are not achieved, possible causes of underperformance or regression may be related to pathologic or surgical electrode-neural interface problems, patient factors, audiologic-habilitative issues, or device issue.

Financial Disclosures: C. Iseli has no financial disclosures. C.A. Buchman serves as a consultant and receives research support from Advanced Bionics, Cochlear, and MedEL Corp.
[a] Department of Otolaryngology-Head & Neck Surgery, University of North Carolina at Chapel Hill, Chapel Hill, NC, USA; [b] 100/30 Wreckyn Street, North Melbourne, Victoria 3051, Australia
* Corresponding author. G190 Physicians Office Building, 170 Manning Drive, Chapel Hill, NC 27599-7600.
E-mail address: buchman@med.unc.edu

Otolaryngol Clin N Am 48 (2015) 995–1010
http://dx.doi.org/10.1016/j.otc.2015.06.004
0030-6665/15/$ – see front matter © 2015 Elsevier Inc. All rights reserved.

Abbreviations	
ABR	Auditory brainstem response
ANSD	Auditory neuropathy spectrum disorder
ASSR	Auditory steady state response
CI	Cochlear implant
CM	Cochlear microphonic
CMV	Cytomegalovirus
CND	Cochlear nerve deficiency
FDA	United States Food and Drug Administration
HA	Hearing aid
HRCT	High-resolution computed tomography
OAE	Otoacoustic emissions
SNHL	Sensorineural hearing loss

OVERVIEW: NATURE OF THE PROBLEM

Severe hearing loss is defined as a pure tone threshold of 71 to 90 dB on hearing level audiogram, whereas profound hearing loss is defined as a pure tone threshold of greater than 90 dB.[1] Approximately 4000 children are born each year in the United States with bilateral severe to profound sensorineural hearing loss (SNHL), which constitutes about one-third to one-fourth of those born with any form of unilateral or bilateral SNHL.[1] In the United Kingdom, the prevalence of children born with any kind of permanent hearing loss is approximately 1 in 1000, with a prevalence of 0.3 in 1000 diagnosed with severe hearing loss and 0.3 in 1000 diagnosed with profound hearing loss.[2] In the United States, these numbers are slightly higher with 3 to 4 per 1000 births with permanent hearing loss and 1 in 1000 with profound hearing loss.[3]

The management of children with severe to profound and profound SNHL is dominated by the need to provide sufficient audibility as well as temporal and spectral resolution capabilities to support expressive and receptive language development. Although hearing aids (HAs) can provide some of the needed information, they are often not sufficient for spoken language development so a cochlear implant (CI) is chosen. Equally important is that auditory information provided by the CI is introduced during a period of sufficient neural plasticity to allow the signal to be integrated into the central pathways and allow connection between the presence of sound and its meaning.

PATIENT EVALUATION OVERVIEW

Assessment to confirm the degree of hearing loss and identify the cause should be carried out as early as is feasible to allow treatment to occur within an appropriate time frame. Ideally, this process begins immediately following the failure result on a newborn infant hearing screening examination or when family members begin to suspect a lack of sound awareness by the child. The management paradigm of such an infant combines formal diagnostic testing of auditory capabilities with a search for a cause and associated medical disorders, education of the family about options for achieving good communication skills, and medical or surgical intervention, all within the first year of life.[4,5] This requires a multidisciplinary approach combining the skills of audiologists, speech pathologists, otolaryngologists, pediatricians, genetic counselors, and early intervention programs, while encouraging the family to be active participants in the health care team (ie, family-centered care). For those with progressive loss that becomes severe to profound in the prelingual period, a similar time frame for evaluation and treatment is ideal. Although postlingual children may not carry the same burden of expediency from a speech and language perspective, a prolonged period of auditory deprivation reduces the child's access to learning opportunities and potentially reduces the efficacy of intervention later on.

Medical Assessment

- History and physical examination should assess
  - The onset, degree, progression, and developmental impact of hearing loss, particularly as it relates to the duration of deafness
  - Risk factors for hearing loss, including perinatal illnesses, prematurity, hypoxia, jaundice, need for neonatal intensive care or intubation, meningitis, exposures to ototoxic drugs, head injury, and family history of hearing loss
  - Other health problems that may preclude or increase the risk of a general anesthetic or may assist in determining if a syndrome is present
  - Other developmental milestones, particularly evidence of cognitive deficits[4]
  - Physical signs of syndromic features, craniofacial anomalies, conductive hearing loss, or otitis media.[4,5]

Audiologic Assessment

To allow early determination of the presence and degree of hearing loss, electrophysiological measures are used when behavioral measures are inappropriate or inaccurate. This should take the form of newborn hearing screening soon after birth, followed by some combination of frequency-specific auditory brainstem response (ABR) testing, auditory steady-state response (ASSR) testing, otoacoustic emission (OAE), and tympanometry. Each test has unique characteristics and a combination of some or all of these are usually required to give the most comprehensive picture of the child's auditory capabilities, including the severity and site of hearing loss. For the population of children with severe to profound SNHL, this early assessment aids in forming an estimate of amplification requirements, mobilization of the care team for close observation of the child's progress, as well as early planning for possible future interventions, thus avoiding treatment delays.[5]

In almost all cases, electrophysiological testing is sufficient to estimate the hearing levels for the purpose of fitting conventional amplification. Importantly, however, such testing methods may have some unique challenges that are critical in managing children with SNHL. Although OAEs are generally absent in children with severe to profound hearing loss, they can be present in children with auditory neuropathy spectrum disorder (ANSD).[6] ANSD affects 10% to 14% of newly diagnosed children with severe to profound bilateral SNHL. These test results, taken in isolation, can inappropriately suggest less severe hearing loss. Similarly, the unique ABR waveforms seen in ANSD often require an experienced clinician to detect.[6-9] Typically, the cochlear microphonic (CM) waveform is present with absent or abnormal ABR waveforms. The CM waveform is distinguished from artifact by demonstration of inversion of the response with inversion of the signal polarity stimulus (**Fig. 1**).[6,10-13] Thus, identification of the CM waveform requires a protocol that includes both rarefaction and condensation stimuli. The CM waveform is further distinguished from artifact by a loss of response when disconnecting the sound tubing. The ANSD phenotype is not diagnosable on ASSR[4,10,14] so ABR is needed to make this diagnosis. Tympanometry can support bone conduction ABR testing and clinical examination in the identification of a conductive component to the hearing loss.

Behavioral testing using visual reinforcement audiometry can accurately confirm the severity of hearing loss in children around 6 to 8 months of age. Behavioral thresholds

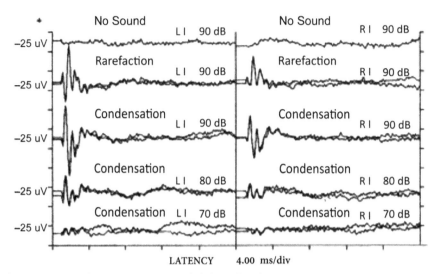

Fig. 1. ABR waveform in a patient with bilateral auditory neuropathy-dyssynchrony. Note presence of CM waveform with absence of the ABR waveform at stimulus levels as high as 90 dB HL. Note also reversal of the CM waveform with change in the signal polarity (condensation vs rarefaction).

are particularly important in children with ANSD because the ABR is unable to determine hearing thresholds for fitting amplification.[9,15] This kind of testing can be challenging in children with severe to profound SNHL due to their lack of familiarity with sound. Those with concurrent global developmental delay can also have less consistent conditioned behavioral responses.[16–18]

Imaging

Imaging is critical in children with significant hearing loss because it can aid in identifying a cause, possibly predict hearing loss progression, and potentially identify those with a poor prognosis for speech development using HAs or CIs.[4] Imaging can take the form of MRI with or without high-resolution computed tomography (HRCT) of the temporal bone structures and brain. Imaging allows anatomic assessment of the labyrinth, cochlea, cochleovestibular, and facial nerves. It also identifies concurrent brain disease. A diagnosis of cochlear nerve deficiency (CND) or significant cochlear or labyrinthine abnormalities may either preclude the use of a CI or predict a low chance of achieving open-set speech perception.[6,8,19–22]

CND is present in approximately 1% of children with bilateral SNHL, most often in the setting of severe to profound thresholds.[13,23,24] Labyrinthine abnormalities have been detected in up to 40% of children with SNHL[25] and can range in severity. Identification of both CND and inner ear malformations allows the treating team to provide realistic expectations to families about outcomes with the various interventions and to maximize communication by augmenting auditory-verbal communication with nonauditory forms. Detecting abnormalities of the facial nerve can help guide safe CI surgery, particularly in the setting of semicircular canal abnormalities (**Fig. 2**).[26]

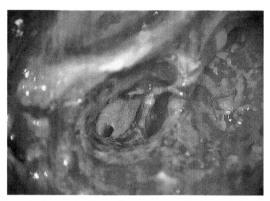

Fig. 2. Intraoperative photograph of a left transmastoid view of the facial nerve running inferior to the stapes superstructure in the setting of an absent lateral semicircular canal.

High-resolution MRI with a 3-dimensional Fourier transformation constructive interference steady-state protocol is the most sensitive for diagnosing CND[19,24] and has the unique ability to assess for concurrent brain disease,[19,27] which may be present in up to 40% of pediatric CI recipients.[28] HRCT is complementary for assessing labyrinthine anomalies (**Fig. 3**),[6,28,29] other temporal bone disease,[26] and the presence and pathway of the fallopian canal.[24] One shortcoming of HRCT as a single imaging modality is that it cannot identify CND in the setting of a normal caliber internal auditory canal.[6,7,11–13,29–31] Both MRI and HRCT are important in assessing cochlear patency in children suffering from hearing loss secondary to meningitis (**Fig. 4**).[32]

Other Common Testing

These tests may be useful in identifying the cause of the hearing loss and risk of transmission to future off spring, associated medical conditions that may require early treatment, and potential prognosis for progression of hearing loss and performance with CIs:

- Electrocardiogram (Jervell and Lange-Nielsen syndrome)
- Cytomegalovirus (CMV) testing of urine and Guthrie card
- Connexin 26 and 30 gene sequencing and other genetic testing
- Urinalysis (Alport syndrome in older children)
- Retinal examination and visual acuity testing[5] (Usher's syndrome)
- Renal ultrasound in children with branchial anomalies (branchio-oto-renal syndrome)
- Investigations for concurrent medical conditions as the history and examination indicate
- Comprehensive, molecular genetic testing.

MANAGEMENT GOALS

Overall, the aim of management in children with severe to profound SNHL is to either introduce adequate sound for the purposes of auditory-verbal speech and language development or teach the child and caregivers alternative communication strategies. Irrespective of approach, intervention should ideally be undertaken as soon as is medically feasible to optimize outcomes.

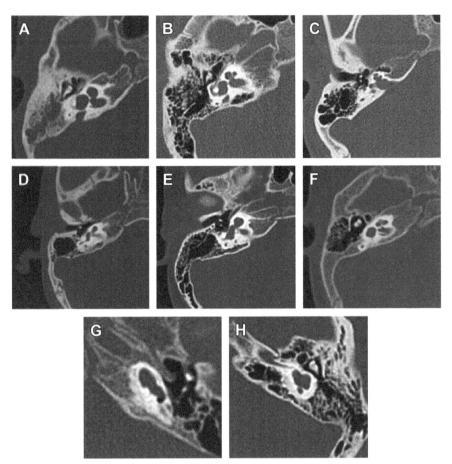

Fig. 3. Labyrinthine malformations (*A–C*) are varieties of cochlear incomplete partitions. (*A, B*) are variations on the spectrum of incomplete partition with enlarged vestibular aqueduct. (*C*) X-linked stapes gusher (deafness) morphology. (*D–F*) Varying degrees of cochlear hypoplasia with or without semicircular dysplasia. (*D*) Marked and (*E*) moderate hypoplasia. (*F*) Cochlear hypoplasia with a small vestibular remnant and absent semicircular canals characteristic of CHARGE association. (*G, H*) Common (cystic) cavity deformities of the cochlea and vestibular vestige.

Communication Options and Intervention

Communication options for children with severe, severe to profound, and profound hearing loss include verbal and nonverbal strategies (ie, sign language). Although nonauditory approaches to verbal communication through lipreading were commonplace in the past, auditory approaches have become more common in recent times, owing to better outcomes. Auditory supplementation through amplification when possible or cochlear implantation allows for improved sound awareness, enhanced lipreading, speech understanding, and vocal control. These are the underpinnings for optimal auditory-oral communication development.

As a matter of ethical and moral obligation to these children, appropriate resources should be made available for learning about verbal and nonverbal communication strategies. Auditory-oral communication supplemented through amplification and/or

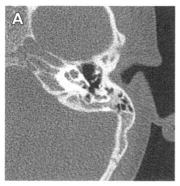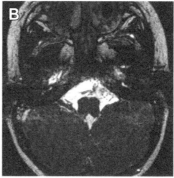

Fig. 4. Hyperdensity on HRCT (A) and loss of hyperintensity on constructive interference in steady state (CISS) MRI sequence (B) in the left basal turn of the cochlea consistent with postmeningitic obstruction and ossification.

cochlear implantation results in the highest levels of educational achievement and employment opportunities for hard-of-hearing and deaf children. Importantly, informed parental choice remains the single most important determinant in such decisions because self-determination is not possible at such an early age. To advocate for a delayed choice at this early age is, by default, a decision for nonverbal communication because delayed intervention, beyond the critical period for speech and language development in the brain, rarely results in age-appropriate auditory-verbal skills. Because 95% of hard-of-hearing and deaf children are born to 2 hearing parents, auditory-oral communication is the dominant choice because this represents a more familiar strategy for these families.

For families that choose to pursue auditory-oral communication for their child, a referral to an appropriate early intervention specialist, and fitting of HAs by a pediatric audiologist should be carried out as early as possible to maximize each child's access to sound. The Joint Committee on Infant Hearing recommends that HA fitting occur before 3 months of age and that an early intervention program is in place by 6 months of age.[5] It is critical that each child be closely observed for speech and language progress by a variety of well-trained professionals (audiologists, speech-language pathologists, pediatricians, and otolaryngologists). By necessity, this patient population requires high-gain amplification with resulting issues of feedback, distortion, cerumen impaction, and occasionally otitis externa. Additionally, otitis media can be problematic in this age group and can add conductive hearing loss to the underling SNHL. Close collaboration between the treating audiologist and otolaryngologist is needed to minimize the impact of these medical issues. If a given child is making adequate progress with HAs alone, then continued close observation is appropriate.[4] In most instances, children with severe to profound SNHL do not make age-appropriate gains[33] despite correctly fitted amplification. In such cases, cochlear implantation should be considered to achieve auditory-verbal language.

COORDINATION OF CARE

Following a failure result on the newborn infant screening examination, there are several medical or surgical and audiologic issues that need careful attention in the early months to mitigate later delays in therapy. These include the need for: (1) diagnostic ABR to identify thresholds for amplification fitting or the ANSD phenotype,

(2) temporal bone and brain imaging to identify anatomic factors that impact on decision-making, and (3) clearance of middle ear fluid (otitis media with effusion) to optimize HA fitting and prepare the ear for later cochlear implantation, if needed. The authors prefer to offer a single coordinated anesthetic for the necessary combination of these procedures. Importantly, this coordination reduces the need for multiple anesthetics and provides much needed information that can mitigate treatment delays resulting from transitions of care. This does require a portable sedation or anesthetic team, cooperative surgeons, audiologists and radiologists, and an environment that is conducive to the minor surgical procedure, imaging, and ABR.

It is important to remedy any conductive component to the hearing loss resulting from otitis media early in the management continuum. Prolonged watchful waiting is inappropriate in children with underlying SNHL. This is accomplished through tympanostomy tube placement. The tubes are placed before ABR testing to remove the middle ear fluid. Great care is taken to avoid bleeding because this can have a negative effect on testing and tube patency in the future. Concurrently with diagnostic ABR testing, ear mold impressions are made for amplification fitting before transporting the patient to the radiology suite.

COCHLEAR IMPLANTATION
Treatment Goals

For most children with severe to profound SNHL pursuing auditory-verbal communication, a CI is the mainstay of treatment. The aim is to restore adequate hearing to allow speech and language development. There is now extensive evidence to show that implantation around 12 months of age offers the greatest chance of significant open-set speech understanding with resulting language acquisition rates that match those of normal hearing peers. Timing of the intervention remains critical, with worse outcomes achieved for those receiving an implant beyond 2 years.[34–36] There is also emerging evidence for the benefit of simultaneous or close bilateral sequential implantation. Bilateral implantation offers the potential for improved sound localization and hearing in noise abilities as well as demonstrating a trend for improved speech and language acquisition.[21,37–42] Presumably, incidental learning is enhanced among those with bilateral CIs. For those with bilateral severe to profound SNHL, it also offers a built-in backup system to avoid complete loss of sound if one device fails or is lost or broken.[4]

Though a thorough discussion about all surgical considerations needed for cochlear implantation is beyond the scope of this article, it is the mainstay of treatment of severe to profound SNHL in children; therefore, the key points are discussed.

Preoperative Planning and Preparation

Preoperative planning requires both the medical work up discussed previously and extensive education of the family to help them understand the process and to have realistic expectations of the time and energy investment required to maximize outcome. Parental involvement is most critical to good outcomes[33,34,41] and this can be maximized through early and ongoing education and empowerment of parents. Preoperative testing, family counseling, and patient preference guide the selection of the device most appropriate for each child.

Preoperative vaccination should be encouraged, when medically safe, due to the increased risk of meningitis in those with hearing loss[43] and particularly those undergoing cochlear implantation.[44,45] The United States Food and Drug Administration (FDA) and the Centers for Disease Control recommend universal vaccination for common pathogens that cause bacterial meningitis, particularly streptococcus pneumoniae and hemophilus influenza type B. The FDA's current advice on vaccination schedule can be found at: http://www.fda.gov/MedicalDevices/Safety/AlertsandNotices/PublicHealthNotifications/ucm062057.htm.

Patient Positioning

The patient undergoes general anesthetic and is then positioned in a supine position with the head turned to the contralateral side. Flexion or extension of the neck may be needed to bring the mastoid cortex and descending facial nerve axis parallel to the floor. Facial nerve monitoring is placed and the integrity of the system checked before proceeding. Prophylactic antibiotics are given at the start of the case, often accompanied by a dose of intravenous steroids.

Procedural Approach

A short curvilinear incision is made through the postauricular skin and subcutaneous tissues down to the level of the temporalis fascia and mastoid periosteum. A C-shaped incision is then made through the periosteum. The resulting anteriorly based, subperiosteal flap is then raised and held forward with a self-retaining retractor. A cortical mastoidectomy is performed and posterior tympanotomy is then made through the facial recess. Wide access is critical to unimpeded round window (RW) dissection and electrode insertion. This is especially critical in cases of inner ear malformation or facial nerve anomaly. The round window niche overhang is routinely drilled off to visualize the round window membrane. A posterosuperior subperiosteal pocket is then created. A seat is fashioned only if the implant body requires recession. Following receiver-stimulator placement, a single suture cinches the periosteum and immobilizes the device. An inferior cochleostomy, round window–related cochleostomy, or round window incision is made, as appropriate to the device being used, and the electrode is slowly advanced into the cochlea.[46] The cochleostomy is packed with small pieces of temporalis fascia and the ground electrode is directed under the periosteum in the region of the zygomatic root. For children with severe to profound hearing loss, with minimal residual hearing, the excess electrode cable is looped under the incus bridge away from the mastoid cortex. The wound is then closed in layers with absorbable sutures, butterfly closures, and a mastoid dressing. Remote intraoperative telemetry confirms an active device, minimizes the risks of multiple electrode shorts or open circuits, and identifies neural response thresholds for use in later programming. A transorbital skull radiograph also confirms expected coiling of the array and the absence of an unexpected tip rollover.

Potential Complications and Management

Complications in cochlear implantation are generally rare. Parents are warned about bleeding, infection, loss of residual hearing, facial nerve injury, dysgeusia, tinnitus, vertigo, meningitis, and device failure.[4] Intraoperative perilymph gushers are more common in those with labyrinthine abnormalities and are managed by forming a large cochleostomy, followed by tight packing with temporalis fascia. An effective seal is confirmed intraoperatively with Valsalva maneuver. Lumbar drainage is unnecessary in these cases. When managed appropriately, studies show the presence of a gusher does not affect outcome with the device.[47]

Postprocedural Care

Children are generally observed in the hospital for a short time after the procedure, then discharged home on the same day in most instances. Children who receive bilateral, simultaneous implants, who are very young, or have other comorbidities, generally stay overnight for observation. The authors advise parents to take the mastoid dressing down around 4 days postoperatively and keep the postauricular wound completely dry until the first postoperative visit at 1 week.

Rehabilitation and Recovery

It is essential that a strong audiologic and speech rehabilitation program using an auditory-verbal focus accompany cochlear implantation. Parental involvement and engagement with this program is critical and can be encouraged with early education and regular empowerment about to the impact of their involvement. The rehabilitation process is an intense period of work with CI audiologists and speech therapists to maximize the output of the implant for each child and help connect the central neural pathways with both the presence and meaning of sound. It requires a deep commitment from families, with regular visits to achieve a stable and appropriate implant map as well as education sessions for the child and family, both with teachers and at home.

Outcomes

Fig. 5 and **Table 1** demonstrate the speech outcomes of 478 pediatric patients, with a wide range of causes necessitating implantation. One outcome measure uses a graduated assessment tool called the modified Speech Reception Index in Quiet (see **Table 1**), which ranks speech perception test measures based on how challenging the test is to perform. It demonstrates that almost all children with implants get some sound awareness and almost all get some form of open-set speech with 12 to 24 months of the implant experience (see **Fig. 5**). Previous studies have shown that the rate of acquisition and the maximum achieved level of both receptive and expressive language is affected by the age at implantation[34–36]; the presence and type of cochlear malformations[21,22,25]; the degree of parental involvement[41]; a diagnosis of perinatal CMV[48–50]; postmeningitis as the cause of hearing loss,[51] particularly when ossification is present[32]; and the presence of other medical comorbidities or developmental delays.[51–53] About one-third of those with significant development delays can develop oral language but this is often at a slower acquisition rate than children without these issues.[17,18,53] Motor delays have less impact than other forms of developmental delay.[16] Autism poses specific issues with both developmental delays and behavioral issues that can form barriers to engaging with education and testing.[53] Those with ANSD are a heterogeneous group with a wide range of outcomes, likely reflecting the wide range of causes that present with this phenotype.[6–9,54,55] ANSD is not a contraindication to CI.

In comparison with those with congenital hearing loss who are implanted in a timely fashion, those with progressive hearing loss generally demonstrate good speech and language outcomes, particularly if hearing loss occurs in the setting of a strong language foundation (provided the duration of profound hearing loss is not prolonged). Evolving understanding of the genetic basis of hearing loss raises the possibility of using genetic testing to add to the predictive arsenal.[56–64] Intraoperative electrocochleography as a measure of cochlear health is also emerging as a way to both predict speech perception scores and explain previously unexplained outcome variability in pediatric CI recipients.[65]

In light of so many variables that can affect outcome, it is helpful for the clinical team to give each family realistic individualized expectations of their child's potential.

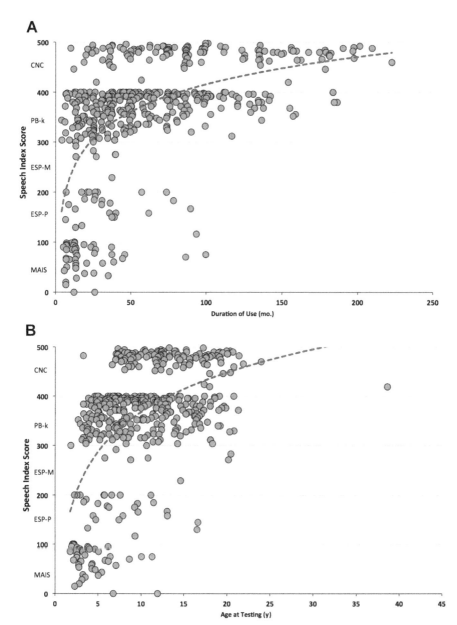

Fig. 5. Best speech recognition score for all patients able to participate in behavioral testing, plotted against duration of CI use in months (A) and age in years (B) on the day of testing. CNC, consonant-nucleus-consonant; ESP-M, early speech perception test–monosyllable; ESP-P, early speech perception test–pattern; MAIS, meaningful auditory integration scale; PB-k, phonetically balanced kindergarten word list.

Table 1
Speech reception index in quiet

Test	Score Range	Type
Meaningful Auditory Integration Scale (MAIS)	0–100	Parental questionnaire
Early Speech Perception Test–Pattern Perception (ESP-P)	100–200	Closed set
Early Speech Perception Test–Monosyllabic Words (ESP-M)	200–300	
Phonetically Balanced Kindergarten Word List (PB-k words)	300–400	Open set
Consonant Nucleus Consonant (CNC) Word List	400–500	

This analysis consists of using the best percentage score achieved for the most difficult test each patient participated in and then hierarchically ranking and stacking these scores in 100-point increments in the following order of difficulty: MAIS, ESP-P, ESP-M, PB-k words, and the CNC word list scores; with a maximum score of 500. These scores can then be plotted against age at testing or duration of use after implantation.

Evaluation of Outcome, Adjustment of Treatment, and Long-Term Recommendations

Once a stable map is achieved and a child is well on his or her way to language acquisition, regular audiometric and speech and language evaluations are required to ensure optimal outcomes. Possible causes of underperformance or regression may be related to missed diagnoses, such as electrode-neural interface problems (CND, inner ear malformation, electrode malposition or extrusion); patient factors, such as poor compliance with wearing the device or educational activities; audiologic issues, such as incorrectly assigned mapping; or device issues, such as individual electrode or complete device failure.

Troubleshooting of such issues requires a complete work up. Based on the clinical scenario, this may include review of preoperative imaging to look for possible missed diagnoses and repeat imaging (HRCT) to ascertain the current device position within the cochlea, audiology assessment for the integrity of the device, adequacy of the map, and the number of hours registered wearing the device per day. If all other reversible factors have been excluded, so-called soft-failures or suspected device malfunction is considered.

AUDITORY BRAINSTEM IMPLANTS

When labyrinthine or cochlear nerve anatomy precludes successful cochlear implantation or results in very poor performance, an emerging alternative is auditory brainstem implantation. Though this is considered an option for only a small proportion of the overall group of children with severe to profound SNHL, it offers sound detection for individuals who did not previously have that possibility. The language acquisition of this group seems to follow a more gradual trajectory but most demonstrate some benefit with the device.[66]

SUMMARY

Children with severe to profound SNHL benefit from a multidisciplinary approach to management and most will gain the best chance for achieving auditory-verbal communication through cochlear implantation and strong audiology and speech rehabilitation. It is critical to the child's success that parents are engaged in the entire process through strong and continuing education.

REFERENCES

1. Smith RJ, Bale JF Jr, White KR. Sensorineural hearing loss in children. Lancet 2005;365(9462):879–90.
2. Fortnum HM, Summerfield AQ, Marshall DH, et al. Prevalence of permanent childhood hearing impairment in the United Kingdom and implications for universal neonatal hearing screening: questionnaire based ascertainment study. BMJ 2001;323(7312):536–40.
3. Available at: http://www.cdc.gov/ncbddd/hearingloss/data.html. Accessed April 1, 2015.
4. Buchman CA, Adunka OF, Jewells V, et al. Hearing loss in children: the otologist's perspective. In: Seewald RC, Bamford JM, editors. A Sound Foundation Through Early Amplification 2007. Proceedings from the 4th international conference. Switzerland: Phonak AG; 2008. p. 63–78.
5. American Academy of Pediatrics, Joint Committee on Infant Hearing. Year 2007 position statement: principles and guidelines for early hearing detection and intervention programs. Pediatrics 2007;120(4):898–921.
6. Buchman CA, Roush PA, Teagle HF, et al. Auditory neuropathy characteristics in children with cochlear nerve deficiency. Ear Hear 2006;27(4):399–408.
7. Walton J, Gibson WP, Sanli H, et al. Predicting cochlear implant outcomes in children with auditory neuropathy. Otol Neurotol 2008;29(3):302–9.
8. Valero J, Blaser S, Papsin BC, et al. Electrophysiologic and behavioral outcomes of cochlear implantation in children with auditory nerve hypoplasia. Ear Hear 2012;33(1):3–18.
9. Teagle HF, Roush PA, Woodard JS, et al. Cochlear implantation in children with auditory neuropathy spectrum disorder. Ear Hear 2010;31(3):325–35.
10. Kang WS, Lee JH, Lee HN, et al. Cochlear implantations in young children with cochlear nerve deficiency diagnosed by MRI. Otolaryngol Head Neck Surg 2010;143(1):101–8.
11. Carner M, Colletti L, Shannon R, et al. Imaging in 28 children with cochlear nerve aplasia. Acta Otolaryngol 2009;129(4):458–61.
12. Adunka OF, Jewells V, Buchman CA. Value of computed tomography in the evaluation of children with cochlear nerve deficiency. Otol Neurotol 2007;28(5):597–604.
13. Adunka OF, Roush PA, Teagle HF, et al. Internal auditory canal morphology in children with cochlear nerve deficiency. Otol Neurotol 2006;27(6):793–801.
14. Warren FM 3rd, Wiggins RH 3rd, Pitt C, et al. Apparent cochlear nerve aplasia: to implant or not to implant? Otol Neurotol 2010;31(7):1088–94.
15. Roland P, Henion K, Booth T, et al. Assessment of cochlear implant candidacy in patients with cochlear nerve deficiency using the P1 CAEP biomarker. Cochlear Implants Int 2012;13(1):16–25.
16. Amirsalari S, Yousefi J, Radfar S, et al. Cochlear implant outcomes in children with motor developmental delay. Int J Pediatr Otorhinolaryngol 2012;76(1):100–3.
17. Lee YM, Kim LS, Jeong SW, et al. Performance of children with mental retardation after cochlear implantation: speech perception, speech intelligibility, and language development. Acta Otolaryngol 2010;130(8):924–34.
18. Youm HY, Moon IJ, Kim EY, et al. The auditory and speech performance of children with intellectual disability after cochlear implantation. Acta Otolaryngol 2013; 133(1):59–69.
19. Pakdaman MN, Herrmann BS, Curtin HD, et al. Cochlear implantation in children with anomalous cochleovestibular anatomy: a systematic review. Otolaryngol Head Neck Surg 2012;146(2):180–90.

20. Buchman CA, Copeland BJ, Yu KK, et al. Cochlear implantation in children with congenital inner ear malformations. Laryngoscope 2004;114(2):309–16.

21. Chadha NK, James AL, Gordon KA, et al. Bilateral cochlear implantation in children with anomalous cochleovestibular anatomy. Arch Otolaryngol Head Neck Surg 2009;135(9):903–9.

22. Loundon N, Rouillon I, Munier N, et al. Cochlear implantation in children with internal ear malformations. Otol Neurotol 2005;26(4):668–73.

23. Wu CM, Ng SH, Wang JJ, et al. Diffusion tensor imaging of the subcortical auditory tract in subjects with congenital cochlear nerve deficiency. AJNR Am J Neuroradiol 2009;30(9):1773–7.

24. Parry DA, Booth T, Roland PS. Advantages of magnetic resonance imaging over computed tomography in preoperative evaluation of pediatric cochlear implant candidates. Otol Neurotol 2005;26(5):976–82.

25. Buchman CA, Teagle HF, Roush PA, et al. Cochlear implantation in children with labyrinthine anomalies and cochlear nerve deficiency: implications for auditory brainstem implantation. Laryngoscope 2011;121(9):1979–88.

26. Roche JP, Huang BY, Castillo M, et al. Imaging characteristics of children with auditory neuropathy spectrum disorder. Otol Neurotol 2010;31(5):780–8.

27. Moon IJ, Kim EY, Park GY, et al. The clinical significance of preoperative brain magnetic resonance imaging in pediatric cochlear implant recipients. Audiol Neurootol 2012;17(6):373–80.

28. Trimble K, Blaser S, James AL, et al. Computed tomography and/or magnetic resonance imaging before pediatric cochlear implantation? Developing an investigative strategy. Otol Neurotol 2007;28(3):317–24.

29. Pagarkar W, Gunny R, Saunders DE, et al. The bony cochlear nerve canal in children with absent or hypoplastic cochlear nerves. Int J Pediatr Otorhinolaryngol 2011;75(6):764–73.

30. Miyanohara I, Miyashita K, Takumi K, et al. A case of cochlear nerve deficiency without profound sensorineural hearing loss. Otol Neurotol 2011; 32(4):529–32.

31. Giesemann AM, Kontorinis G, Jan Z, et al. The vestibulocochlear nerve: aplasia and hypoplasia in combination with inner ear malformations. Eur Radiol 2012; 22(3):519–24.

32. Nichani J, Green K, Hans P, et al. Cochlear implantation after bacterial meningitis in children: outcomes in ossified and nonossified cochleas. Otol Neurotol 2011; 32(5):784–9.

33. Novaes BC, Versolatto-Cavanaugh MC, Figueiredo Rde S, et al. Determinants of communication skills development in children with hearing impairment. J Soc Bras Fonoaudiol 2012;24(4):335–41.

34. Ching TY, Dillon H, Day J, et al. Early language outcomes of children with cochlear implants: interim findings of the NAL study on longitudinal outcomes of children with hearing impairment. Cochlear Implants Int 2009;10(Suppl 1): 28–32.

35. Dettman SJ, Pinder D, Briggs RJ, et al. Communication development in children who receive the cochlear implant younger than 12 months: risks versus benefits. Ear Hear 2007;28(2 Suppl):11S–8S.

36. Yoshinaga-Itano C, Sedey AL, Coulter DK, et al. Language of early- and later-identified children with hearing loss. Pediatrics 1998;102(5):1161–71.

37. Chadha NK, Papsin BC, Jiwani S, et al. Speech detection in noise and spatial unmasking in children with simultaneous versus sequential bilateral cochlear implants. Otol Neurotol 2011;32(7):1057–64.

38. Scherf F, Van Deun L, van Wieringen A, et al. Three-year postimplantation auditory outcomes in children with sequential bilateral cochlear implantation. Ann Otol Rhinol Laryngol 2009;118(5):336–44.

39. Scherf F, Van Deun L, van Wieringen A, et al. Subjective benefits of sequential bilateral cochlear implantation in young children after 18 months of implant use. ORL J Otorhinolaryngol Relat Spec 2009;71(2):112–21.

40. Scherf FW, van Deun L, van Wieringen A, et al. Functional outcome of sequential bilateral cochlear implantation in young children: 36 months postoperative results. Int J Pediatr Otorhinolaryngol 2009;73(5):723–30.

41. Sarant J, Harris D, Bennet L, et al. Bilateral versus unilateral cochlear implants in children: a study of spoken language outcomes. Ear Hear 2014;35(4): 396–409.

42. Kim LS, Jeong SW, Lee YM, et al. Cochlear implantation in children. Auris Nasus Larynx 2010;37(1):6–17.

43. Parner ET, Reefhuis J, Schendel D, et al. Hearing loss diagnosis followed by meningitis in Danish children, 1995–2004. Otolaryngol Head Neck Surg 2007;136(3): 428–33.

44. Reefhuis J, Honein MA, Whitney CG, et al. Risk of bacterial meningitis in children with cochlear implants. N Engl J Med 2003;349(5):435–45.

45. Biernath KR, Reefhuis J, Whitney CG, et al. Bacterial meningitis among children with cochlear implants beyond 24 months after implantation. Pediatrics 2006; 117(2):284–9.

46. Basura GJ, Adunka OF, Buchman CA. Scala tympani cochleostomy for cochlear implantation. In: McKinnon BJ, editor. Operative Techniques in Otolaryngology. Atlanta (GA): Elsevier; 2010. p. 218–22.

47. Adunka OF, Teagle HF, Zdanski CJ, et al. Influence of an intraoperative perilymph gusher on cochlear implant performance in children with labyrinthine malformations. Otol Neurotol 2012;33(9):1489–96.

48. Yamazaki H, Yamamoto R, Moroto S, et al. Cochlear implantation in children with congenital cytomegalovirus infection accompanied by psycho-neurological disorders. Acta Otolaryngol 2012;132(4):420–7.

49. Lee DJ, Lustig L, Sampson M, et al. Effects of cytomegalovirus (CMV) related deafness on pediatric cochlear implant outcomes. Otolaryngol Head Neck Surg 2005;133(6):900–5.

50. Matsui T, Ogawa H, Yamada N, et al. Outcome of cochlear implantation in children with congenital cytomegalovirus infection or GJB2 mutation. Acta Otolaryngol 2012;132(6):597–602.

51. Janeschik S, Teschendorf M, Bagus H, et al. Influence of etiologic factors on speech perception of cochlear-implanted children. Cochlear Implants Int 2013; 14(4):190–9.

52. Oghalai JS, Caudle SE, Bentley B, et al. Cognitive outcomes and familial stress after cochlear implantation in deaf children with and without developmental delays. Otol Neurotol 2012;33(6):947–56.

53. Cruz I, Vicaria I, Wang NY, et al. Language and behavioral outcomes in children with developmental disabilities using cochlear implants. Otol Neurotol 2012; 33(5):751–60.

54. Peterson A, Shallop J, Driscoll C, et al. Outcomes of cochlear implantation in children with auditory neuropathy. J Am Acad Audiol 2003;14(4):188–201.

55. Breneman AI, Gifford RH, Dejong MD. Cochlear implantation in children with auditory neuropathy spectrum disorder: long-term outcomes. J Am Acad Audiol 2012;23(1):5–17.

56. Yan YJ, Li Y, Yang T, et al. The effect of GJB2 and SLC26A4 gene mutations on rehabilitative outcomes in pediatric cochlear implant patients. Eur Arch Otorhinolaryngol 2013;270(11):2865–70.

57. Wu CC, Lee YC, Chen PJ, et al. Predominance of genetic diagnosis and imaging results as predictors in determining the speech perception performance outcome after cochlear implantation in children. Arch Pediatr Adolesc Med 2008;162(3): 269–76.

58. Vivero RJ, Fan K, Angeli S, et al. Cochlear implantation in common forms of genetic deafness. Int J Pediatr Otorhinolaryngol 2010;74(10):1107–12.

59. Kawasaki A, Fukushima K, Kataoka Y, et al. Using assessment of higher brain functions of children with GJB2-associated deafness and cochlear implants as a procedure to evaluate language development. Int J Pediatr Otorhinolaryngol 2006;70(8):1343–9.

60. Jatana KR, Thomas D, Weber L, et al. Usher syndrome: characteristics and outcomes of pediatric cochlear implant recipients. Otol Neurotol 2013;34(3):484–9.

61. Cullen RD, Zdanski C, Roush P, et al. Cochlear implants in Waardenburg syndrome. Laryngoscope 2006;116(7):1273–5.

62. Cullen RD, Buchman CA, Brown CJ, et al. Cochlear implantation for children with GJB2-related deafness. Laryngoscope 2004;114(8):1415–9.

63. Connell SS, Angeli SI, Suarez H, et al. Performance after cochlear implantation in DFNB1 patients. Otolaryngol Head Neck Surg 2007;137(4):596–602.

64. Bauer PW, Geers AE, Brenner C, et al. The effect of GJB2 allele variants on performance after cochlear implantation. Laryngoscope 2003;113(12):2135–40.

65. Formeister EJ, McClellan JH, Merwin WH 3rd, et al. Intraoperative round window electrocochleography and speech perception outcomes in pediatric cochlear implant recipients. Ear Hear 2015;36(2):249–60.

66. Colletti L, Zoccante L. Nonverbal cognitive abilities and auditory performance in children fitted with auditory brainstem implants: preliminary report. Laryngoscope 2008;118(8):1443–8.

Management of Children with Unilateral Hearing Loss

Judith E.C. Lieu, MD, MSPH

KEYWORDS

- Unilateral hearing loss • Speech-language development • Children • Amplification
- Quality of life

KEY POINTS

- Lack of binaural input results in difficulties with sound localization and understanding speech in noisy backgrounds.
- Children with unilateral hearing loss (UHL) are at risk for speech-language delay, poor academic performance, and decreased quality of life compared with children with normal hearing.
- As yet, no study has shown any specific intervention that can definitely mitigate the negative effects of UHL.
- Because evidence-based guidelines are lacking, individual patient and family needs and preferences must be considered to recommend interventions for children with UHL.
- Interventions may include preferential seating in class, individualized education program (IEP) or 504(c) plan, frequency-modulated (FM) systems, amplification devices (hearing aids or contralateral routing of signal [CROS] devices), osseointegrated bone conduction hearing devices, or cochlear implantation, tailored to fit the needs of the child and to set the child up for success in academic and social settings.

INTRODUCTION AND BACKGROUND
Epidemiology

The prevalence of UHL is estimated at 1 per 1000 children at birth,[1] increasing with age due to delayed-onset congenital hearing loss and acquired hearing loss. Because the prevalence of UHL can vary significantly according to the definition applied, it is useful to consider that at least one-third of all children born with hearing loss have UHL; epidemiologically, an estimated 3% to 6% of school-aged children in the United States have UHL.[2] By adolescence, the prevalence of UHL is as high as 14.0% if

Disclosures: The author has no financial or intellectual conflicts of interest to disclose.
Department of Otolaryngology – Head and Neck Surgery, Washington University School of Medicine, 660 South Euclid Avenue, Campus Box 8115, St Louis, MO 63110, USA
E-mail address: lieuj@ent.wustl.edu

Otolaryngol Clin N Am 48 (2015) 1011–1026
http://dx.doi.org/10.1016/j.otc.2015.07.006
0030-6665/15/$ – see front matter © 2015 Elsevier Inc. All rights reserved.

oto.theclinics.com

Abbreviations

BHL   Bilateral hearing loss
CI   Cochlear implantation
CT   Computed tomography
FM   Frequency modulated
IEP   Individualized educational program
QOL   Quality of life
UHL   Unilateral hearing loss

---

thresholds greater than 15 dB are considered and 2.7% if only thresholds 25 dB or higher are considered.[3] Furthermore, approximately 10% of children born with UHL eventually develop bilateral hearing loss (BHL).[4,5]

Etiology and Evaluation

The incidence of temporal bone anomalies in congenital UHL is high compared with congenital BHL. Enlarged vestibular aqueduct (EVA) and cochlear nerve aplasia or hypoplasia are increasingly identified using high-resolution computed tomography (CT) and MRI. Among children with severe to profound UHL, the prevalence of cochlear nerve aplasia or hypoplasia approaches 50%.[6,7] Other temporal bone abnormalities commonly reported include enlarged vestibular aqueduct, Mondini deformity, cochlear and vestibular malformations, and common cavity malformation, although the likelihood of identifying an abnormality may depend on the severity of UHL, with more severe losses associated with a greater percentage of anatomic abnormalities.[5,8,9] Although genetic causes are predominant for BHL, this is not true for UHL. Investigators have identified variants of genes associated with BHL, including Pendred syndrome (SLC26A4) associated with EVA, but have not found them to be major determinants of UHL.[8,10,11] Although families with sensorineural UHL have been reported, the genetic mutations associated with them have not been identified.[12–14] Other syndromic causes of childhood hearing loss may initially present, or simply be associated with, a unilateral loss, for example, branchio-otorenal syndrome and Waardenburg syndrome.

Other important causes of sensorineural UHL include congenital cytomegalovirus (CMV) infections, meningitis, and trauma. Although children with symptomatic congenital CMV infection are more likely to have BHL, children with asymptomatic CMV infection are more likely to have UHL.[15] Congenital mumps and measles are infrequent in the developed world because of childhood immunization schedules but should be considered for families who choose not to immunize their children or for children adopted without clear immunization history. Temporal bone trauma, as a result of motor vehicle accidents, falls, or other head trauma, is a common cause of acquired postlingual UHL.

Important causes of conductive UHL include unilateral aural atresia, cholesteatoma, chronic otitis media, otosclerosis, ossicular discontinuity, and congenital ossicular malformations. Otitis media, labyrinthitis, and cholesteatoma are possible causes for UHL, usually mild to moderate in severity, diagnosed on physical examination. Hearing loss associated with these entities must be evaluated by audiogram. Congenital ossicular malformations can be identified on high-resolution temporal bone CT scans, and otosclerosis or ossicular discontinuity can be verified at the time of a middle ear exploration or planned stapedectomy or ossicular reconstruction.

As noted in the diagnostic algorithm suggested by Preciado and colleagues,[16] temporal bone imaging is the most likely test that reveals a cause in children with UHL.

Whether CT or MRI scan is the best modality is still under debate. Pragmatically, deciding which scan to order may depend on the age of the child, family history, type and severity of hearing loss, and other presenting symptoms. A child who could stay still in the scanner for 15 minutes but not 45 minutes might be better having a CT scan and forgo the sedation needed for a longer MRI sequence, but an infant/toddler may have an MRI with sedation out of concern for radiation exposure to the head. If another member of the family is known to have enlarged vestibular aqueduct, the sibling with hearing loss should also undergo an imaging study (CT or MRI, although CT seems to show this anomaly a bit more readily).[17] A CT scan may also be more helpful in a child with conductive or mixed UHL, but an MRI would rule out a brainstem lesion in a child with UHL and ataxia.

Advantages of Binaural Hearing

The audiologic disability resulting from lack of binaural hearing can be summarized as difficulty picking out a desired signal in the midst of background noise and trouble with identifying the source of a signal in 2- or 3-dimensional space. The combination of binaural summation, binaural release of masking, and the head shadow effect phenomena contribute to the ease of listening and comprehension enjoyed by those with bilateral normal hearing. These concepts, along with sound localization, are described in more detail in the following section.

Bilateral summation refers to a listener's greater sensitivity to sound when 2 ears hear simultaneously rather than just 1 ear, stemming from central auditory processing.[18] Experimental data show that this summation is 2 to 3 dB at threshold, when sounds are just detectable[19] and increases up to 10 dB at 90 dB sensation level.[20] Because speech discrimination scores improve at a rate of 6% per dB, 2 to 3 dB can result in improved speech discrimination score of 12% to 18%. However, binaural summation may not occur when the hearing levels of the 2 ears differ by as little as 6 dB.[19] But it is clear that many derive benefit from bilateral hearing aids or bilateral cochlear implants, and binaural summation may be part of this added improvement in hearing.

Binaural release of masking or squelch allows for understanding spoken language in the midst of background noise or conversation. For a pure-tone signal at 500 Hz, the advantage of 2 ears over 1 ear is 12 to 15 dB; for speech signals, the advantage is typically 3 to 8 dB.[20] Improvement in signal to noise ratios (SNRs) of 3 dB improves word recognition scores about 18%.[20] Empiric studies have documented that binaural hearing benefits speech intelligibility particularly when there are multiple spoken interferences at different locations from the listener.[21]

The head shadow effect results from sound being attenuated by the head sitting between the 2 ears. Empirically, there is a 6.4-dB reduction of speech intensity from one side of the head to the other.[22] For pure tones, the head shadow effect is greatest in high frequencies, 20 dB for 5000 to 6000 Hz. For those with UHL, the head shadow effect results in a bad ear side and good ear side depending on whether the sound signal originates from the side with the UHL (bad ear side) or normal hearing (good ear side). Children with UHL often describe awkward social moments when they are completely unaware of others speaking to them from the bad ear side; unless they develop compensatory behaviors to cope, they may be accused of not paying attention or ignoring others.

Sound localization in the horizontal plane depends on interaural time and level (or intensity) differences and is much more easily accomplished by 2 ears than 1 ear. Low-frequency sounds are localized with interaural time differences, whereas high-frequency sounds are localized with interaural level differences. In general, children with UHL have difficulty identifying a sound source and make more errors on tests of sound localization, but there is a great deal of variability.[23,24] Some are able to learn how to use vertical interaural level differences using the spectral cues that result from the shape of the pinna or residual high-frequency hearing to retain the ability to localize sound.[25–27]

Children with hearing loss in general are known to experience increased fatigue from the extra cognitive effort expended to detect, decode, process, and comprehend speech.[28,29] They also experience more difficulty with learning new words and multitasking, which can result in possible negative results in school settings.[30] In addition, infants and young children require a greater signal to noise ratio than adults to comprehend speech sounds in the presence of masking noise.[31] Thus, young children with UHL may experience more difficulty with speech in noise than adults with UHL and certainly more difficulty than their normal-hearing peers.

CONSEQUENCES OF UNILATERAL HEARING LOSS
Educational Impact

In their landmark study, Bess and Tharpe[32] reported that children with UHL had a 10-fold rate of repeating grades (35%) compared with a 3% rate for typical school children, usually in kindergarten and first grade. Their findings were corroborated by other investigators who found 22% to 24% rates of failing at least 1 grade compared with district-wide averages of 2% to 3%.[23,33] In addition, 12% to 41% of children with UHL were noted to receive additional educational assistance, and a high rate had educational or behavioral problems (20%–59%).[23,32–34] Using the Screening Instrument for Targeting Educational Risks, a teacher-based questionnaire to screen for educational difficulties, investigators documented that children with UHL had more academic problems than the normal-hearing controls and even children with moderate to severe BHL.[35,36] One possible explanation for these findings is that because the children did not receive any acknowledgment that UHL might handicap their learning, they did not receive extra services that helped the children with moderate to severe BHL.[36] Subsequently, children with aural atresia and conductive hearing loss unilaterally have also been found to require more speech therapy and educational resources in school.[37,38] These findings are alarms challenging the status quo assumptions that hearing with 1 ear is sufficient for normal development of speech and language and thus educational attainment.

Speech and Language Consequences

Additional studies have documented delays in speech and language in children with UHL since the reports from the 1980s and 1990s. There are limited data regarding the effects of UHL on speech-language development in preschool children but more in elementary school children. Kiese-Himmel[39] reported that among the 31 children with UHL in her study, the average age of first word spoken was not delayed (mean 12.7 months, range 10–33 months), but the average of first 2-word phrase spoken was delayed (mean 23.5 months, range 18–48 months). Compared with children with normal hearing, fifty-eight 4- to 6-year-old children with UHL had significantly delayed language in Sweden.[40] Another study comparing preschool children with UHL or mild BHL (n = 10) with children with moderate to profound BHL (n = 19) and normal-hearing controls (n = 74) similarly found that all children with hearing loss had lower comprehension and expressive language scores.[41] Furthermore, there were no statistically significant differences between the 2 groups of children with hearing loss.

Among school-aged children, a series of controlled studies have documented a robust, negative effect of UHL on speech-language scores. Compared with 74 normal-hearing siblings, 74 children with UHL were found to have significantly poorer scores on the Oral and Written Language Scales, a 2.6 greater odds of having received speech therapy, and a 4.4 greater odds of receiving extra help at school via an IEP.[42] Verbal intelligence quotient (IQ) scores were also lower among the children with UHL. A subsequent study with a larger group confirmed these findings (**Fig. 1**).[43] On following up a subgroup of these children with UHL, their language and verbal IQ scores improved significantly with time but their school performance and need for IEPs or extra help did not diminish.[44] In a small study of adolescents that included some of the earlier studied children with UHL, Fischer and Lieu[45] reported that the gap in language scores between those with UHL and normal-hearing siblings did not diminish with time but perhaps even widened. Thus, speech-language development seems to be delayed or diminished in children with UHL on average.

Cognition and Executive Functions

Concerns about the potential effect of UHL on cognition began to appear as children with UHL were reported to have lower IQ scores, usually among children with profound or right-sided UHL.[46,47] Several studies have found lower scores on standardized cognitive tests in children with UHL compared with children with normal hearing (see **Fig. 1**).[43,45] A pilot study of working memory and phonological processing suggested deficits in executive function in children with UHL compared with their normal-hearing siblings.[48] These studies suggest that unilateral auditory stimulation of central pathways may result in altered central cortical processing.

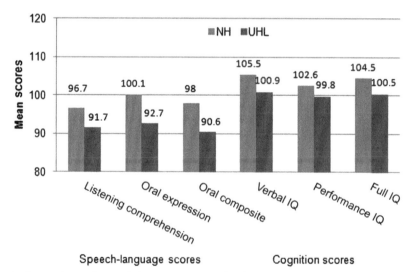

Fig. 1. Comparison of speech-language scores (Oral and Written Language Scales) and cognition scores (Wechsler Abbreviated Scale of Intelligence) between 107 children with unilateral hearing loss (UHL) and 94 siblings with normal hearing (NH).[49] Differences in language comprehension and oral composite speech-language scores were statistically significant at the $P<.01$ level, the difference in oral expression was significant at the $P<.001$ level, and the difference in verbal IQ was significant at the $P<.05$ level. (*Data from* Lieu JE, Karzon RK, Ead B, et al. Do audiologic characteristics predict outcomes in children with unilateral hearing loss? Otol Neurotol 2013;34(9):1703–10.)

MRI studies of children with UHL, including functional MRI (fMRI), resting state functional connectivity MRI (rs-fcMRI), and diffusion tension imaging, have been used to show differences in the gray and white matter of brains of children with UHL compared with children with normal hearing. Task-based fMRI studies have demonstrated that in response to noise chirps at different frequencies delivered to the poorer-hearing ear, children with UHL have decreased activation of auditory regions and no activation of auditory association areas and attention networks.[50] In addition, speech-in-noise tasks activated only the secondary auditory processing areas in the left hemisphere, whereas in controls, these areas were activated bilaterally. A subsequent fMRI study that evaluated cross-modal processing with the visual system noted that children with UHL displayed decreased activation in visual processing areas and reduced deactivation of the default mode network compared with normal-hearing peers.[51] They also increased activation of the left posterior superior temporal gyrus, which is involved in secondary auditory processing. A study of passive rs-fcMRI showed that resting-state brain connections were altered in the presence of UHL, particularly in areas that are thought to be involved with task-based executive functions.[52] Finally, even white-matter connections within the brain were found to be significantly altered in the setting of UHL, differences that were associated with some educational outcome variables.[53]

Impact on Quality of Life

For many years, it has been acknowledged that adults with acquired UHL experience significant social and emotional decrements in quality of life (QOL) because UHL disrupts their ability to interact with others.[54,55] Qualitative reports of how UHL affects QOL include social interactions (ie, one-on-one preferred to group interactions) and difficulty with conversations (eg, pretending to hear what was said, concentrating really hard to understand, or misunderstanding words).[56] Studies have shown that children and adolescents with UHL report their own hearing-related QOL to be significantly poorer than children and adolescents with normal hearing (**Figs. 2** and **3**).[57,58] Moreover, their level of QOL was similar to that reported by children and adolescents with BHL. The only domain where adolescents with UHL had statistically better QOL than BHL was in the social interactions domain.[57]

A few studies have suggested that amplification of the worse-hearing ear may benefit QOL in children with UHL. For children with mild to moderate UHL, use of conventional digital hearing aids resulted in large improvements in hearing-related QOL.[59] For children with profound UHL, the CROS hearing aid may offer some benefit, although children may not take to these devices because the perceived benefit may be low; they do not aid in sound localization and they may make speech perception worse in noise.[60] Use of osseointegrated bone conducting implants in children and adolescents with severe to profound UHL seems to have a beneficial effect on hearing in noise, as measured by Hearing in Noise Test (HINT), and ease of listening, as measured by the Children's Home Inventory for Listening Difficulties questionnaire.[61] Use of a cochlear implant in 3 children with postlingual profound UHL suggests improvements in child-adapted Speech, Spatial, and Qualities scale (SSQ) and parent-reported SSQ after cochlear implantation (CI).[62]

MANAGEMENT GOALS

As with any child with BHL, the goals for management of children with UHL should include the following:

- Minimize or eliminate speech-language delay, both receptive and expressive language, as well as speech articulation deficits

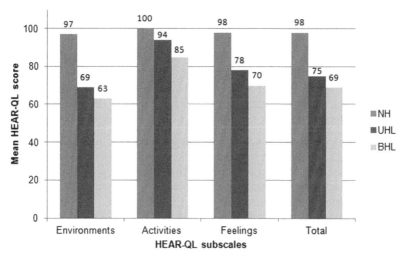

Fig. 2. Comparison of Hearing Environments and Reflection on Quality of Life (HEAR-QL) scores for children 7 to 12 years old with normal hearing (NH, n = 35), unilateral hearing loss (UHL, n = 35), and bilateral hearing loss (BHL, n = 45). All differences between NH and UHL or BHL were statistically significant at the $P<.001$ level. The activities score was significantly different between children with UHL and BHL ($P<.05$). (*Data from* Umansky AM, Jeffe DB, Lieu JE. The HEAR-QL: quality of life questionnaire for children with hearing loss. J Am Acad Audiol 2011;22(10):644–53.)

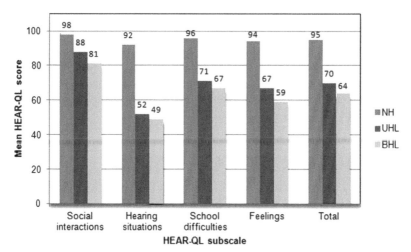

Fig. 3. Comparison of Hearing Environments and Reflection on Quality of Life (HEAR-QL) scores for adolescents 13 to 18 years old with normal hearing (NH, n = 54), unilateral hearing loss (UHL, n = 63), and bilateral hearing loss (BHL, n = 109). All differences between NH and UHL or BHL were statistically significant at the $P<.001$ level. The Social Interactions score was significantly different between adolescents with UHL and BHL at the $P<.05$ level. (*Data from* Rachakonda T, Jeffe DB, Shin JJ, et al. Validity, discriminative ability, and reliability of the hearing-related quality of life questionnaire for adolescents. Laryngoscope 2014;124(2):570–8.)

- Optimize cognitive development, educational learning, and academic performance
- Maximize hearing function, including sound localization abilities for both safety and social reasons, and ability to comprehend speech in noisy situations
- Optimize hearing-related QOL, including communication, social engagement, and participation in activities.

TREATMENT OPTIONS

Because there are no definitive evidence-based guidelines for how children with UHL should be treated, a collaborative/team approach, involving parents, audiologists, speech therapists, educators, pediatricians, and the child when he or she is old enough to have an opinion, is recommended. **Table 1** summarizes the available and to-be-evaluated treatment options.

Families may have strong opinions about the approach to their infant child; some parents will have observed no apparent problem with hearing in their baby and are happy to observe only, but others want to be as aggressive as possible, enrolling in parent-infant programs and fitting hearing aids. For those who prefer a wait-and-watch approach, observation and screening for speech-language delay is a reasonable option; there is no alternative treatment that is proved to result in better outcomes. However, educating parents to optimize the home environment for language learning is a potentially valuable benefit to the child. Not only should parents keep background noise to a minimum but they should also interact and converse with their children as much as possible. Investigators have shown that the number of words that young children speak is highly correlated to the number of words that their parents spoke to them, which is later correlated with vocabulary and later school performance.[63–65] The number of words that young children hear from adults is thought to be a major mediating factor in the association between socioeconomic status and child language development. These associations have led to social experiments in Chicago, Illinois, and Providence, Rhode Island, where programs have been developed to teach parents how to talk and read to their toddlers and how to engage toddlers in more conversation.[66,67] Along similar lines, Glanemann and colleagues[68] developed a program to enhance parental communication skills toward their infant-toddler children, with the intent of improving overall language skills in their children with hearing loss.

Table 1		
Options for management of children with UHL		
Nonmedical	**Amplification**	**Surgical**
Observation	Conventional hearing aid	BAHA System
First Steps/Birth-to-Three program referral	Contralateral routing of signal aid	Sophono
Parental education/training	TransEar	Cochlear implant
Preferential seating in class	—	Auditory brainstem implant
Frequency-modulated devices	—	—
Auditory rehabilitation	—	—

BAHA System, Cochlear Americas, Centennial, CO, USA.
Sophono, Sophono, Inc, Boulder, CO, USA.
TransEar, Ear Technology Corp, Johnson City, TN, USA.

Other parents opt for early auditory rehabilitation with amplification from hearing aids.[69] These caregivers can also benefit from the education that parent-infant programs can provide. Although there have been no studies showing direct benefit to language outcomes, studies suggest that binaural hearing is possible with the use of hearing aids in children with UHL. In terms of sound localization, Johnstone and colleagues[70] found that younger children with UHL (6–9 year olds) improved their ability to localize sound with the use of hearing aids, whereas older children (10–14 year olds) experienced a decrement in their ability to localize sound.

Before the advent of newborn hearing screening, the most common age for identification of UHL in children coincided with preschool or kindergarten hearing screening programs, about the age of 5 years. Preferential seating in school, placing the child in the front of the classroom with the better-hearing ear directed toward the teacher, was an easy accommodation from the perspective of schools and teachers. It is still a reasonable option, particularly for children who do not use an amplification device.

For children with UHL or BHL, many families pursue an IEP, a plan or program developed with the school system to ensure that a child who has a disability identified under the law and is attending an elementary or secondary educational institution receives specialized instruction and related services (http://www.washington.edu/doit/what-difference-between-iep-and-504-plan). If specialized instruction is not necessary, families can request a 504(c) plan, a plan developed to ensure that a child who has a disability identified under the law and is attending an elementary or secondary educational institution receives accommodations that ensure their academic success and access to the learning environment (http://www.washington.edu/doit/what-difference-between-iep-and-504-plan).

FM systems are another well-established school-based intervention that has some support from small studies showing that children with UHL performed better on speech-in-noise tests using FM systems than with analog hearing aids or CROS aids.[71,72] The FM system can be an excellent solution in the classroom setting. The teacher wears a microphone, and the receiver should be applied to the child's better hearing ear so that the student can directly hear the teacher's voice.

Use of conventional digital hearing aids is another useful option that does not carry a recommendation for the optimal fitting age. Because studies of children with profound and mild to moderate BHL have shown benefit of early amplification and remediation in speech-language development and educational performance, it is tempting to extrapolate benefits for children with UHL.[73,74] However, no study has yet been performed to show that the benefits of a hearing aid for a young child with UHL outweigh the nuisance of trying to keep that child from pulling the hearing aid off. One pilot study has shown that school-aged children with mild-to-moderate sensorineural UHL can experience significant benefit in subjective hearing situations and QOL when conventional digital hearing aids were fitted.[59] Unlike earlier studies, which used analog hearing aids, the investigators found no decrement in performance in speech-in-noise tests. Although there is no documentation of an upper age limit or duration of UHL when no benefit from amplification is expected, theoretically there might be a time when an amplification trial might be considered futile. If neural plasticity results in the reassignment of formerly auditory central pathways to other functions, amplification may result in interference of comprehension to the normal-hearing ear.

For children with conductive UHL, such as from unilateral aural atresia or ossicular malformation, surgical implantation of an osseointegrated bone conduction hearing device has been shown to improve binaural hearing, although not in all patients. Because the auditory neural pathways are intact, equivalent or near-equal sound levels from both ears have the potential to result in true binaural hearing. However, for children with severe to profound sensorineural UHL, an osseointegrated implanted device does not improve the ability to localize sound.[75] Furthermore, all studies of these implanted devices have been short term and have not yet demonstrated that long-term outcomes of language development and educational performance can be improved.

CI is the current research and clinical frontier for children with severe to profound UHL. Hassepass and colleagues[62] in Germany reported favorable outcomes of CI in 3 children, 2 of whom had postlingual profound UHL. Other centers around the world are conducting pilot studies in small numbers of children. One extremely important limitation to CI in this population of children is the high prevalence of cochlear nerve aplasia and hypoplasia. Therefore, it is imperative to image the temporal bone, preferably MRI, to confirm the presence of a cochlear nerve or to rule out a narrow cochlear nerve canal or internal auditory canal on CT scan. If no cochlear nerve is identified, CI is not expected to be beneficial, and an auditory brainstem implant would have to be considered the final possible option. Given the current state of auditory brainstem implant technology, however, it would be extremely unlikely that parents of a child with 1 normal-hearing ear would choose that option today.

TREATMENT RESISTANCE OR COMPLICATIONS
Hearing Rehabilitation

In contrast to adults who lose hearing in 1 ear and are acutely aware of the deficiency of binaural hearing, children with congenital UHL have never experienced binaural hearing and thus do not recognize what they miss. Placement of a hearing aid may thus result in too much sound from the worse-hearing ear, which the brain has difficulty integrating, and may result in aversion to using the hearing aid. Because neural plasticity allows for attainment of binaural integration of sound signals, time for compensation is required before full acceptance and adherence to use occurs. Even when a child experiences progressive hearing loss, hearing aid fitting often requires time for adjustment, just as with bilateral hearing aids, and may require time for neural plasticity to adjust to binaural hearing.

Reluctance to Acknowledge Unilateral Hearing Loss as a Problem for Children

Both parents and children may evince reluctance to acknowledge UHL as a problem. In contrast to adults who lose hearing in 1 ear and are acutely aware of the deficiency, children with congenital UHL never experience binaural hearing and thus do not recognize what they miss. Older children and adolescents may avoid admitting to any difficulty with hearing to be as typical as possible and not be different from peers. Because selective hearing in children is a ubiquitous parental complaint, parents may not recognize that their child is displaying a true hearing problem rather than a behavior. Parents may not notice that their child avoids large groups of friends and attribute their tendency to seek one-on-one interactions to the child's personality rather than to problems associated with UHL.

Medical professionals often fail to acknowledge that UHL can be a real disability for children. Many physicians, audiologists, and health professionals may still hold onto the belief that UHL is not a significant issue for a child. Thus, if an infant does not pass newborn hearing screening in 1 ear, a child may not have diagnostic auditory brainstem response testing in a timely fashion or parents may be advised not to worry about a UHL if one is diagnosed. In this author's experience, about one-third of children with UHL were never referred to an otolaryngologist for further evaluation of their hearing loss. Many primary care physicians may be unaware of the more recent research regarding the difficulties children with UHL have with speech-language development and continue to consider UHL to be a trivial problem, not a true disability.

Schools and educators also tend to resist the notion that UHL might affect learning in children. In the United States, children with significant hearing loss have access to additional services and resources in public schools through the Individuals with Disabilities Education Act (IDEA) enacted in 1975. However, eligibility for services is determined by each state, so that children with UHL are not automatically eligible for Early Intervention through the First Steps or Birth to Three programs (Part C of IDEA) or preschool or school IEPs (Part B of IDEA), as are children with BHL.[76,77] Schools may exhibit reluctance to identify UHL as a significant hearing impairment when it results in a request for a school-provided FM system.

EVALUATION OF OUTCOME

The outcomes to be evaluated change with time as the child grows older. Short-term outcomes, proximal to the time of diagnosis of UHL, are audiologic ones (eg, speech and pure tone thresholds, word recognition scores). Medium-term outcomes, in the 1- to 5-year perspective, include speech and language outcomes, social engagement, participation, and QOL. Long-term outcomes (>5 years) include educational achievement, cognitive outcomes, and QOL, as the child's listening needs, preferences, and personality develop and change. Eventually, the highest educational attainment and occupational outcomes will need to be evaluated in children who have or have not had intervention for their UHL.

As for children with BHL, regular-interval audiograms for apparently stable hearing and urgent audiograms on noting acute changes in hearing ability are indicated. Monitoring hearing in the normal-hearing ear, in addition to evaluating for progression in the worse-hearing ear, is important particularly for young children who do not have the words to indicate that their hearing has changed. BHL may develop in 10% to 15% of children initially diagnosed with UHL, and progression of hearing loss may occur in 15% to 20% in the impaired ear over time, especially in children with enlarged vestibular aqueduct or undiagnosed congenital CMV infections. Speech perception tests are important to perform as soon as a child can cooperate with them. Word recognition scores in the worse-hearing ear in quiet and noise may be helpful, as well as speech in noise tests, such as the HINT or Bamford-Kowal-Bench Speech-in-Noise test (BKB-SIN).[78] Sound localization tests are not standard clinical tests and thus may only be available in research settings.

Speech-language development in young children should be monitored carefully. For young children who show any suggestion of delay, a speech evaluation can be helpful. Infants and toddlers may not display obvious speech-language delay, and thus may not show any problem with UHL. However, as they enter preschool and school, they may begin to experience difficulty with hearing teachers in a noisy classroom. Teachers may begin to comment about behavioral issues, such as not paying attention or speaking in a very loud voice, and suggest evaluation for attention-deficit hyperactivity disorder. The challenges experienced by the patient with UHL need reassessment with each return visit, as their listening and communication needs develop and change. Some children may become frustrated when they begin playing organized sports, having difficulty with team play because they cannot localize the sounds of their teammates, whereas others will have no apparent problem.

As children progress through school, additional outcomes to monitor include behavior, QOL, and educational performance. Parents may notice changes in the patterns of social interactions, such as avoiding large group outings and preferring smaller circles of friends. A teenager who used to wear a hearing aid daily may begin leaving it at home, and grades may begin to decline. QOL questionnaires can be helpful to allow children to communicate with professionals and parents about what they perceive and how they feel related to their hearing but do not easily voice. Annual visits are recommended for this purpose. Ultimately, future studies ought to monitor the level of the highest educational attainment, as well as difficulty with completing secondary education and matriculating to college.

SUMMARY

Among children with UHL there is a general concern for speech-language delay, with high rates of speech therapy and needing academic assistance in schools. QOL as reported by children with UHL is similar to QOL reported by children with BHL, suggesting that intervention can be beneficial. A paucity of evidence for the benefits or risks of treatment limits recommendations; thus, rigorous comparative studies are needed before guidelines can be promulgated. Until there is better evidence, treatments for UHL in children should be guided by the needs, values, and preferences of the child and family.

REFERENCES

1. Johnson JL, White KR, Widen JE, et al. A multicenter evaluation of how many infants with permanent hearing loss pass a two-stage otoacoustic emissions/automated auditory brainstem response newborn hearing screening protocol. Pediatrics 2005;116(3):663–72.
2. Ross DS, Visser SN, Holstrum WJ, et al. Highly variable population-based prevalence rates of unilateral hearing loss after the application of common case definitions. Ear Hear 2009;31(1):126–33.
3. Shargorodsky J, Curhan SG, Curhan GC, et al. Change in prevalence of hearing loss in US adolescents. JAMA 2010;304(7):772–8.
4. Declau F, Boudewyns A, Van den EJ, et al. Etiologic and audiologic evaluations after universal neonatal hearing screening: analysis of 170 referred neonates. Pediatrics 2008;121(6):1119–26.
5. Uwiera TC, DeAlarcon A, Meinzen-Derr J, et al. Hearing loss progression and contralateral involvement in children with unilateral sensorineural hearing loss. Ann Otol Rhinol Laryngol 2009;118(11):781–5.
6. Clemmens CS, Guidi J, Caroff A, et al. Unilateral cochlear nerve deficiency in children. Otolaryngol Head Neck Surg 2013;149(2):318–25.
7. Nakano A, Arimoto Y, Matsunaga T. Cochlear nerve deficiency and associated clinical features in patients with bilateral and unilateral hearing loss. Otol Neurotol 2013;34(3):554–8.
8. Dodson KM, Georgolios A, Barr N, et al. Etiology of unilateral hearing loss in a national hereditary deafness repository. Am J Otolaryngol 2012;33(5):590–4.
9. Ghogomu N, Umansky A, Lieu JE. Epidemiology of unilateral sensorineural hearing loss with universal newborn hearing screening. Laryngoscope 2014;124(1):295–300.
10. Chattaraj P, Reimold FR, Muskett JA, et al. Use of SLC26A4 mutation testing for unilateral enlargement of the vestibular aqueduct. JAMA Otolaryngol Head Neck Surg 2013;139(9):907–13.
11. Jonard L, Niasme-Grare M, Bonnet C, et al. Screening of SLC26A4, FOXI1 and KCNJ10 genes in unilateral hearing impairment with ipsilateral enlarged vestibular aqueduct. Int J Pediatr Otorhinolaryngol 2010;74(9):1049–53.

12. Dikkers FG, Verheij JB, van Mechelen M. Hereditary congenital unilateral deafness: a new disorder? Ann Otol Rhinol Laryngol 2005;114(4):332–7.

13. Dodson KM, Kamei T, Sismanis A, et al. Familial unilateral deafness and delayed endolymphatic hydrops. Am J Med Genet A 2007;143A(14):1661–5.

14. Patel N, Oghalai JS. Familial unilateral cochlear nerve aplasia. Otol Neurotol 2006;27(3):443–4.

15. Goderis J, De LE, Smets K, et al. Hearing loss and congenital CMV infection: a systematic review. Pediatrics 2014;134(5):972–82.

16. Preciado DA, Lawson L, Madden C, et al. Improved diagnostic effectiveness with a sequential diagnostic paradigm in idiopathic pediatric sensorineural hearing loss. Otol Neurotol 2005;26(4):610–5.

17. Karchniarz B, Chen JX, Gilani S, et al. Diagnostic yield of MRI for pediatric hearing loss. Otolaryngol Head Neck Surg 2015;152(1):5–22.

18. Litovsky R, Parkinson A, Arcaroli J, et al. Simultaneous bilateral cochlear implantation in adults: a multicenter clinical study. Ear Hear 2006;27(6):714–31.

19. Pollack I. Monaural and binaural threshold sensitivity for tones and for white noise. J Acoust Soc Am 1948;20(1):52–7.

20. Bess FH, Tharpe AM. An introduction to unilateral sensorineural hearing loss in children. Ear Hear 1986;7(1):3–13.

21. Hawley ML, Litovsky RY, Culling JF. The benefit of binaural hearing in a cocktail party: effect of location and type of interferer. J Acoust Soc Am 2004;115(2):833–43.

22. Tillman TW, Kasten RN, Horner JS. Effect of head shadow on reception of speech. ASHA 1963;5:778–9.

23. Bovo R, Martini A, Agnoletto M, et al. Auditory and academic performance of children with unilateral hearing loss. Scand Audiol Suppl 1988;30:71–4.

24. Humes LE, Allen SK, Bess FH. Horizontal sound localization skills of unilaterally hearing-impaired children. Audiology 1980;19(6):508–18.

25. Agterberg MJ, Snik AF, Hol MK, et al. Contribution of monaural and binaural cues to sound localization in listeners with acquired unilateral conductive hearing loss: improved directional hearing with a bone-conduction device. Hear Res 2012; 286(1–2):9–18.

26. Agterberg MJ, Hol MK, Van Wanrooij MM, et al. Single-sided deafness and directional hearing: contribution of spectral cues and high-frequency hearing loss in the hearing ear. Front Neurosci 2014;8:188.

27. Otte RJ, Agterberg MJ, Van Wanrooij MM, et al. Age-related hearing loss and ear morphology affect vertical but not horizontal sound-localization performance. J Assoc Res Otolaryngol 2013;14(2):261–73.

28. Bess FH, Hornsby BW. Commentary: listening can be exhausting–fatigue in children and adults with hearing loss. Ear Hear 2014;35(6):592–9.

29. Kuppler K, Lewis M, Evans AK. A review of unilateral hearing loss and academic performance: is it time to reassess traditional dogmata? Int J Pediatr Otorhinolaryngol 2013;77(5):617–22.

30. McFadden B, Pittman A. Effect of minimal hearing loss on children's ability to multitask in quiet and in noise. Lang Speech Hear Serv Sch 2008;39(3):342–51.

31. Nozza RJ, Wagner EF, Crandell MA. Binaural release from masking for a speech sound in infants, preschoolers, and adults. J Speech Hear Res 1988;31(2):212–8.

32. Bess FH, Tharpe AM. Unilateral hearing impairment in children. Pediatrics 1984; 74(2):206–16.

33. Oyler RF, Oyler AL, Matkin ND. Unilateral hearing loss: demographics and educational impact. Lang Speech Hear Serv Sch 1988;19:201–10.

34. Brookhouser PE, Worthington DW, Kelly WJ. Unilateral hearing loss in children. Laryngoscope 1991;101(12 Pt 1):1264–72.

35. Dancer J, Burl NT, Waters S. Effects of unilateral hearing loss on teacher responses to the SIFTER. Screening Instrument for Targeting Educational Risk. Am Ann Deaf 1995;140(3):291–4.

36. Most T. Assessment of school functioning among Israeli Arab children with hearing loss in the primary grades. Am Ann Deaf 2006;151(3):327–35.

37. Jensen DR, Grames LM, Lieu JE. Effects of aural atresia on speech development and learning: retrospective analysis from a multidisciplinary craniofacial clinic. JAMA Otolaryngol Head Neck Surg 2013;139(8):797–802.

38. Kesser BW, Krook K, Gray LC. Impact of unilateral conductive hearing loss due to aural atresia on academic performance in children. Laryngoscope 2013;123(9):2270–5.

39. Kiese-Himmel C. Unilateral sensorineural hearing impairment in childhood: analysis of 31 consecutive cases. Int J Audiol 2002;41(1):57–63.

40. Borg E, Edquist G, Reinholdson AC, et al. Speech and language development in a population of Swedish hearing-impaired pre-school children, a cross-sectional study. Int J Pediatr Otorhinolaryngol 2007;71(7):1061–77.

41. Vohr B, Topol D, Girard N, et al. Language outcomes and service provision of preschool children with congenital hearing loss. Early Hum Dev 2012;88(7):493–8.

42. Lieu JE, Tye-Murray N, Karzon RK, et al. Unilateral hearing loss is associated with worse speech-language scores in children. Pediatrics 2010;125(6):e1348–55.

43. Lieu JE, Karzon RK, Ead B, et al. Do audiologic characteristics predict outcomes in children with unilateral hearing loss? Otol Neurotol 2013;34(9):1703–10.

44. Lieu JE, Tye-Murray N, Fu Q. Longitudinal study of children with unilateral hearing loss. Laryngoscope 2012;122(9):2088–95.

45. Fischer C, Lieu J. Unilateral hearing loss is associated with a negative effect on language scores in adolescents. Int J Pediatr Otorhinolaryngol 2014;78(10):1611–7.

46. Bess FH. Children with unilateral hearing loss. Jara 1982;15:116–30.

47. Niedzielski A, Humeniuk E, Blaziak P, et al. Intellectual efficiency of children with unilateral hearing loss. Int J Pediatr Otorhinolaryngol 2006;70(9):1529–32.

48. Ead B, Hale S, DeAlwis D, et al. Pilot study of cognition in children with unilateral hearing loss. Int J Pediatr Otorhinolaryngol 2013;77(11):1856–60.

49. Carrow-Woolfolk E. Oral and Written Language Scales. Bloomington (MN): Pearson Assessments; 1995.

50. Propst EJ, Greinwald JH, Schmithorst V. Neuroanatomic differences in children with unilateral sensorineural hearing loss detected using functional magnetic resonance imaging. Arch Otolaryngol Head Neck Surg 2010;136(1):22–6.

51. Schmithorst VJ, Plante E, Holland S. Unilateral deafness in children affects development of multi-modal modulation and default mode networks. Front Hum Neurosci 2014;8:164.

52. Tibbetts K, Ead B, Umansky A, et al. Interregional brain interactions in children with unilateral hearing loss. Otolaryngol Head Neck Surg 2011;144(4):602–11.

53. Rachakonda T, Shimony JS, Coalson RS, et al. Diffusion tensor imaging in children with unilateral hearing loss: a pilot study. Front Syst Neurosci 2014;8:87.

54. Giolas TG, Wark DJ. Communication problems associated with unilateral hearing loss. J Speech Hear Disord 1967;32(4):336–43.

55. Newman CW, Jacobson GP, Hug GA, et al. Perceived hearing handicap of patients with unilateral or mild hearing loss. Ann Otol Rhinol Laryngol 1997;106(3):210–4.

56. Borton SA, Mauze E, Lieu JEC. Quality of life in children with unilateral hearing loss: a pilot study. Am J Audiol 2010;19(1):61–72.

57. Rachakonda T, Jeffe DB, Shin JJ, et al. Validity, discriminative ability, and reliability of the hearing-related quality of life questionnaire for adolescents. Laryngoscope 2014;124(2):570–8.

58. Umansky AM, Jeffe DB, Lieu JE. The HEAR-QL: quality of life questionnaire for children with hearing loss. J Am Acad Audiol 2011;22(10):644–53.

59. Briggs L, Davidson L, Lieu JE. Outcomes of conventional amplification for pediatric unilateral hearing loss. Ann Otol Rhinol Laryngol 2011;120(7):448–54.

60. Updike CD. Comparison of FM auditory trainers, CROS aids, and personal amplification in unilaterally hearing impaired children. J Am Acad Audiol 1994;5:204–9.

61. Christensen L, Richter GT, Dornhoffer JL. Update on bone-anchored hearing aids in pediatric patients with profound unilateral sensorineural hearing loss. Arch Otolaryngol Head Neck Surg 2010;136(2):175–7.

62. Hassepass F, Aschendorff A, Wesarg T, et al. Unilateral deafness in children: audiologic and subjective assessment of hearing ability after cochlear implantation. Otol Neurotol 2013;34(1):53–60.

63. Hart B, Risley T. Meaningful differences in the everyday experience of young American children. Baltimore (MD): Brookes Publishing; 1995.

64. Hoff E. The specificity of environmental influence: socioeconomic status affects early vocabulary development via maternal speech. Child Dev 2003;74(5): 1368–78.

65. Walker D, Greenwood C, Hart B, et al. Prediction of school outcomes based on early language production and socioeconomic factors. Child Dev 1994;65(2 Spec No):606–21.

66. Leffel K, Suskind D. Parent-directed approaches to enrich the early language environments of children living in poverty. Semin Speech Lang 2013;34(4): 267–78.

67. Rosenberg T. The power of talking to your baby. The New York Times 2013.

68. Glanemann R, Reichmuth K, Matulat P, et al. Muenster Parental Programme empowers parents in communicating with their infant with hearing loss. Int J Pediatr Otorhinolaryngol 2013;77(12):2023–9.

69. McKay S, Gravel JS, Tharpe AM. Amplification considerations for children with minimal or mild bilateral hearing loss and unilateral hearing loss. Trends Amplif 2008;12(1):43–54.

70. Johnstone PM, Nabelek AK, Robertson VS. Sound localization acuity in children with unilateral hearing loss who wear a hearing aid in the impaired ear. J Am Acad Audiol 2010;21(8):522–34.

71. Kenworthy OT, Klee T, Tharpe AM. Speech recognition ability of children with unilateral sensorineural hearing loss as a function of amplification, speech stimuli and listening condition. Ear Hear 1990;11(4):264–70.

72. Updike CD. Comparison of FM auditory trainers, CROS aids, and personal amplification in unilaterally hearing impaired children. J Am Acad Audiol 1994;5(3): 204–9.

73. Ching TY, Day J, Seeto M, et al. Predicting 3-year outcomes of early-identified children with hearing impairment. B-ENT 2013;(Suppl 21):99–106.

74. Tomblin JB, Oleson JJ, Ambrose SE, et al. The influence of hearing aids on the speech and language development of children with hearing loss. JAMA Otolaryngol Head Neck Surg 2014;140(5):403–9.

75. Battista RA, Mullins K, Wiet RM, et al. Sound localization in unilateral deafness with the Baha or TransEar device. JAMA Otolaryngol Head Neck Surg 2013; 139(1):64–70.

76. State EHDI/UNHS mandates: summary table. National Center for Hearing Assessment and Management (NCHAM) 1998 November 4. Available at: http://www.infanthearing.org/legislative/summary/index.html. Accessed July 3, 2012.

77. Holstrum WJ, Gaffney M, Gravel JS, et al. Early intervention for children with unilateral and mild bilateral degrees of hearing loss. Trends Amplif 2008;12(1): 35–41.

78. Etymotic Research: Bamford-Kowal-Bench Speech-in-Noise Test (Version 1.03 Audio CD). Elk Grove Village, Etymotic Research 2005.

Auditory Neuropathy/Dys-Synchrony Disorder

Diagnosis and Management

Linda J. Hood, PhD[a,b,*]

KEYWORDS

- Auditory • Neuropathy • Dys-synchrony • Diagnosis • Management
- Cochlear implant • Characteristics

KEY POINTS

- Effect, directly or indirectly, is on neural processing of auditory stimuli.
  - Physiologic measures are needed to accurately characterize patients with auditory neuropathy spectrum disorder (ANSD).
  - Clinical behavioral responses vary greatly and are not useful diagnostic measures.
- Patients with ANSD have greater difficulty listening in noise than those with other types of hearing disorders.
  - Separating detection ability from discrimination ability is critical in considering various management approaches.
- Without clear auditory input, visual information is needed for auditory communication and speech/language development.
- Many patients benefit from cochlear implants; fewer benefit from hearing aids.
- Patients should be followed closely, as changes in auditory function may occur over time.

Auditory neuropathy (AN),[1] auditory neuropathy/dys-synchrony (AN/AD),[2] and, more recently, auditory neuropathy spectrum disorder (ANSD) are variable terms used to describe an auditory disorder seen in patients ranging in age from infants to adults. With knowledge of the inherent problems presented by each term, ANSD

Disclosure: The author has nothing to disclose.
Research related to auditory neuropathy/dys-synchrony supported by the NIH National Institute on Deafness and Other Communication Disorders (NIDCD), Oberkotter Foundation, Vanderbilt University.
[a] Department of Hearing and Speech Sciences, Vanderbilt University, 1215 21st Avenue South, MCE South Tower, Room 8310, Nashville, TN 37232-8242, USA; [b] School of Rehabilitation Sciences, University of Queensland, Brisbane, Queensland, Australia
* Department of Hearing and Speech Sciences, Vanderbilt University, 1215 21st Avenue South, MCE South Tower, Room 8310, Nashville, TN 37232-8242.
E-mail address: linda.j.hood@vanderbilt.edu

Otolaryngol Clin N Am 48 (2015) 1027–1040
http://dx.doi.org/10.1016/j.otc.2015.06.006
0030-6665/15/$ – see front matter © 2015 Elsevier Inc. All rights reserved.

oto.theclinics.com

Abbreviations	
ABR	Auditory brainstem response
AN	Auditory neuropathy
AN/AD	Auditory neuropathy/auditory dys-synchrony
ANSD	Auditory neuropathy spectrum disorder
APD	Auditory processing disorder
CM	Cochlear microphonic
EVA	Enlarged vestibular aqueduct
FM	Frequency modulation
HMSN	Hereditary motor sensory neuropathy
IHC	Inner hair cells
MEMR	Middle-ear muscle reflex
MOCR	Medial olivocochlear reflex
NICU	Neonatal intensive care unit
OAE	Otoacoustic emission
OHC	Outer hair cells
OTOF	Otoferlin
SNHL	Sensorineural hearing loss

is used here with the understanding that no one term is completely definitive or descriptive.

OVERVIEW OF CHARACTERISTICS

ANSD is characterized by evidence of intact outer hair cell (OHC) function, shown by the presence of otoacoustic emissions (OAEs) and/or cochlear microphonics (CMs), accompanied by poor eighth nerve–brainstem responses, demonstrated by absent or highly abnormal auditory brainstem responses (ABRs).[3] Further evidence of effects on neural function is demonstrated by absent or elevated middle-ear muscle reflexes (MEMRs)[4] and abnormal medial olivocochlear reflexes (MOCRs).[5] Although understanding of speech in noise is poorer than that observed in sensorineural hearing loss (SNHL), word recognition in quiet is highly variable, and thresholds for pure tones range from normal to profound losses. Most ANSD patients show bilateral characteristics, although function may be asymmetric between ears, and patients with unilateral ANSD have been documented.

Despite fairly similar findings on auditory physiologic measures, patients vary considerably in functional communication abilities.[6,7] Clinical presentation typically includes difficulty listening in noise, may include fluctuating hearing ability, and, in the case of infants and children, most often involves delays in speech and language development. Patients with ANSD typically demonstrate poor temporal resolution[8] and may have neural deficits in other systems.

INCIDENCE

ANSD occurs in about 10% of individuals who have a dys-synchronous ABR, or an ABR consistent with an estimate of severe or profound hearing loss. This estimate is based on data from several sources that include screening of more than 1000 children enrolled in schools for the d/Deaf in North America,[9] a similar smaller-scale study in Hong Kong,[10] a hospital-based study of children in Australia,[11] and a multicenter newborn screening study in the United States.[12] A higher incidence of 17.3% and 15.4%, respectively, was reported among children identified with hearing loss following newborn hearing screening.[13,14] In the neonatal intensive care unit (NICU), rates of ANSD physiologic characteristics ranged from 24% to 40% of infants who failed ABR testing in one or both ears.[15,16]

CLINICAL FINDINGS

Physiologic measures that assess cochlear active processes related to OHC and mechanical activity and peripheral neural function of the eighth nerve and brainstem pathways most accurately describe patients with ANSD. Cochlear processes are evidenced by the presence of OAEs and CMs. Clinical tests specifically sensitive to auditory nerve dysfunction are the ABR, MEMRs, and the MOCR. Of these measures, OAEs and ABR together form the most sensitive combination. A summary of physiologic and behavioral audiologic test results in patients with ANSD is shown in **Table 1**.

Hair Cell Responses: Otoacoustic Emissions and Cochlear Microphonics

OAEs provide a measure of cochlear active processes related to OHC function and cochlear mechanics. The presence of ANSD is typically established based on presence of these responses when peripheral neural responses are absent or significantly reduced. In the absence of middle-ear disorders, OAEs are typically present in patients with ANSD. Because OAEs are low-amplitude acoustic signals, even small middle-ear changes can be sufficient to reduce OAE amplitude or prevent the OAE from being recorded. The effect of even minor middle-ear problems and the high incidence of otitis media in infants and children can confound identification of ANSD.

Cochlear function can also be evaluated using the CM.[3,11,17] Because the CM is an electrical response, it does not depend on reverse transmission through the middle ear system. A key factor in distinguishing CM from neural responses is the reversal of the electrical response with presentation of condensation versus rarefaction stimuli. The CM will invert with stimulus polarity reversal, whereas neural responses to clicks typically do not completely invert (**Fig. 1**).[3]

Neural Responses: Auditory Brainstem Response

ABRs are most often absent in patients with ANSD, although some patients demonstrate small evidence of neural synchrony for high-level stimuli. In the germinal article defining AN, Starr and colleagues[1] reported absent ABRs in 9 of 10 patients and an abnormal ABR characterized by Wave V responses only to high-intensity stimuli in 1 patient. A subsequent review[7] of ABR data for 186 patients with ANSD indicated that approximately 75% of patients had absent ABRs while 25% showed abnormal

Table 1 Typical physiologic and behavioral audiologic test results in ANSD patients	
Test	Outcome
Otoacoustic emissions	Typically present
Middle-ear muscle reflexes	Typically absent
Cochlear microphonic	Present (inverts with stimulus polarity reversal)
Auditory brainstem response	Absent or severely abnormal
Pure-tone thresholds	Normal to severe/profound hearing loss
Word recognition in quiet	Variable; slightly reduced to greatly reduced
Word recognition in noise	Generally poor
Medial olivocochlear reflex	Typically absent

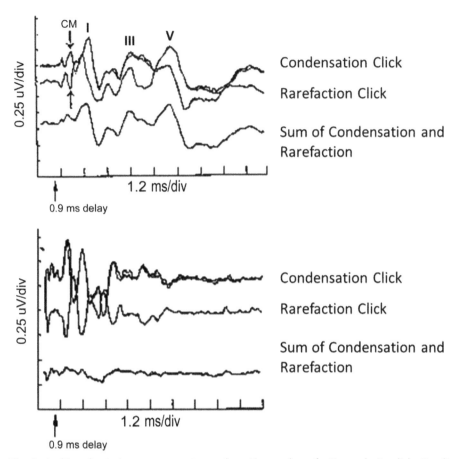

Fig. 1. Auditory brainstem responses to condensation and rarefaction polarity click stimuli in an individual with normal auditory function (*upper*) and an ANSD patient (*lower*). Note the inverting CM in both figures and the lack of a neural response in the lower figure. I, Wave I of the ABR; III, Wave III of the ABR; V, Wave V of the ABR.

responses characterized by the presence of low-amplitude Wave V only at high stimulus levels (75–90 dB nHL).

The absence or abnormality of all components of the ABR including Wave I suggests that the distal portion of the eighth nerve is affected, either directly or indirectly, in ANSD. This characteristic distinguishes patients with ANSD from those with space-occupying lesions affecting the eighth nerve where ABR Wave I is present. Imaging studies (MRI, computed tomography) are characteristically normal in patients with ANSD. Neural changes in ABR are attributed to demyelinating and axonal neuropathies.[1]

Neural Responses: Efferent Acoustic Reflexes

Both ipsilaterally and contralaterally elicited MEMRs are most often absent in these patients, although a small percentage (about 10%) of patients may display MEMRs at elevated levels or in combination with absent responses.[4,18] The MOCR assesses changes in OAEs when the olivocochlear neural pathway, terminating at the cochlear

OHCs, is activated. Although patients with ANSD typically demonstrate the presence of OAEs, they consistently show no or minimal suppression of transient OAEs for binaural, ipsilateral, and contralateral suppressor stimuli.[1,5] Abnormalities in both reflexes seem to be related to poor afferent auditory input, based on both the ability to elicit nonacoustic reflexes and studies in patients with unilateral ANSD.

Behavioral Findings: Pure-Tone Thresholds and Speech Recognition

Pure-tone thresholds and speech recognition, particularly in quiet, are the least informative measures in the evaluation of ANSD. Pure-tone thresholds range from normal sensitivity to severe or profound hearing loss.[1,7,19,20] Some patients show rising or unusual configurations with possible asymmetry between ears.[7] When OAEs are present and pure-tone thresholds are poorer than expected for the presence of OAEs, this combination may provide a clue to the presence of ANSD or another type of neural disorder that warrants further investigation.

Speech recognition in ANSD patients is typically poorer than expected based on pure-tone thresholds,[1,8] but performance varies widely across individuals. Some patients with ANSD demonstrate word-recognition ability in quiet in ranges similar to those with SNHL, whereas word-recognition ability in noise is clearly below that expected in SNHL.[1,7,21] Of 68 patients aged 4 years and older in whom word recognition was measurable using standardized tests, more than half had no word-recognition ability, even in quiet. Of the remaining patients, 30 had word-recognition scores greater than 0% in quiet and only 5 patients had measurable word recognition in noise.[7] This widely varying ability presents a particular challenge in both understanding ANSD and planning appropriate management.

UNDERLYING MECHANISMS

The set of clinical test results observed in patients with ANSD can occur as a result of absence or disruption of inner hair cell (IHC) activity, disorders of the auditory nerve, or abnormalities at the synapses of the IHCs and auditory nerve. IHC abnormalities could result from a lack of development, traumatic insult, or a loss over time. Selective IHC loss was observed in several premature newborns who failed ABR testing.[22] Hypoxia and toxic insults specific to IHCs are other possible explanations.[23,24] Direct effects on auditory nerve activity have been implicated in patients with concomitant peripheral neuropathies such as Charcot-Marie-Tooth disease, Friedreich ataxia, Mohr-Tranebjaerg syndrome who also display characteristics of ANSD.[1,25] Study of underlying mechanisms is enhanced through efforts to distinguish presynaptic versus postsynaptic responses using electrocochleography.[26–28]

Links between ANSD and genetic mutations are well documented with evidence of recessive, dominant, and mitochondrial inheritance patterns, and occurrence in syndromic and nonsyndromic hearing loss (see Ref.[26] for review). An example is the *OTOF* gene that encodes otoferlin, whose mutations are associated with nonsyndromic recessive ANSD.[29–31] Otoferlin plays a role in neurotransmitter release at the synapse between the IHCs and the auditory nerve.

In some patients with ANSD, fluctuations in auditory function have been linked to fluctuations in body temperature (as little as 1°C) and an apparent temperature-sensitive form of ANSD. Several reports implicate *OTOF* gene mutations and other mechanisms, possibly autoimmune disorders, whereby auditory function varies with changes in body temperature.[19,32,33] ANSD is also reported in infants with potential risk factors that include hypoxia and hyperbilirubinemia.[7,11,15]

DIFFERENTIAL DIAGNOSIS

Although the test protocols necessary to diagnose ANSD are now well established, dysfunction of the IHCs and their synapses can lead to a hearing disorder that is difficult to distinguish clinically from an auditory nerve disorder. Identifying concomitant peripheral neuropathies or radiologic abnormalities is helpful in distinguishing among various conditions.

Association with Other Neurologic Abnormalities

Several neurologic problems are identified in patients with ANSD, including hereditary motor sensory neuropathy (HMSN), Charcot-Marie-Tooth disease, Friedreich ataxia, Mohr-Tranebjaerg syndrome, gait ataxia, loss of deep tendon reflexes, or motor system disturbances.[1,7,34] The motor neural system may be affected without accompanying sensory problems involving the auditory system. When the auditory system is affected, characteristics such as absent or highly abnormal ABRs with preserved OAEs provide evidence consistent with ANSD. Broad variation in auditory characteristics such as speech understanding exists, likely related to underlying genetic characteristics in addition to the stage in the progression of the disorder.

Cochlear Nerve Deficiency

Absent or hypoplastic auditory nerves are not uncommon,[35] and these conditions resemble ANSD when OHC responses are present.[36,37] Audiologic management in these patients is problematic because a cochlear implant cannot work when the nerve is absent, and might not work well when the cochlear nerve is hypoplastic.[38]

Enlarged Vestibular Aqueduct

Patients with an enlarged vestibular aqueduct (EVA) present with a wide variety of audiometric thresholds and physiologic results, and may demonstrate clinical characteristics consistent with ANSD.[39,40] EVA is associated with SNHL, onset from birth to adolescence, progression, fluctuation, the possibility of other congenital ear anomalies, and contributing factors such as head trauma. Not all cases of EVA will show clinical test results consistent with ANSD.

DIAGNOSTIC AND MANAGEMENT DILEMMAS
Variation Among Patients with Auditory Neuropathy Spectrum Disorder

ANSD varies in age of onset, presence or absence of associated neurologic abnormalities, etiology, progression or fluctuation over time, and unilateral versus bilateral involvement. Furthermore, some patients, regardless of age, have no known risk factors or associated neurologic disorders. Progressive worsening of hearing ability is observed in some patients and may involve factors such as loss of OAEs and CM over time in infants, and progressive decreases in speech recognition or hearing sensitivity related to the progressive nature of some HMSNs. Other patients demonstrate stable physiologic responses and behavioral audiometric thresholds over many years.

Berlin and colleagues[7] describe a continuum of functional communication ability among patients with ANSD. A few patients at one extreme exhibit no delays in language development or auditory complaints until adulthood, or until they are first evaluated with MEMRs or ABR. These patients generally demonstrate the greatest residual speech recognition ability in quiet, although they report difficulty in noise. At the other extreme are ANSD patients who exhibit a total lack of sound awareness. The largest group of patients falls between these 2 extremes and may demonstrate inconsistent auditory responses, managing better in quiet and poorly in noise. Their audiograms may be inconsistent with other test results. The ABR is desynchronized and MEMRs are absent. From a clinical management perspective, visual language is helpful without cochlear implantation, unless the family prefers cultural Deafness.

Auditory Neuropathy Spectrum Disorder in Infants

With the implementation of universal newborn hearing screening programs, infants with ANSD characteristics are identified at birth in those programs utilizing ABR as the screening tool. Programs that use OAEs as the screening tool will miss infants with ANSD, who will be identified later when parental concern about delays in speech and language development arises. To address this issue, the Joint Committee on Infant Hearing[41] issued a recommendation for ABR protocols in NICU settings based on the higher risk for ANSD in this population. The growing number of infants with ANSD underscores the heterogeneity of this population. Numerous causes (hereditary, infectious, and metabolic) and risk factors (hypoxia and hyperbilirubinemia, among others) have been suggested to have an association with ANSD. Nevertheless, at least half of the patients cannot be assigned a cause and do not seem to present any concomitant disorders.

Infants who refer on an initial screening ABR and then show the presence of OAEs and poor or absent ABR on follow-up testing may be considered at risk for ANSD. A diagnostic dilemma here relates to the fact that the ABR continues to mature through the first 12 to 18 months of age. Some infants who show ANSD characteristics at birth develop an ABR over the first year of life[42,43]; however, the number of infants showing these characteristics remains a minority. A further consideration is whether having an absent or poor ABR at birth places an infant at risk for later auditory problems. More information is needed to adequately understand the reasons for poor synchrony and the factors that may contribute to later development of the ABR in these infants. In the meantime, it is important to closely monitor infants over at least the first year of life both with ABR and other indices of auditory development.

Unilateral Auditory Neuropathy Spectrum Disorder

Although most patients with ANSD are bilateral though often asymmetric, some have unilateral ANSD whereby the pattern of test results is consistent with ANSD only in one ear. Some patients with unilateral ANSD are found to have cochlear nerve dysplasia on imaging studies.[44] Auditory function in the other ear ranges from normal hearing to varying degrees of cochlear hearing losses, with ABR, MEMR, and OAE results consistent with behavioral results, patient complaint and history, and other aspects of auditory status. Functionally, patients with unilateral ANSD may have some of the same listening difficulties as patients with other types of unilateral hearing loss, although some patients report interference from sound in the ANSD ear.

Central Auditory Processing Disorder

Individuals with a centrally based auditory processing disorder (APD) typically can detect pure tones and speech in quiet, but fail to hear well in the presence of competing speech or background noise.[45] Some persons with ANSD also demonstrate good detection of sound and possibly good speech recognition in quiet, but difficulty in understanding speech in noisy environments. Although the 2 disorders share some characteristics, differences are determined through physiologic testing. Eighth nerve and brainstem responses in patients with ANSD (ABR, MEMR) will be absent or highly abnormal. By contrast, patients with an APD typically have normal MEMR thresholds and normal ABR responses. This fact underscores the importance of MEMR testing for all children suspected of having an APD. The presence of OAEs would be expected in both groups as long as middle-ear function was normal. If MEMRs are absent or elevated, an ABR recorded with both click polarities can then accurately determine the type of hearing disorder.

MANAGEMENT APPROACHES AND OUTCOMES

Variation in clinical presentation across individuals with ANSD dictates the need for individual management approaches along with the ability to refine these approaches based on changes in an individual's auditory function and needs. Visual information, through communication systems such as cued speech or sign language, facilitates language development in infants and children, and captioning and other visual assistance is useful in children and adults.[46] Use of visual information is critical in the absence of clear auditory signals. Many patients are able to use auditory input as their primary communication method after cochlear implantation, but may continue to use visual information in difficult listening situations.

Amplification

Given the reported variation in benefit with amplification across ANSD patients, a trial of amplification is typically undertaken. Challenges exist in determining threshold sensitivity in young infants because reliable behavioral threshold testing is difficult in infants younger than 5 to 6 months of age, and clinicians typically rely on ABR data in this age group. Recent studies using cortical responses show promise.[47,48] Amplification is fit to targets to assure audibility of signals. A key to assessment of benefit involves improved sound discrimination, which is necessary to facilitate speech and language development and to support auditory communication. Reports of benefit are variable, ranging from benefit in only a minority of patients with ANSD, even with appropriately audible signals,[7,49] to benefit from amplification in some ANSD patients.[50,51] Despite the lack of clear evidence at present,[52] general practice is to provide an amplification trial that provides appropriately audible signals for ANSD patients who display reduced threshold sensitivity.

Frequency Modulation Systems

Use of a frequency modulation (FM) system (alone or with other devices) is helpful to persons with ANSD in noisy settings such as a classroom, car, or restaurant. Providing a clearer signal to an auditory system that cannot cope with interference from noise, as occurs in ANSD, can be particularly helpful in those patients with some residual word recognition in quiet.[53]

Cochlear Implants

Both children and adults with ANSD demonstrate improved speech perception and significant benefit from cochlear implants.[54–58] Improvement is observed related to sensitivity, speech perception in quiet and in noise, in addition to evidence of synchronous neural responses in electrical ABRs and neural response telemetry. It is logical that ANSD patients with IHC loss or synaptic disorders may have more intact neural function and would derive benefit from cochlear implants. Some patients with demyelinating disease have also received benefit from cochlear implants, although sufficient data are not available to assess the impact of differences among underlying mechanisms on outcomes of cochlear implantation. As may be expected, more favorable speech perception scores after cochlear implantation are reported for ANSD subjects with intact cochlear nerves when compared with those with cochlear nerve deficiencies.[35,59]

Sound Detection Versus Discrimination

In assessing benefit from various management strategies while making decisions and recommendations related to proceeding from amplification to cochlear implantation, it is critical to separate the ability to detect sound from the ability to discriminate sound. This aspect is particularly important for speech signals. It is not unusual for a child (or adult) to become more aware of the presence of sound when amplification is fitted. However, a key determinant is whether this sound will facilitate speech and language development and communication ability. Following the guideline for at least 3 months' progress in language development in a period of 3 calendar months is recommended. If a child is not meeting this mark, particularly after several months of hearing aid use, a cochlear implant may be recommended for a patient and family to consider.

Two Patients Highlighting Detection Versus Discrimination

Two patients highlight differences between detection and discrimination in the management of ANSD. Both patients have present OAEs, absent ABR, absent MEMRs, minimal or no word recognition in quiet, and no word recognition in noise. Patient A presented at age 2 years with very poor sound detection and no speech discrimination. Her pre–cochlear implant audiogram is shown in **Fig. 2**. She would fit into the usual audiometric criteria for a cochlear implant. She derived no benefit from amplification and received a cochlear implant at age 3 years. Her post–cochlear implant threshold sensitivity is consistent with other cochlear implant patients. She entered school fully mainstreamed, is an auditory communicator, is an excellent student, and now has a second cochlear implant.

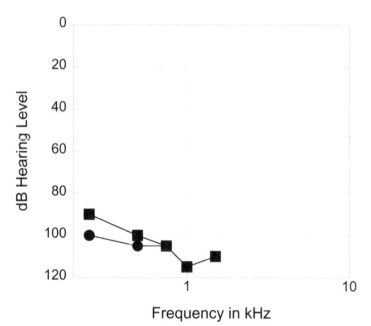

Fig. 2. Test results for ANSD cochlear implant patient A. Right ear, filled circles; left ear, filled squares. See text for other test results.

Patient B has had hearing sensitivity similar to that shown on her audiogram in **Fig. 3** since she was a young child. Her word recognition progressively worsened over time, and at 15 years old was 8% and 10% in the left and right ears, respectively, in quiet, and 0% in noise. She had twice tried to use amplification with no success. With pure-tone thresholds in the range of normal to mild hearing loss in the higher frequencies, she would not typically be considered a candidate for a cochlear implant. The decision to recommend a cochlear implant was based on inability to discriminate auditory signals sufficient for communication, basing decisions on discrimination rather than detection. After cochlear implantation, word recognition ability was 96% in quiet (preimplant 8%–10%) and 74% in noise at a +10 signal-to-noise ratio (preimplant 0%). This patient underscores the importance of considering discrimination, not detection, in evaluating candidacy for a cochlear implant in ANSD.

A Team Approach

Collaboration among audiologists, otolaryngologists, neurologists, speech-language pathologists, other physicians and health care professionals, and early interventionists and teachers of the d/Deaf, is of great value to patients and their families. Although an audiologist is often one of the first professionals to encounter a patient with ANSD, management should focus on medical needs and development of global communication skills and abilities needed to acquire language, become literate, and be self-sufficient. If one modality (eg, amplification of sound) is insufficient in meeting the communication needs of the child, the team should discuss and make recommendations for a different course of action (eg, FM system or cochlear implantation).

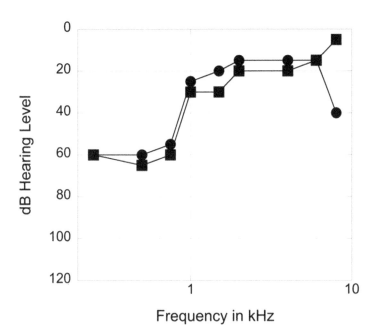

Fig. 3. Test results for ANSD cochlear implant patient B. Right ear, filled circles; left ear, filled squares. See text for other test results.

SUMMARY

The observed variation among patients with ANSD underscores the importance of accurately distinguishing among its various forms, underlying mechanisms, and functional differences. Progress in these areas will include discoveries in genetics, medical and imaging advances, improved sensitivity of physiologic responses, inclusion of auditory cortical responses, and further exploration of psychophysical tasks. Future research and clinical assessment should involve greater utilization of novel stimuli and paradigms, more sensitive approaches, and development of clinically feasible methods using these advances. Even within various forms of ANSD one should expect that variation will exist, underscoring the need to understand the range of variation and contributing factors.

Advances in understanding various forms of ANSD should guide us toward more focused and appropriate management strategies, ability to predict outcomes, and ability to predict who will develop speech/language with minimal intervention despite poor neural synchrony. Guidelines for fitting and programming hearing aids, FM systems, and cochlear implants are needed, in addition to understanding of whether protocols should differ between patients with ANSD and those with SNHL. Patient and parent education is critical as we learn more about ANSD and use our knowledge to guide our patients and their families in making informed decisions.

ACKNOWLEDGMENTS

Significant contributions to research on auditory neuropathy come from many colleagues including Charles I. Berlin PhD, Thierry Morlet PhD, Bronya Keats PhD, Diane Wilensky MA, and Cathrine Hayes AuD.

REFERENCES

1. Starr A, Picton TW, Sininger Y, et al. Auditory neuropathy. Brain 1996;119:741–53.
2. Berlin C, Hood L, Rose K. On renaming auditory neuropathy as auditory dys-synchrony: implications for a clearer understanding of the underlying mechanisms and management options. Audiology Today 2001;13:15–7.
3. Berlin CI, Bordelon J, St John P, et al. Reversing click polarity may uncover auditory neuropathy in infants. Ear Hear 1998;19:37–47.
4. Berlin CI, Hood LJ, Morlet T, et al. Absent or elevated middle ear muscle reflexes in the presence of normal otoacoustic emissions: a universal finding in 136 cases of auditory neuropathy/dys-synchrony. J Am Acad Audiol 2005;16:546–53.
5. Hood LJ, Berlin CI, Bordelon J, et al. Patients with auditory neuropathy/dys-synchrony lack efferent suppression of transient evoked otoacoustic emissions. J Am Acad Audiol 2003;14:302–13.
6. Starr A, Sininger YS, Pratt H. The varieties of auditory neuropathy. J Basic Clin Physiol Pharmacol 2000;11:215–30.
7. Berlin CI, Hood LJ, Morlet T, et al. Multi-site diagnosis and management of 260 patients with auditory neuropathy/dys-synchrony (auditory neuropathy spectrum disorder). Int J Audiol 2010;49:30–43.
8. Zeng FG, Oba S, Garde S, et al. Temporal and speech processing deficits in auditory neuropathy. Neuroreport 1999;10:3429–35.
9. Berlin CI, Hood LJ, Morlet T, et al. The search for auditory neuropathy patients and connexin 26 patients in schools for the Deaf. ARO Abstr 2000;23:23.
10. Lee JS, McPherson B, Yuen KC, et al. Screening for auditory neuropathy in a school for hearing impaired children. Int J Pediatr Otolaryngol 2001;61:39–46.

11. Rance G, Beer DE, Cone-Wesson B, et al. Clinical findings for a group of infants and young children with auditory neuropathy. Ear Hear 1999;20:238–52.
12. Sininger YS. Auditory neuropathy in infants and children: implications for early hearing detection and intervention programs. Audiology Today 2002;14:16–21.
13. Ngo RY, Tan HK, Balakrishnan A, et al. Auditory neuropathy/auditory dys-synchrony detected by universal newborn hearing screening. Int J Pediatr Otorhinolaryngol 2006;70:1299–306.
14. Kirkim G, Serbetcioglu B, Erdag TK, et al. The frequency of auditory neuropathy detected by universal newborn hearing screening program. Int J Pediatr Otorhinolaryngol 2008;72:1461–9.
15. Berg AL, Spitzer SB, Towers HM, et al. Newborn hearing screening in the NICU: profile of failed auditory brainstem response/passed otoacoustic emission. Pediatrics 2005;116:933–8.
16. Rea PA, Gibson WP. Evidence for surviving outer hair cell function in congenitally deaf ears. Laryngoscope 2003;113:2030–4.
17. Santarelli R, Arslan E. Electrocochleography in auditory neuropathy. Hear Res 2002;170:32–47.
18. Stein LK, Tremblay K, Pasternak J, et al. Auditory brainstem neuropathy and elevated bilirubin levels. Sem Hear 1996;17:197–213.
19. Gorga MP, Stelmachowicz PG, Barlow SM, et al. Case of recurrent, reversible, sudden sensorineural hearing loss in a child. J Am Acad Audiol 1995;6:163–72.
20. Kaga K, Nakamura M, Shinogami M, et al. Auditory nerve disease of both ears revealed by auditory brainstem responses, electrocochleography and otoacoustic emissions. Scand Audiol 1996;25:233–8.
21. Rance G, Barker E, Mok M, et al. Speech perception in noise for children with auditory neuropathy/dys-synchrony type hearing loss. Ear Hear 2007;28:351–60.
22. Amatuzzi MG, Northrop C, Liberman MC, et al. Selective inner hair cell loss in premature infants and cochlea pathological patterns from neonatal intensive care unit autopsies. Arch Otolaryngol Head Neck Surg 2001;127:629–36.
23. Shirane M, Harrison RV. The effects of hypoxia on sensory cells of the cochlea in the chinchilla. Scanning Microsc 1987;1:1175–83.
24. Takeno S, Harrison RV, Mount RJ, et al. Induction of selective inner hair cell damage by carboplatin. Scanning Microsc 1994;8:97–106.
25. Merchant SN, McKenna MJ, Nadol JB Jr, et al. Temporal bone histopathologic and genetic studies in Mohr-Tranebjaerg syndrome (DFN-1). Otol Neurotol 2001;22:506–11.
26. Santarelli R. Information from cochlear potentials and genetic mutations helps localize the lesion site in auditory neuropathy. Genome Med 2010;2:91–100.
27. McMahon CM, Patuzzi RB, Gibson WP, et al. Frequency-specific electrocochleography indicates that presynaptic and postsynaptic mechanisms of auditory neuropathy exist. Ear Hear 2008;29:314–25.
28. Stuermer KJ, Beutner D, Foerst A, et al. Electrocochleography in children with auditory synaptopathy/neuropathy: diagnostic findings and characteristic parameters. Int J Pediatr Otorhinolaryngol 2015;79:139–45.
29. Yasunaga S, Grati M, Cohen-Salmon M, et al. A mutation in *OTOF*, encoding otoferlin, A FER-1-like protein, causes DFNB9, a nonsyndromic form of deafness. Nat Genet 1999;21:362–9.
30. Varga R, Kelley PM, Keats BJ, et al. Non-syndromic recessive auditory neuropathy is the results of mutations in the otoferlin (*OTOF*) gene. J Med Genet 2003;40:45–50.

31. Rodríguez-Ballesteros M, Reynoso R, Olarte M, et al. A multicenter study on the prevalence and spectrum of mutations in the otoferlin gene (*OTOF*) in subjects with nonsyndromic hearing impairment and auditory neuropathy. Hum Mut 2008;29:823–31.

32. Starr A, Sininger Y, Winter M, et al. Transient deafness due to temperature-sensitive auditory neuropathy. Ear Hear 1998;19:169–79.

33. Marlin S, Feldmann D, Nguyen Y, et al. Temperature-sensitive auditory neuropathy associated with an otoferlin mutation: deafening fever! Biochem Biophys Res Commun 2010;394:737–42.

34. Butinar D, Zidar J, Leonardis L, et al. Hereditary auditory, vestibular, motor, and sensory neuropathy in a Slovenian Roma (Gypsy) kindred. Ann Neurol 1999;46: 36–44.

35. Buchman CA, Roush PA, Teagle HF, et al. Auditory neuropathy characteristics in children with cochlear nerve deficiency. Ear Hear 2006;27:399–408.

36. Roche JP, Huang BY, Castillo M, et al. Imaging characteristics of children with auditory neuropathy spectrum disorder. Otol Neurotol 2010;31:780–8.

37. Levi J, Ames J, Bacik K, et al. Clinical characteristics of children with cochlear nerve dysplasias. Laryngoscope 2013;123:752–6.

38. Teagle HF, Roush PA, Woodard JS, et al. Cochlear implantation in children with auditory neuropathy spectrum disorder. Ear Hear 2010;31:325–35.

39. Morlet T, O'Reilly R, Morlet S. Enlarged vestibular aqueduct in infants and children: what is the appropriate test battery? NHS meeting. Como (Italy), June 19–21, 2008.

40. Ahmmed A, Brockbank C, Adshead J. Cochlear microphonics in sensorineural hearing loss: lesson from newborn hearing screening. Int J Pediatr Otorhinolaryngol 2008;72:1281–5.

41. Joint Committee on Infant Hearing. Year 2007 position statement: principles and guidelines for early hearing detection and intervention programs. Pediatrics 2007;120:898–921.

42. Attias J, Raveh E. Transient deafness in young candidates for cochlear implants. Audiol Neurotol 2007;12:325–33.

43. Dowley AC, Whitehouse WP, Mason SM, et al. Auditory neuropathy: unexpectedly common in a screening newborn population. Dev Med Child Neurol 2009;51: 642–6.

44. Mohammadi A, Walker P, Gardner-Berry K. Unilateral auditory neuropathy spectrum disorder: retrocochlear lesion in disguise? J Laryngol Otol 2015;129:S38–44.

45. Chermak GD. Deciphering auditory processing disorders in children. Otolaryngol Clin North Am 2002;35:733–49.

46. Berlin CI, Li L, Hood LJ, et al. Auditory neuropathy/dys-synchrony: after the diagnosis, then what? Sem Hear 2002;23:209–14.

47. Gardner-Berry K, Purdy SC, Ching TYC, et al. The audiological journey and early outcomes of twelve infants with auditory neuropathy spectrum disorder from birth to two years of age. Int J Audiol 2015;54:524–35.

48. He S, Grose JH, Teagle HF, et al. Acoustically evoked auditory change complex in children with auditory neuropathy spectrum disorder: a potential objective tool for identifying cochlear implant candidates. Ear Hear 2015;36:289–301.

49. Raveh E, Buller N, Badrana O, et al. Auditory neuropathy: clinical characteristics and therapeutic approach. Am J Otol 2007;28:302–8.

50. Rance G, Barker EJ. Speech and language outcomes in children with auditory neuropathy/dys-synchrony managed with either cochlear implants or hearing aids. Int J Audiol 2009;48:313–20.

51. Ching TY, Day J, Dillon H, et al. Impact of the presence of auditory neuropathy spectrum disorder (ANSD) on outcomes of children at three years of age. Int J Audiol 2013;52:S55–64.

52. Roush P, Frymark T, Venediktov R, et al. Audiologic management of auditory neuropathy spectrum disorder in children: a systematic review of the literature. Am J Audiol 2011;20:159–70.

53. Hood LJ, Wilensky D, Li L, et al. The role of FM technology in the management of patients with auditory neuropathy/dys-synchrony. Chicago: Proc Int Conf FM Technology; 2004.

54. Trautwein P, Sininger Y, Nelson R. Cochlear implantation of auditory neuropathy. J Am Acad Audiol 2000;11:309–15.

55. Peterson A, Shallop J, Driscoll C, et al. Outcomes of cochlear implantation in children with auditory neuropathy. J Am Acad Audiol 2003;14:188–201.

56. Zeng FG, Liu S. Speech perception in individuals with auditory neuropathy. J Speech Lang Hear Res 2006;49:367–80.

57. Breneman AI, Gifford RH, Dejong MD. Cochlear implantation in children with auditory neuropathy spectrum disorder: long-term outcomes. J Am Acad Audiol 2012;23:5–17.

58. Budenz CL, Starr K, Arnedt C, et al. Speech and language outcomes of cochlear implantation in children with isolated auditory neuropathy versus cochlear hearing loss. Otol Neurotol 2013;34:1615–21.

59. Walton J, Gibson WP, Sanli H, et al. Predicting cochlear implant outcomes in children with auditory neuropathy. Otol Neurotol 2008;29:302–9.

Genetics of Hearing Loss

Syndromic

Tal Koffler, MSc, Kathy Ushakov, MSc, Karen B. Avraham, PhD*

KEYWORDS

- Deafness • Hearing loss • Genetics • Genome • Sequencing

KEY POINTS

- Syndromic hearing loss (SHL) is a form of hearing loss (HL) accompanied by additional clinical features in the visual, nervous system, endocrine, and other systems. The most prevalent syndromes are Usher, Waardenburg, and Pendred.
- Genetic diagnostics can detect pathogenic variants and provide an answer regarding the cause of the HL, as well as the associated clinical symptoms of the SHL, to care for patients.
- Linkage analysis with DNA markers and polymerase chain reaction diagnostics is often used to detect these variants in clinical settings. High-throughput sequencing methods, focusing on specific genes, the exons of genes, or the entire genome of a patient, are moving into the clinic to provide more cost-effective and efficient methods for diagnostics.

INTRODUCTION

Hearing loss (HL) is the most prevalent sensory impairment in both childhood and adulthood.[1,2] According to the last update of the World Health Organization (WHO), approximately 360 million people worldwide, equaling 5% of the world's population, have a disabling HL (**Table 1**). Most of these people live in low- and middle-income countries where treatments for HL are more difficult to obtain and consanguinity increases the risk of recessive disease. HL is an etiologically heterogeneous pathology caused by different genetic and environmental factors, with half of the cases estimated to be genetic.[3] HL can also be a result of infections, injuries, and exposure to excessive noise.

Disclosures: None.

Research in the K.B. Avraham laboratory is supported by the National Institutes of Health (NIH)/NIDCD R01DC011835, I-CORE Gene Regulation in Complex Human Disease Center No. 41/11, Israel Science Foundation 1320/11, Human Frontier Science Program RGP0012/2012, and United States-Israel Binational Science Foundation (BSF) 2013027.

Department of Human Molecular Genetics and Biochemistry, Sackler Faculty of Medicine and Sagol School of Neuroscience, Tel Aviv University, Tel Aviv 6997801, Israel

* Corresponding author. Department of Human Molecular Genetics, Sackler Faculty of Medicine, Room 1003, Tel Aviv 6997801, Israel.

E-mail address: karena@post.tau.ac.il

Abbreviations

ASHA	American Speech-Language-Hearing Association
ATP	Adenosine triphosphate
BOR	Branchio-oto-renal
bp	Base pair
CHARGE	Coloboma, heart defect, atresia choanae, retarded growth and development, genital hypoplasia, ear anomalies/deafness syndrome
DFN	Deafness
DFNA	Nonsyndromic deafness, autosomal dominant
DFNB	Nonsyndromic deafness autosomal recessive
DFNX	Nonsyndromic deafness, X-linked
HARS	Histidyl tRNA synthetase
HL	Hearing loss
IHC	Inner hair cell
JLNS	Jervell and Lange-Nielsen syndrome
MPS	Massive parallel sequencing
NGS	Next-generation sequencing
NIDCD	National Institute on Deafness and Other Communication Disorders
NSHL	Nonsyndromic hearing loss
OHC	Outer hair cell
OMIM	Online Mendelian Inheritance in Man
PCR	Polymerase chain reaction
PRLTS1	Perrault syndrome 1
SHL	Syndromic hearing loss
SNHL	Sensorineural hearing loss
SNP	Single nucleotide polymorphism
SNV	Single nucleotide variant
STL1	Type I Stickler syndrome
UCSC	University of California, Santa Cruz
USH1, 2, 3	Usher syndrome 1, 2, 3
WES	Whole-exome sequencing
WGS	Whole-genome sequencing
WHO	World Health Organization
WS1, 2, 3, 4	Waardenburg syndrome 1, 2, 3, 4

HEARING LOSS

Our ability to hear is orchestrated by the auditory system. The vestibular system is responsible for balance, 3-dimensional orientation, and gravity perception. The ear is a 3-chambered organ divided into the external, the middle, and the inner ear, which are all essential for the intact activity of the auditory and the vestibular systems. The external and middle ear are responsible for collecting and conducting the sound wave's energy to the inner ear.[4,5] The sensorineural end organ of hearing is the snail-shaped organ of Corti that resides in the inner ear. It is composed of a single row of inner hair cell (IHC), 3 rows of outer hair cells (OHCs), and supporting cells. The IHC act as sensory transducers, capturing stimulus energy, interpreting it as electrical responses and sending the impulses to the brain through the auditory nerve. The OHCs are responsible for enhancing the signal.[6]

According to the American Speech-Language-Hearing Association (ASHA) (see **Table 1**), normal hearing occurs in the range of −10 to 15 dB, with a slight HL if the range of loss is within 16 to 25 dB. Mild HL occurs when the HL ranges between 26 and 40 dB; moderate HL is when the HL ranges between 41 and 55 dB; moderate to severe HL ranges between 56 and 70 dB. Individuals with HL in these ranges are considered to be hard of hearing and can benefit from hearing aids and assistive

Table 1 Informative Web sites for SHL	
WHO	http://www.who.int/topics/deafness/en/
ASHA	http://www.asha.org/public/hearing/Degree-of-Hearing-Loss/
NIDCD	http://www.nidcd.nih.gov/health/statistics/Pages/quick.aspx
Hereditary Hearing Loss Homepage	http://hereditaryhearingloss.org/
Deafness Variation database	http://deafnessvariationdatabase.org/
Leiden Open Variation Database	http://grenada.lumc.nl/LOVD2/WS/
Genetics Home Reference	http://ghr.nlm.nih.gov/
Online Mendelian Inheritance in Man	http://www.ncbi.nlm.nih.gov/omim/
UCSC Genome Browser	https://genome.ucsc.edu/
Genome Reference Consortium	http://www.ncbi.nlm.nih.gov/projects/genome/assembly/grc/
GATK	https://www.broadinstitute.org/gatk/
GenVec	http://www.genvec.com/product-pipeline/cgf-166-hearing-loss

Abbreviations: ASHA, American Speech-Language-Hearing Association; GATK, Genome Analysis Toolkit; NIDCD, National Institute on Deafness and Other Communication Disorders; UCSC, University of California, Santa Cruz.

listening devices. With severe or profound HL, one is considered to be deaf, when HL ranges between 71 and 90 dB in the former case or profound when the HL range is greater than 91 dB. Individuals with this kind of HL may benefit only from cochlear implants.[7]

HL is the most common neurosensory disorder in humans. It can be a congenital, caused by genetic factors or by complications during pregnancy and childbirth. It can also be acquired later in life, at any age. Acquired HL can be caused by infectious diseases, physical injuries, the use of ototoxic drugs, and genetic pathogenic variants or mutations. Congenital HL is the most commonly occurring condition for which new-borns are screened for, with about 1 out of 1000 infants born affected.

Nearly 1 in 5 individuals aged 12 years and older suffer from unilateral or bilateral HL in the United States alone.[8] Age-related HL is the most prevalent sensory deficit in the elderly,[9] with nearly 25% of those aged 65 to 74 years and 50% of those who are aged 75 years and older suffering from a disabling HL in the United States alone, according to the National Institute on Deafness and Other Communication Disorders (NIDCD; see **Table 1**). Half of the HL cases are estimated to be genetically related[3] and account for about 50% to 60% of childhood HL cases in developed countries.[2] Over the years, more than 100 deafness-related loci and their associated genes have been identified and studied, revealing the genetic basis of different deafness-related pathologies.[10]

The diversity of ear disease pathologies is classified according to the cause of the case, which can be genetically related or from environmental causes. If the pathology is genetically related, it is further classified according to the pattern of inheritance (dominant, recessive, X-linked or Y-linked). HL is also classified according to the onset of the pathology, the type, the severity, unilateral or bilateral, and the association with other disorders as syndromic HL (SHL) versus non-SHL (NSHL).[11]

For NSHL, HL loci are classified and named according to their mode of inheritance, with a prefix of *DFN* (for *deafness*) (Hereditary Hearing Loss Homepage; see **Table 1**).

DFNA refers to autosomal dominant inheritance; DFNB refers to autosomal recessive inheritance; and DFNX refers to an X-linked mode of inheritance. Furthermore, Y-chromosome–linked genes and maternal inheritance linked to mitochondria have also been identified.[12] Each locus name also contains a number that represents the order in which these loci were identified in association with deafness. In many cases, the genes for the DFN loci have subsequently been identified[13] (Hereditary Hearing Loss Homepage, Deafness Variation Database; see **Table 1**).

As HL is one of the most common birth defects in developed countries, newborn screening for hearing defects has an important role in treatment and rehabilitation strategies, such as cochlear implantation.[14] The early diagnosis of the cause of a child's HL can allow the monitoring of possible complications and can indicate which therapy is the most suitable and effective one. It also allows for more accurate genetic counseling for parents who want to have more children.[10]

SYNDROMIC HEARING LOSS

SHL is a form of HL accompanied by additional clinical features. Approximately 30% of the genetic cases of HL are considered to be syndromic.[11] SHL consists of HL that presents with anomalies of the eye, kidney, the musculoskeletal and the nervous systems, as well as pigmentary disorders and others[15] (**Fig. 1**). Among the well-known syndromes are Usher, Waardenburg, and Pendred. Of these syndromes, Pendred and Usher syndromes are the most common.[10] Several genes associated with SHL (**Fig. 2**) are also involved with NSHL, as in the case of *SLC26A4* mutations leading to Pendred syndrome and DFNB4.[10] The genes associated with SHL are represented in **Table 1** and **Fig. 1**.

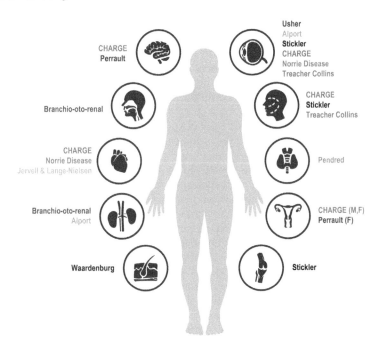

Fig. 1. Different organs are involved in the clinical symptoms of patients with SHL in addition to the phenotype in the inner ear. The organs affected in each syndrome are indicated. F, female genitals; M, male genitals.

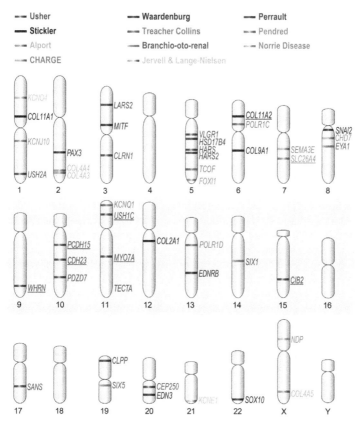

Fig. 2. The chromosomal location of genes associated with SHL. The genes are color coded according to the syndrome they are associated with. The genes associated with both SHL and NSHL are underlined. (*Adapted from* Dror AA, Avraham KB. Hearing impairment: a panoply of genes and functions. Neuron 2010;68:295; with permission.)

FORMS OF SYNDROMIC HEARING LOSS
Usher Syndrome

The eye and the ear are the sensory organs responsible for vision, balance, and hearing in mammals. These organs are essential for both communication and environmental perception.[16,17] Diseases affecting the inner ear and retina of the eye can cause major impairments for human communication systems. Syndromes that include symptoms of both blindness and hearing impairment are widely known. In humans, there are approximately 40 syndromes that include both impairments; about half of the affected cases are caused by mutations attributed to Usher syndrome.[18] Usher syndrome is an autosomal recessive genetic disease with clinically and genetically heterogeneous characteristics. In humans, it is defined by congenital, bilateral deafness and a later onset of vision impairment caused by retinitis pigmentosa.[16] Epidemiologic studies have estimated that the prevalence of Usher syndrome ranges from 1 per 6000 to 1 per 10,000.[19,20] Usher syndrome is subclassified into 3 clinical types, USH1, USH2, and USH3, based on the severity of the sensorineural HL (SNHL), the presence or absence of vestibular dysfunction, and the age at onset of retinitis pigmentosa. Patients with USH1 have severe to profound congenital bilateral

HL accompanied by congenital vestibular dysfunction. In terms of retinitis pigmentosa symptoms, night blindness may be detected during childhood, followed by a narrowing of the visual field, which progresses to severe blindness.[16,21] Patients with USH2 have moderate to severe congenital HL with no vestibular abnormalities. Retinitis pigmentosa is usually diagnosed between 10 and 40 years of age.[22] In patients with USH3, hearing impairment begins before the third decade of life and is characterized by variable progression. In most cases, patients eventually become profoundly deaf. Vestibular defects are variable, and retinitis pigmentosa usually begins from 20 years of age.[22] Early symptoms of retinitis pigmentosa are night blindness and loss of peripheral vision. This form of Usher syndrome is the least common in the general population[23] but is more prevalent in the Finnish and Ashkenazi Jewish populations.[24,25]

To date, 16 independent loci on different chromosomes are known to be associated with Usher syndrome. These loci are further divided into *USH1A-G*, *USH2A-C*, and *USH3A*. Moreover, 13 genes have been identified. The *USH1* genes are *MYO7A* for the *USH1B* locus, encoding the motor protein myosin VIIA.[26] *USH1C* encodes harmonin[27,28] and *USH1G* encodes SANS,[29] both of which are scaffold proteins. *CDH23* mutations are responsible for USH1D, which encodes cadherin 23,[30] *PCDH15* mutations lead to USH1F and encodes protocadherin 15,[31] both of which are cell adhesion molecules. *CIB2* mutations are the cause of USH1J, which encodes calcium and integrin-binding protein 2.[32] The *USH2* genes are *USH2A*, encoding usherin[33] and *ADGRV1* for USH2C, encoding adhesion G protein–coupled receptor VI, also referred to as *GPCR98* or *VLGR1*.[34,35] Both genes are transmembrane proteins that are involved in signaling. Another gene associated with USH2 is *WHRN*, encoding whirlin for USH2D.[36] The *USH3* genes are *CLRN1* for USH3A, encoding clarin 1, and *HARS* (histidyl tRNA synthetase).[24,37–39] Moreover, another 2 Usher syndrome genes have recently been identified. *PDZD7* encodes the protein PDZ domain containing 7 and *CEP250* encodes centrosome-associated protein 250. Usher syndrome has recently been proposed to be an oligogenic disease because of the digenic inheritance of *PDZD7* and *USH2A* or *ADGRV1* in patients with Usher syndrome. Two genes have been proposed to lead to variable phenotypes of Usher syndrome, depending on the dosage. *CEP250* is associated with early onset HL and severe retinitis pigmentosa in conjunction with 2 mutant alleles of *C2orf71*. The patients have mild HL and retinal degeneration with one mutant allele of *C2or71*.[40,41] *C2orf71* mutations are associated with retinitis pigmentosa and proposed to encode a ciliary protein.[42] Importantly, many of the genes listed earlier have been reported to cause NSHL (see **Fig. 1**). For example, different mutations in *MYO7A* are known to cause recessive deafness DFNB2 and dominant deafness DFNA11.[43,44]

Waardenburg Syndrome

Waardenburg syndrome was considered to be an autosomal dominant inherited disease of the neural crest cells, but this syndrome is more clinically and genetically heterogeneous than originally known.[45] Waardenburg syndrome is characterized mostly by SNHL and pigmentation abnormalities that can occur in the eyes, hair, skin, and the cochlear stria vascularis. Other features can be found in a subset of patients. These features are used for clinical classification of the syndrome. Waardenburg syndrome is estimated to have a prevalence of 1 per 42,000 and is responsible for 1% to 3% of all congenital HL cases.[45] During embryonic development, the pluripotent neural crest cells migrate from the neural tube and give rise to different cell types, among them melanocytes of the skin and inner ear, glia, neurons of the peripheral and enteric nervous systems, and some of the skeletal tissue. The symptoms associated with Waardenburg syndrome result from an abnormal proliferation, survival, and migration or differentiation of neural crest-derived melanocytes.[45] Waardenburg syndrome is subdivided into 4 subtypes, WS1, WS2, WS3, and WS4, by the presence or absence of additional symptoms.[46] WS1 is further characterized by dystopia canthorum, an appearance of wide-set eyes caused by a prominent broad nasal root, whereas WS2 has no further significant features. WS1 and WS2 are the most frequent among the 4 subtypes. WS3 is further characterized by dystopia canthorum and musculoskeletal abnormalities of the upper limbs. WS4 is associated with Hirschsprung disease, characterized by a blockage of the large intestine caused by improper muscular bowel movement and neurologic defects. Neurologic features were also observed in a subset of patients with WS2.[47] Among the symptoms of this syndrome, the SNHL is the most frequent one, with 60% in WS1 to 90% in WS2.[48] Six genes are associated with this syndrome: paired box 3 (*PAX3*),[49] microphthalmia-associated transcription factor (*MITF*),[50] endothelin receptor type B (*EDNBR*),[51] endothelin 3 (*EDN3*),[52] SRY box10 (*SOX10*),[53] and snail homolog 2 (*SNAI2*).[54] These genes are known to be involved in the regulation of melanocyte differentiation.[45] A database for the Waardenburg syndrome–associated genes can be found at the Leiden Open Variation Database (see **Table 1**).

Pendred Syndrome

Pendred syndrome is one of the most common autosomal recessive syndromic causes of HL. The audiological phenotype is quite broad, ranging from mild to profound, and can be congenital or with a later onset and be progressive.[55] A common feature among patients is an enlarged vestibular aqueduct, a common radiological malformation of the inner ear. In addition to SNHL, patients who have this syndrome also show features of congenital and severe to profound temporal bone abnormalities, in addition to goiter partial iodine organification defects resulting in a positive perchlorate discharge test from the goiter, usually in late childhood to early adulthood. Pendred syndrome also features thyroid dysfunction, ranging from euthyroid to hypothyroidism,[56,57] and vestibular dysfunction, demonstrated in approximately 65% of affected individuals. The vestibular dysfunction can range from mild unilateral canal paresis to gross bilateral absence of function.[58]

The estimated prevalence of Pendred syndrome is 7.5 per 100,000 newborns and it accounts for approximately 1% to 8% of the cases of congenital deafness.[59] Approximately half of the Pendred syndrome cases are caused by a mutation in one of 3 genes. *SLC26A4*, encoding the protein pendrin, is an iodide-chloride transporter. Mutations in this gene are responsible for both Pendred syndrome and DFNB4, a form of NSHL. Pendrin is expressed in the kidneys, the inner ear, and thyroid.[59] Approximately 50% Pendred syndrome–affected individuals have a mutation in this gene (Genetics Home Reference, see **Table 1**). Less than 2% of the rest of the affected individuals have mutations in *FOXI1* encoding Forkhead box protein I1 or *KCNJ10* encoding the ATP-sensitive inward rectifier potassium channel 10.[58] More than 280 *SLC26A4*-Pendred syndrome and DFNB4-causing mutations have been identified; but in different ethnic groups, unique pathogenic alleles are found more frequently than others, reflecting a few prevalent founder mutations.[58]

Additional Syndromes

In addition to the aforementioned syndromes, there are more than 700 genetic syndromes that have been described with features of hearing impairment.[15] Alport syndrome is characterized by renal defects, SNHL, and ocular abnormalities[60] with a prevalence of 1 in 50,000 (Genetics Home Reference). Three genes are associated with this syndrome: *COL4A3* encoding collagen, type IV, alpha 3, and *COL4A4* encoding collagen, type IV, alpha 4 for the autosomal inherited types[61,62] and *COL4A5* encoding collagen, type IV, alpha 5 for the X-linked type.[63]

Branchio-oto-renal (BOR) syndrome is an autosomal dominant disease, characterized by defects in the development of the tissues in the neck and malformations of the ear and kidney.[64] It is estimated that the prevalence of this syndrome is 1 in 40,000 (Genetics Home Reference). Approximately 40% of the individuals affected test positive for mutations in the *EYA1* gene encoding the eyes absent homolog 1. An additional 5% and 4% of affected individuals have a mutation in *SIX5* encoding the homeobox protein SIX5 and *SIX1* encoding the homeobox protein SIX1, respectively.[64]

CHARGE syndrome is an autosomal dominant syndrome that features coloboma, heart defect, atresia choanae, retarded growth and development, genital hypoplasia, ear anomalies/deafness. It is estimated that the prevalence of CHARGE syndrome is 1 in 8500 to 10,000 individuals (Genetics Home Reference). This syndrome is mostly caused by mutations in the *CHD7* gene encoding Chromodomain-helicase-DNA-binding protein 7, an ATP-dependent chromatin remodeling protein.[65]

Jervell and Lange-Nielsen syndrome is an autosomal recessive disease with features of arrhythmia, SNHL, and a significantly higher risk of fainting and sudden death as a result of prolongation of the corrected QT interval.[66] This syndrome is estimated to affect 1.6 to 6.0 per 1,000,000 people worldwide, with a higher frequency in Denmark (Genetics Home Reference; see **Table 1**). The genes associated with this syndrome are *KCNQ1* encoding the potassium channel, voltage-gated KQT-like subfamily Q, member 1 and *KCNE1* encoding potassium channel, and voltage-gated subfamily E regulatory beta subunit 1.[66–68] Approximately 90% of the cases are caused by a mutation in the *KCNQ1* gene, with the rest of the cases caused by mutations in *KCNE1*.[69,70]

Norrie disease is characterized by a spectrum of fibrous vascular changes of the retina at birth that progresses to visual impairment with age. About 30 to 50% of males with Norrie disease have developmental delays or other forms of intellectual disability, behavioral abnormalities, or psychoticlike features. Moreover, most of the males also develop HL. This syndrome is X-linked, recessively inherited, and caused by mutations in the *NDP* gene encoding the norrin protein. Mutations in this gene are responsible for about 95% of the affected individuals.[71] The prevalence of this syndrome is unknown, and it is not associated with any racial or ethnic group (Genetics Home Reference, see **Table 1**).

Stickler syndrome can be both dominant and recessive and is characterized by ocular, skeletal, orofacial, and auditory abnormalities.[72,73] The prevalence of this syndrome is about 1 in 7500 to 1 in 9000 newborns (Genetics Home Reference; see **Table 1**). Stickler syndrome is subdivided into 5 subtypes based on its underlying genetic collagen defect. For the autosomal dominant form of Stickler syndrome, 3 genes have been identified. Type I Stickler syndrome (STL1) is associated with mutations in *COL2A1* encoding collagen, type II, alpha-1.[74] Moreover, mutations in *COL11A1* encoding collagen, type XI, alpha-1 are associated with type II (STL2)[75] and mutations in *COL11A2* encoding collagen, type XI, alpha-2 are associated with type III (STL3).[76] The autosomal recessive forms of Stickler syndrome are STL4 and STL5; their identified related genes are *COL9A1* encoding collagen, type IX, alpha-1 and *COL9A2* encoding collagen, type IX, alpha-2, respectively.[77,78] There is a degree of variability in HL frequency and severity in the different types of this syndrome, even within the same family.[79]

Treacher-Collins syndrome is usually an autosomal dominant syndrome that affects the development of the bones and other tissues of the face. These abnormalities contribute to speech and language difficulties, visual impairment, conductive HL, and breathing difficulties. The symptoms of this syndrome can range from undetectable to severe. Half of the affected individuals have HL caused by defects of the 3 bones of the middle ear or defects in the development of the ear canal. One in 50,000 people will have this syndrome (Genetics Home Reference; see **Table 1**), caused by mutations in 3 genes: *TCOF1* encoding the treacle protein, *POLR1C* encoding polymerase I polypeptide C, and POLR1D encoding polymerase I polypeptide D. Most patients have a mutation in *TCOF1*, with 1% of the cases caused by a recessive form of this syndrome, with mutations in *POLR1C*.[80]

Perrault syndrome is an autosomal recessive disease characterized by SNHL in both sexes and ovarian dysfunction in females. The HL symptoms are bilateral and range from moderate with early childhood onset to profound at birth. Moreover, the early childhood form can be progressive. The ovarian dysfunction symptoms can also vary; affected females also show, in some cases, neurologic features, such as developmental delay and cerebellar ataxia. Less than 100 affected individuals have been documented (Genetics Home Reference; see **Table 1**), most probably because of the difficulties in diagnosis. Four genes have been associated with this syndrome: *HARS2* encoding histidyl-tRNA synthetase 2, HSD17B4 encoding hydroxysteroid (17-beta) dehydrogenase 4, LARS2 encoding leucyl-tRNA synthetase 2, and CLPP encoding the caseinolytic mitochondrial matrix peptidase proteolytic subunit. This syndrome is subdivided into 4 types: type I, II, III, and IV, also called PRLTS1, 2, 3, and 4, respectively. The classification of the subtypes is determined according to the neurologic involvement and its state, progressive or nonprogressive. This classification is now being reconsidered, as mutations in *CLPP* were found to include both types of cases, with or without neurologic symptoms.[81] The clinical features and the molecular genetic information of these syndromes are comprehensively described in the Online Mendelian Inheritance in Man (OMIM) database (see **Table 1**).

GENETICS OF HEARING LOSS

Single-gene disorders may be inherited in an autosomal recessive or dominant mode, carried on the X-chromosome, or inherited through the mitochondria. Each form of inheritance may have implications for the number of children to manifest the disease in each case or whether one or both sexes will be affected. As a result, an accurate and thorough family history is essential on examining patients.

Diseases inherited in a recessive manner are often the most severe in nature and are expressed at birth (congenital) or soon thereafter. As recessive inheritance skips a generation, and depends on 2 carriers of the pathogenic variant, there is often no family history in patients with a recessively inherited disease (**Fig. 3**A). In other cases, multiply affected patients in every other generation are very clear signs of recessive diseases (see **Fig. 3**B). Consanguinity, whereby parents are related, may increase the incidence of recessive disease and is more prevalent in regions of the world such as the Middle East, India, and Pakistan (see **Fig. 3**A, B). Both females and males are affected in equal proportions. Many forms of SHL are inherited in a recessive manner, including Jervell and Lange syndrome, Usher syndrome, Pendred syndrome, Perrault syndrome, and some forms of Alport and Waardenburg syndrome (**Table 2**).

Dominant inheritance tends to involve the onset of the disease phenotype later in life and may be less severe than recessively inherited diseases (see **Fig. 3**C). Only one parent needs to carry the pathogenic variant and is also affected by the disease. Complications in diagnosis may arise because of reduced penetrance, whereby a patient harbors the genotype but not the phenotype of the disease.

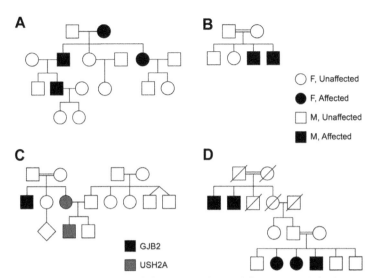

Fig. 3. Representative pedigrees of families with HL. (*A*) Recessive inheritance with no previous family history. After biallelic variants were found in the child, the parents were each found to be carriers of the variant, validating the recessive pattern of inheritance. (*B*) Recessive inheritance with family history. The family represented in the pedigree presented with symptoms of USH1, with 5 affected individuals. The chromosomal critical region was defined by the use of microsatellite DNA markers, pinpointing the locus to chromosome 15q22.[85] Several years later, *CIB2* was found to be the pathogenic variant responsible for this new form of Usher syndrome, USH1J.[32] (*C*) Dominant inheritance, with an affected individual in 3 out of 4 generations, which may be observed for Waardenburg syndrome with a *PAX3, SNAI2,* or *MITF* mutation. (*D*) A family with both SHL and NSHL. Two patients have USH2, with pathogenic variants in the *USH2A* gene. One patient has NSHL caused by biallelic pathogenic variants in the *GJB2* gene.[110] (*Data from* Refs.[32,85,110])

It is important to note that several syndromes may be inherited in either a recessive or dominant fashion, depending on the gene and variant involved. Furthermore, families may harbor mutations in more than one gene, leading to the presence of more than one disease in an extended family (see **Fig. 3**D).

A more complex scenario arises because of the oligogenic nature of some diseases. It has become clearer in recent years that the phenotype of patients, even with what seems to be a single-gene disorder, may be caused by multiple variants. An example is described earlier for Usher syndrome.[40,41]

DIAGNOSIS OF HEARING LOSS

Screening and identifying the cause of HL is extremely important to provide the best opportunities for care and rehabilitation in children. The introduction of newborn screening for HL in developed countries has led to earlier diagnosis and improvement in ascertainment and potential outcomes,[82] as treatment strategies are examined and applied sooner. Determining the cause of HL is even more crucial in cases of SHL, as the associated clinical features are usually more severe.[10] Early diagnosis can help predict the progression of the HL in patients and the prescribed course of action in treating patients as well as provide warnings for future potentially life-threatening abnormalities.

Table 2
SHL-associated genes

Syndrome	Gene	Protein	OMIM Entry
Alport syndrome	COL4A5	Collagen, type IV, alpha 5	303630
	COL4A3	Collagen, type IV, alpha 3	120070
	COL4A4	Collagen, type IV, alpha 4	120131
BOR syndrome	EYA1	Eyes absent homolog 1	601653
	SIX5	Homeobox protein SIX5	600963
	SIX1	Homeobox protein SIX1	601205
CHARGE syndrome	SEMA3E	Semaphorin 3E	608166
	CHD7	Chromodomain-helicase-DNA-binding protein 7	608892
Jervell & Lange-Nielsen syndrome	KCNQ1	Potassium channel, voltage-gated KQT-like subfamily Q, member 1	607542
	KCNE1	Potassium channel, voltage-gated subfamily E regulatory beta subunit 1	176261
Norrie disease	NDP	Norrie disease protein	300658
Pendred syndrome	SLC26A4	Pendrin	605646
	FOXI1	Forkhead box protein I1	601093
	KCNJ10	ATP-sensitive inward rectifier potassium channel 10	602208
Stickler syndrome	COL2A1	Collagen, type II, alpha-1	120140
	COL11A1	Collagen, type XI, alpha-1	120280
	COL11A2	Collagen, type XI, alpha-2	120290
	COL9A1	Collagen, type IX, alpha-1	120210
	COL9A2	Collagen, type IX, alpha-2	120260
Treacher Collins syndrome	TCOF1	Treacher Collins-Franceschetti syndrome 1	606847
	POLR1D	Polymerase I polypeptide D	613715
	POLR1C	Polymerase I polypeptide C	610060
Usher syndrome	MYO7A	Myosin VIIA	276903
	USH1C	Harmonin	605242
	CDH23	Cadherin 23	605516
	PCDH15	Protocadherin 15	605514
	SANS	Scaffold protein containing ankyrin repeats and sam domain	607696
	CIB2	Calcium and integrin binding protein 2	605564
	USH2A	Usherin	608400
	VLGR1	Very large G-coupled protein receptor isoform b	602851
	WHRN	Whirlin	607928
	CLRN1	Clarin 1	606397
	HARS	Histidyl tRNA synthetase	142810
	PZDZ7	PDZ domain containing 7	NA
	CEP250	Centrosome associated protein 250	NA
Waardenburg syndrome	PAX3	Paired box 3	606567
	SNAI2	Snail homolog 2	602150
	EDN3	Endothelin 3	131242
	EDNRB	Endothelin receptor type B	131244
	MITF	Microphthalmia-associated transcription factor	156845
	SOX10	SRY box10	602229

(continued on next page)

Table 2 (continued)			
Syndrome	Gene	Protein	OMIM Entry
Perrault syndrome	HSD17B4	Hydroxysteroid (17-beta) dehydrogenase 4	601860
	HARS2	Histidyl-tRNA synthetase 2	600783
	CLPP	Caseinolytic mitochondrial matrix peptidase proteolytic subunit	601119
	LARS2	Leucyl-tRNA synthetase 2	604544

Abbreviation: NA, not available.

A continuing challenge in medical genetics has been to determine the cause of each disease. For example, the presence of SLC26A4 mutations in a child may help predict whether the child will develop goiter and hypothyroidism after puberty or be more susceptible to acute HL following head trauma.[10] Patients with Jervell and Lange-Nielsen syndrome will be more sensitive to syncope and are at risk for sudden death.[10] As a result, being aware that a child has a KCNQ1 mutation can be extremely informative for his or her health. Today, mutations in at least 45 genes are known to be associated with SHL, providing an opportunity for patients with these mutations to benefit from this knowledge. Most of these discoveries have only been made in the last 2 decades, and some even more recently. Despite this progress, the underlying genetic cause of hundreds of inherited syndromes is still unknown, and the continuing challenge is to uncover the cause for the affected children and adults.

Identifying Disease Genes Through Linkage Mapping with Genetic Markers

The large size of the genome and the high number of genes it contains made the identification of disease-associated genes a tedious task from a historical perspective. Before the Human Genome Project was completed in 2001,[83] researchers used various techniques for identifying and mapping genes associated with Mendelian and single-gene inherited disorders. Linkage mapping, the most common technique used, was aimed at finding the approximate location of the disease gene relative to a DNA segment with a known chromosomal location, a genetic marker.[84] The process included scanning the genomes of members of an affected family and using highly polymorphic DNA markers to identify regions linked with the disease. The affected family members shared specific variants of the DNA markers more frequently than in the general population, suggesting linkage with the presence of a nearby disease gene. To focus on the disease gene, multiple markers in the linked region were further genotyped to define the critical region. DNA markers were generally in the form of microsatellites, repetitive DNA elements present every 1000 base pair (bp) in the human genome. Their polymorphic nature and presence of multiple alleles in the population rendered these markers to be extremely useful. The most commonly used ones were (CA)n repeats, which could be purchased commercially and could be used for automated genotyping as they were labeled with fluorescent markers. The next generation of DNA markers involved single nucleotide polymorphisms (SNPs). Although they are less polymorphic, having only 2 alleles per SNP, they are more frequent in the genome, at every 100 to 300 bp, and facilitate linkage analysis. As most of the human genes are annotated, examination of the region using genome browsers, such as the University of California, Santa Cruz (UCSC) Genome Browser (see **Table 1**), can provide a list of the genes in the region. The challenge is then to identify the pathogenic variant that leads to the disease under study. Oftentimes there was a gap of years from identification of the chromosomal location of the putative gene, to identification and validation of the pathogenic variant. For example, several families with USH1 from Pakistan were studied by linkage analysis with microsatellite markers.[85] Years later, one of the families in this group was found to harbor a mutation in *CIB2*, defining a new form of Usher syndrome, USH1J (pedigree in **Fig. 3**B). Most genes for SHL were identified in this way.

Validation of the pathogenic variant is subsequently performed using capillary Sanger sequencing, which allows for sequencing of regions of approximately 800 to 1000 bp. A comparison of patients' sequence with unaffected family members can help define the critical variant. However, additional criteria are required for the variant to be defined as the disease causing change in the DNA. Functional analysis, by replicating the variant in cell culture, may help define the pathogenicity further. For example, the *SLC26A4* variant c.1458_1459insT, when replicated in COS7, was mislocalized, providing further evidence that this is a pathogenic variant.[86] Finally, reduction of a particular gene in an animal model can provide the most compelling circumstantial evidence of pathogenicity as well as demonstrate the mechanisms involved. *CIB2*, a candidate for Usher syndrome, was shown to be essential for mechanosensory hair cell function in zebrafish.[32] Gene-targeted mutagenesis of *Slc26a4* in the mouse revealed that pendrin, the protein encoded by this gene, is important for the development of the inner ear and provided an understanding of the cause for deafness in patients with Pendred syndrome.[87] An additional *Slc26a4* mutation in mice, *Slc26a4* [loop/loop], had symptoms of deafness but without the enlarged thyroid gland symptoms that characterizes Pendred syndrome.[88] However, histologic analysis of the thyroid tissue showed morphologic defects and the inner ear showed molecular and morphologic defects consistent with the symptoms seen in patients with disrupted thyroid hormone activity. This study led to the proposal that thyroid hormone deprivation, caused by this *Slc26a4* mutation, contributes to the deafness in this mouse model.

Identifying Disease Genes Through High-Throughput Sequencing

The development of high-throughput sequencing technology has revolutionized both the discovery and diagnosis of pathogenic variants for disease. Massive parallel sequencing (MPS), also known as next-generation sequencing (NGS), enables a more rapid and low-cost method of DNA sequencing. Compared with the traditional capillary or Sanger sequencing, these methods perform large-scale sequencing, generating a billion bases within a single run.[89] The MPS output is aligned to the human reference genome, a consensus representation of the genome (Genome Reference Consortium; see **Table 1**), enabling the identification of differences between the reads of the current genome being sequenced and the reference genome. Bioinformatics tools, such as the Genome Analysis Toolkit software package (see **Table 1**), are next used for detecting the variants, examining whether the variant is unique, the frequency of this variant, and the potential damage of this variant to the protein structure and function. Moreover, the sequence conservation is also examined as well as the mode of inheritance, which should match the one of the disease analyzed. The potential pathogenic variants are then screened for segregation in the affected family. This analysis is less complicated if the variant detected is a known deafness mutation, whereas variants in genes not previously associated with deafness are more challenging to prove.[90]

The development of MPS changed gene sequencing, enabling multiple genomes to be sequenced simultaneously. However, the complexity of genomic analysis for the large number of variants that arise, in particular from noncoding regions of the genome, remains challenging. To circumvent this problem, researchers studying highly heterogeneous diseases, such as Usher syndrome,[91,92] inherited eye diseases,[93] or deafness,[94,95] have screened only for genes already known to be associated with the disease under study. In cases when pathogenic variants are not found using a select number of genes, whole-exome sequencing (WES) becomes the next option. As the costs are decreasing, WES is sometimes the first approach.[96] In this method, only coding exons of genes are sequenced, alleviating the need to analyze noncoding regions, with a substantial savings of cost. Whole-genome sequencing (WGS) has been used for identification of human disease genes in severe cases of neonatal disease.[97] Although considerably more costly, WGS is considered to be the most comprehensive method for detecting all variants, in particular copy number variants that may be involved in disease.[97] Furthermore, linkage analysis, described earlier, may be used in conjunction with WGS to facilitate localization of the pathogenic variant.[97] Overall, currently, NGS technology has a molecular diagnostic success rate of 25%[98] and is predicted to solve the genetic basis of 60% of mendelian inherited disorders in the near future.[99]

The Importance of Genetic Research in Understanding the Processes Involved in Hearing and Deafness

To date there are several different treatments available for hearing impairment. These treatments include amplification of sound using hearing aids and cochlear or auditory brain stem implants that stimulate the cochlear nerve or the nuclei, respectively.[11] Although the physical structure and activity of the ear are well understood, the specific part of the ear that each deafness-associated gene functions in is not fully characterized. Defining the genes and pathways responsible for normal hearing are paving the way toward developing new treatments for hearing impairments. Among the different approaches for newly developed hearing impairment treatments are the regeneration of inner ear sensory cells[100,101] and the use of viral vectors for gene therapy.[102] These potential treatments will be helpful for both genetically and environmentally related HL.[11]

PROSPECTS OF FUTURE TREATMENT MODALITIES FOR HEARING LOSS

Although hearing aids and cochlear implants are far from being ideal, HL treatments today rely mostly on these approaches. With the aim of providing more optimal treatments for patients with HL, the research for alternative treatments has progressed toward different fields, including the use of gene therapy. Understanding the genetic basis of the HL and advances in DNA delivery methods are both essential for achieving the goal of gene therapy development for HL and also for others disorders.[103] One approach for HL therapy is the use of antisense oligonucleotides. These oligonucleotides were successfully used in a mouse model with a loss-of-function mutation in *USH1C*, which correlates with the human Acadian *USH1C* mutation.[104] This specific mutation leads to defects in splicing of the *USH1C* messenger RNA, encoding the harmonin protein. Antisense oligonucleotides can modulate posttranscriptional regulation by gene silencing or alteration of RNA metabolism.[103] In this case, the oligonucleotides were used to restore the correct splicing of the gene, enabling expression of the protein. The most effective results were achieved when 3- to 5-day-old mutant mice were injected intraperitoneally with the antisense oligonucleotides. Although high-frequency hearing was not developed in these mice at this stage, low- and midfrequency hearing levels were the same as those measured in nonmutant mice. These results were maintained for 6 months.[104] Implementing this treatment for humans is more complex. Human newborns can hear, which might require gene therapy intervention during gestation. Moreover, the delayed onset of hearing development in mice makes comparisons with humans difficult. Nevertheless, these initial results are promising, providing hope for the future.[103,105]

Another possible approach to rescue HL is the use of hair cell regenerative treatments, as most HL cases are caused by irreversible damage to hair cells.[105] As mammalian cochlear hair cells do not regenerate naturally, different strategies are being used to regenerate or transplant hair cells. The basis of regenerative research relies on the observation that hair cell regeneration is possible in birds, fish, and amphibians.[100] Regenerative research is aimed at discovering the exact formula of reagents that will trigger the regeneration of mammalian cochlear hair cells from precursor cells. Transplantation focuses on coaxing either inner-ear stem cells or even pluripotent stem cells into hair cell lineage. These cells may subsequently be transplanted into the inner ear. Although very promising, both strategies are in very early stages for HL treatment.[105,106] Novartis and GenVec are currently implementing the first clinical trial using the *Atoh1* gene, which can induce the differentiation of sensory cells in the inner ear (see **Table 1**).

Efforts are also being made in the pharmacologic field with the aim of discovering novel drugs for HL. This field is not limited to orally delivered pharmacologic compounds. The use of noninvasive intratympanic or invasive intracochlear routes are also options being examined.[107] Animal models, including zebrafish and mice, are widely used as preclinical models for drug use, both in vivo and in vitro with cochlear cultures.[108,109] Although there is potential in HL drug treatments, to date, there are no Food and Drug Administration–approved drugs on the market.[105]

SUMMARY

Determining the cause of deafness in patients with SHL is a key goal in order to provide optimal rehabilitation options. In the future, understanding the mechanisms of HL caused by each genetic mutation will pave the way for therapeutic delivery. Alleviating the isolation caused by deafness will greatly improve the quality of life of these patients. The recent development and implementation of new high-throughput sequencing technology will facilitate a significant improvement in identification of novel SHL and NSHL-associated pathogenic variants and genes.

REFERENCES

1. Quaranta N, Coppola F, Casulli M, et al. Epidemiology of age related hearing loss: a review. Hearing Balance Commun 2015;13:77–81.
2. Morton CC, Nance WE. Newborn hearing screening–a silent revolution. N Engl J Med 2006;354:2151–64.
3. Nance WE. The genetics of deafness. Ment Retard Dev Disabil Res Rev 2003;9: 109–19.
4. Dror AA, Avraham KB. Hearing impairment: a panoply of genes and functions. Neuron 2010;68:293–308.
5. Ross M, Pawlina W. Histology: A Text and Atlas, with Correlated Cell and Molecular Biology. 6th edition. Wolters Kluwer, Philadelphia: Paperback; 2010.
6. Raphael Y, Altschuler RA. Structure and innervation of the cochlea. Brain Res Bull 2003;60:397–422.
7. Clark JG. Uses and abuses of hearing loss classification. ASHA 1981;23: 493–500.

8. Lin FR, Thorpe R, Gordon-Salant S, et al. Hearing loss prevalence and risk factors among older adults in the United States. J Gerontol A Biol Sci Med Sci 2011;66:582–90.

9. Huang Q, Tang J. Age-related hearing loss or presbycusis. Eur Arch Otorhino-laryngol 2010;267:1179–91.

10. Parker M, Bitner-Glindzicz M. Genetic investigations in childhood deafness. Arch Dis Child 2015;100(3):271–8.

11. Kalatzis V, Petit C. The fundamental and medical impacts of recent progress in research on hereditary hearing loss. Hum Mol Genet 1998;7:1589–97.

12. Petit C, Levilliers J, Hardelin JP. Molecular genetics of hearing loss. Annu Rev Genet 2001;35:589–646.

13. Vona B, Nanda I, Hofrichter MA, et al. Non-syndromic hearing loss gene identi-fication: a brief history and glimpse into the future. Mol Cell Probes 2015. [Epub ahead of print].

14. Pimperton H, Kennedy CR. The impact of early identification of permanent child-hood hearing impairment on speech and language outcomes. Arch Dis Child 2012;97:648–53.

15. Toriello HV, Reardon W, Gorlin RJ. Hereditary hearing loss and its syndromes. Oxford (United Kingdom): Oxford University Press; 2004.

16. Reiners J, Nagel-Wolfrum K, Jurgens K, et al. Molecular basis of human Usher syn-drome: deciphering the meshes of the Usher protein network provides insights into the pathomechanisms of the Usher disease. Exp Eye Res 2006;83:97–119.

17. Mathur P, Yang J. Usher syndrome: hearing loss, retinal degeneration and asso-ciated abnormalities. Biochim Biophys Acta 2015;1852:406–20.

18. Vernon M. Usher's syndrome–deafness and progressive blindness. Clinical cases, prevention, theory and literature survey. J Chronic Dis 1969;22:133–51.

19. Kimberling WJ, Hildebrand MS, Shearer AE, et al. Frequency of Usher syn-drome in two pediatric populations: implications for genetic screening of deaf and hard of hearing children. Genet Med 2010;12:512–6.

20. Hope CI, Bundey S, Proops D, et al. Usher syndrome in the city of Birmingham–prevalence and clinical classification. Br J Ophthalmol 1997;81:46–53.

21. van Soest S, Westerveld A, de Jong PT, et al. Retinitis pigmentosa: defined from a molecular point of view. Surv Ophthalmol 1999;43:321–34.

22. El-Amraoui A, Petit C. The retinal phenotype of Usher syndrome: pathophysio-logical insights from animal models. C R Biol 2014;337:167–77.

23. Millan JM, Aller E, Jaijo T, et al. An update on the genetics of usher syndrome. J Ophthalmol 2011;2011:417217.

24. Joensuu T, Hamalainen R, Yuan B, et al. Mutations in a novel gene with trans-membrane domains underlie Usher syndrome type 3. Am J Hum Genet 2001;69:673–84.

25. Ness SL, Ben-Yosef T, Bar-Lev A, et al. Genetic homogeneity and phenotypic variability among Ashkenazi Jews with Usher syndrome type III. J Med Genet 2003;40:767–72.

26. Weil D, Blanchard S, Kaplan J, et al. Defective myosin VIIA gene responsible for Usher syndrome type 1B. Nature 1995;374:60–1.

27. Verpy E, Leibovici M, Zwaenepoel I, et al. A defect in harmonin, a PDZ domain-containing protein expressed in the inner ear sensory hair cells, underlies Usher syndrome type 1C. Nat Genet 2000;26:51–5.

28. Bitner-Glindzicz M, Lindley KJ, Rutland P, et al. A recessive contiguous gene deletion causing infantile hyperinsulinism, enteropathy and deafness identifies the Usher type 1C gene. Nat Genet 2000;26:56–60.

29. Weil D, El-Amraoui A, Masmoudi S, et al. Usher syndrome type I G (USH1G) is caused by mutations in the gene encoding SANS, a protein that associates with the USH1C protein, harmonin. Hum Mol Genet 2003;12:463–71.

30. Bolz H, von Brederlow B, Ramirez A, et al. Mutation of CDH23, encoding a new member of the cadherin gene family, causes Usher syndrome type 1D. Nat Genet 2001;27:108–12.

31. Ahmed ZM, Riazuddin S, Ahmad J, et al. *PCDH15* is expressed in the neurosensory epithelium of the eye and ear and mutant alleles are responsible for both USH1F and DFNB23. Hum Mol Genet 2003;12:3215–23.

32. Riazuddin S, Belyantseva IA, Giese AP, et al. Alterations of the CIB2 calcium- and integrin-binding protein cause Usher syndrome type 1J and nonsyndromic deafness DFNB48. Nat Genet 2012;44:1265–71.

33. Eudy JD, Weston MD, Yao S, et al. Mutation of a gene encoding a protein with extracellular matrix motifs in Usher syndrome type IIa. Science 1998;280:1753–7.

34. Kremer H, van Wijk E, Marker T, et al. Usher syndrome: molecular links of pathogenesis, proteins and pathways. Hum Mol Genet 2006;15(Spec No 2):R262–70.

35. Weston MD, Luijendijk MW, Humphrey KD, et al. Mutations in the *VLGR1* gene implicate G-protein signaling in the pathogenesis of Usher syndrome type II. Am J Hum Genet 2004;74:357–66.

36. Ebermann I, Scholl HP, Charbel Issa P, et al. A novel gene for Usher syndrome type 2: mutations in the long isoform of whirlin are associated with retinitis pigmentosa and sensorineural hearing loss. Hum Genet 2007;121:203–11.

37. Puffenberger EG, Jinks RN, Sougnez C, et al. Genetic mapping and exome sequencing identify variants associated with five novel diseases. PLoS One 2012;7:e28936.

38. Adato A, Vreugde S, Joensuu T, et al. *USH3A* transcripts encode clarin-1, a four-transmembrane-domain protein with a possible role in sensory synapses. Eur J Hum Genet 2002;10:339–50.

39. Fields RR, Zhou G, Huang D, et al. Usher syndrome type III: revised genomic structure of the USH3 gene and identification of novel mutations. Am J Hum Genet 2002;71:607–17.

40. Ebermann I, Phillips JB, Liebau MC, et al. *PDZD7* is a modifier of retinal disease and a contributor to digenic Usher syndrome. J Clin Invest 2010;120:1812–23.

41. Khateb S, Zelinger L, Mizrahi-Meissonnier L, et al. A homozygous nonsense CEP250 mutation combined with a heterozygous nonsense C2orf71 mutation is associated with atypical Usher syndrome. J Med Genet 2014;51:460–9.

42. Nishimura DY, Baye LM, Perveen R, et al. Discovery and functional analysis of a retinitis pigmentosa gene, *C2ORF71*. Am J Hum Genet 2010;86:686–95.

43. Liu XZ, Walsh J, Mburu P, et al. Mutations in the myosin VIIA gene cause non-syndromic recessive deafness. Nat Genet 1997;16:188–90.

44. Liu XZ, Walsh J, Tamagawa Y, et al. Autosomal dominant non-syndromic deafness caused by a mutation in the myosin VIIA gene. Nat Genet 1997;17:268–9.

45. Pingault V, Ente D, Dastot-Le Moal F, et al. Review and update of mutations causing Waardenburg syndrome. Hum Mutat 2010;31:391–406.

46. Read AP, Newton VE. Waardenburg syndrome. J Med Genet 1997;34:656–65.

47. Bondurand N, Dastot-Le Moal F, Stanchina L, et al. Deletions at the *SOX10* gene locus cause Waardenburg syndrome types 2 and 4. Am J Hum Genet 2007;81:1169–85.

48. Newton V. Hearing loss and Waardenburg's syndrome: implications for genetic counselling. J Laryngol Otol 1990;104:97–103.

49. Tassabehji M, Read AP, Newton VE, et al. Waardenburg's syndrome patients have mutations in the human homologue of the Pax-3 paired box gene. Nature 1992;355:635–6.

50. Tassabehji M, Newton VE, Read AP. Waardenburg syndrome type 2 caused by mutations in the human microphthalmia (*MITF*) gene. Nat Genet 1994;8:251–5.

51. Attie T, Till M, Pelet A, et al. Mutation of the endothelin-receptor B gene in Waardenburg-Hirschsprung disease. Hum Mol Genet 1995;4:2407–9.

52. Edery P, Attie T, Amiel J, et al. Mutation of the endothelin-3 gene in the Waardenburg-Hirschsprung disease (Shah-Waardenburg syndrome). Nat Genet 1996;12:442–4.

53. Pingault V, Bondurand N, Kuhlbrodt K, et al. *SOX10* mutations in patients with Waardenburg-Hirschsprung disease. Nat Genet 1998;18:171–3.

54. Sanchez-Martin M, Rodriguez-Garcia A, Perez-Losada J, et al. *SLUG (SNAI2)* deletions in patients with Waardenburg disease. Hum Mol Genet 2002;11: 3231–6.

55. King KA, Choi BY, Zalewski C, et al. SLC26A4 genotype, but not cochlear radiologic structure, is correlated with hearing loss in ears with an enlarged vestibular aqueduct. Laryngoscope 2010;120:384–9.

56. Reardon W, Trembath RC. Pendred syndrome. J Med Genet 1996;33:1037–40.

57. Masindova I, Varga L, Stanik J, et al. Molecular and hereditary mechanisms of sensorineural hearing loss with focus on selected endocrinopathies. Endocr Regul 2012;46:167–86.

58. Alasti F, Van Camp G, Smith RJH. Pendred syndrome/DFNB4. In: Pagon RA, Adam MP, Ardinger HH, et al, editors. GeneReviews(R). Seattle (WA): University of Washington. p. 1993–2015.

59. Hone SW, Smith RJ. Genetic screening for hearing loss. Clin Otolaryngol Allied Sci 2003;28:285–90.

60. Alport AC. Hereditary familial congenital haemorrhagic nephritis. Br Med J 1927;1:504–6.

61. Lemmink HH, Mochizuki T, van den Heuvel LP, et al. Mutations in the type IV collagen alpha 3 (COL4A3) gene in autosomal recessive Alport syndrome. Hum Mol Genet 1994;3:1269–73.

62. Mochizuki T, Lemmink HH, Mariyama M, et al. Identification of mutations in the alpha 3(IV) and alpha 4(IV) collagen genes in autosomal recessive Alport syndrome. Nat Genet 1994;8:77–81.

63. Barker DF, Hostikka SL, Zhou J, et al. Identification of mutations in the COL4A5 collagen gene in Alport syndrome. Science 1990;248:1224–7.

64. Smith RJH. Branchiootorenal spectrum disorders. In: Pagon RA, Adam MP, Ardinger HH, et al, editors. GeneReviews(R). Seattle (WA): University of Washington. p. 1993–2015.

65. Martin DM. Epigenetic developmental disorders: CHARGE syndrome, a case study. Curr Genet Med Rep 2015;3:1–7.

66. Neyroud N, Tesson F, Denjoy I, et al. A novel mutation in the potassium channel gene *KVLQT1* causes the Jervell and Lange-Nielsen cardioauditory syndrome. Nat Genet 1997;15:186–9.

67. Tyson J, Tranebjaerg L, Bellman S, et al. IsK and KvLQT1: mutation in either of the two subunits of the slow component of the delayed rectifier potassium channel can cause Jervell and Lange-Nielsen syndrome. Hum Mol Genet 1997;6: 2179–85.

68. Schulze-Bahr E, Wang Q, Wedekind H, et al. *KCNE1* mutations cause Jervell and Lange-Nielsen syndrome. Nat Genet 1997;17:267–8.

69. Tyson J, Tranebjaerg L, McEntagart M, et al. Mutational spectrum in the cardioauditory syndrome of Jervell and Lange-Nielsen. Hum Genet 2000;107: 499–503.

70. Schwartz PJ, Spazzolini C, Crotti L, et al. The Jervell and Lange-Nielsen syndrome: natural history, molecular basis, and clinical outcome. Circulation 2006;113:783–90.

71. Sims KB. NDP-related retinopathies. In: Pagon RA, Adam MP, Ardinger HH, et al, editors. GeneReviews(R). Seattle (WA): University of Washington. p. 1993–2015.

72. Rose PS, Levy HP, Liberfarb RM, et al. Stickler syndrome: clinical characteristics and diagnostic criteria. Am J Med Genet A 2005;138A:199–207.

73. Temple IK. Stickler's syndrome. J Med Genet 1989;26:119–26.

74. Ahmad NN, Ala-Kokko L, Knowlton RG, et al. Stop codon in the procollagen II gene (*COL2A1*) in a family with the Stickler syndrome (arthro-ophthalmopathy). Proc Natl Acad Sci U S A 1991;88:6624–7.

75. Richards AJ, Yates JR, Williams R, et al. A family with Stickler syndrome type 2 has a mutation in the *COL11A1* gene resulting in the substitution of glycine 97 by valine in alpha 1 (XI) collagen. Hum Mol Genet 1996;5:1339–43.

76. Vikkula M, Mariman EC, Lui VC, et al. Autosomal dominant and recessive osteo-chondrodysplasias associated with the *COL11A2* locus. Cell 1995;80:431–7.

77. Van Camp G, Snoeckx RL, Hilgert N, et al. A new autosomal recessive form of Stickler syndrome is caused by a mutation in the *COL9A1* gene. Am J Hum Genet 2006;79:449–57.

78. Mayne R, Brewton RG, Mayne PM, et al. Isolation and characterization of the chains of type V/type XI collagen present in bovine vitreous. J Biol Chem 1993;268:9381–6.

79. Acke FR, Dhooge IJ, Malfait F, et al. Hearing impairment in Stickler syndrome: a systematic review. Orphanet J Rare Dis 2012;7:84.

80. Kadakia S, Helman SN, Badhey AK, et al. Treacher Collins syndrome: the genetics of a craniofacial disease. Int J Pediatr Otorhinolaryngol 2014;78: 893–8.

81. Jenkinson EM, Rehman AU, Walsh T, et al. Perrault syndrome is caused by recessive mutations in *CLPP*, encoding a mitochondrial ATP-dependent chambered protease. Am J Hum Genet 2013;92:605–13.

82. Choo D, Meinzen-Derr J. Universal newborn hearing screening in 2010. Curr Opin Otolaryngol Head Neck Surg 2010;18:399–404.

83. Lander ES, Linton LM, Birren B, et al. Initial sequencing and analysis of the human genome. Nature 2001;409:860–921.

84. Weber JL, May PE. Abundant class of human DNA polymorphisms which can be typed using the polymerase chain reaction. Am J Hum Genet 1989;44: 388–96.

85. Ahmed ZM, Riazuddin S, Khan SN, et al. USH1H, a novel locus for type I Usher syndrome, maps to chromosome 15q22-23. Clin Genet 2009;75:86–91.

86. Brownstein ZN, Dror AA, Gilony D, et al. A novel SLC26A4 (PDS) deafness mutation retained in the endoplasmic reticulum. Arch Otolaryngol Head Neck Surg 2008;134:403–7.

87. Everett LA, Belyantseva IA, Noben-Trauth K, et al. Targeted disruption of mouse Pds provides insight about the inner-ear defects encountered in Pendred syndrome. Hum Mol Genet 2001;10:153–61.

88. Dror AA, Lenz DR, Shivatzki S, et al. Atrophic thyroid follicles and inner ear defects reminiscent of cochlear hypothyroidism in Slc26a4-related deafness. Mamm Genome 2014;25:304–16.

89. Shendure J, Ji H. Next-generation DNA sequencing. Nat Biotechnol 2008;26: 1135–45.

90. Brownstein Z, Bhonker Y, Avraham KB. High-throughput sequencing to decipher the genetic heterogeneity of deafness. Genome Biol 2012; 13:245.

91. Bujakowska KM, Consugar M, Place E, et al. Targeted exon sequencing in Usher syndrome type I. Invest Ophthalmol Vis Sci 2014;55:8488–96.

92. Aparisi MJ, Aller E, Fuster-Garcia C, et al. Targeted next generation sequencing for molecular diagnosis of Usher syndrome. Orphanet J Rare Dis 2014;9:168.

93. Consugar MB, Navarro-Gomez D, Place EM, et al. Panel-based genetic diagnostic testing for inherited eye diseases is highly accurate and reproducible, and more sensitive for variant detection, than exome sequencing. Genet Med 2015;17:253–61.

94. Shearer AE, DeLuca AP, Hildebrand MS, et al. Comprehensive genetic testing for hereditary hearing loss using massively parallel sequencing. Proc Natl Acad Sci U S A 2010;107:21104–9.

95. Brownstein Z, Friedman LM, Shahin H, et al. Targeted genomic capture and massively parallel sequencing to identify genes for hereditary hearing loss in Middle Eastern families. Genome Biol 2011;12:R89.

96. Riahi Z, Bonnet C, Zainine R, et al. Whole exome sequencing identifies mutations in usher syndrome genes in profoundly deaf Tunisian patients. PLoS One 2015;10:e0120584.

97. Saunders CJ, Miller NA, Soden SE, et al. Rapid whole-genome sequencing for genetic disease diagnosis in neonatal intensive care units. Sci Transl Med 2012; 4:154ra135.

98. Yang Y, Muzny DM, Reid JG, et al. Clinical whole-exome sequencing for the diagnosis of mendelian disorders. N Engl J Med 2013;369:1502–11.

99. Gilissen C, Hoischen A, Brunner HG, et al. Disease gene identification strategies for exome sequencing. Eur J Hum Genet 2012;20:490–7.

100. Rubel EW, Furrer SA, Stone JS. A brief history of hair cell regeneration research and speculations on the future. Hear Res 2013;297:42–51.

101. Liu Q, Chen P, Wang J. Molecular mechanisms and potentials for differentiating inner ear stem cells into sensory hair cells. Dev Biol 2014;390:93–101.

102. Chien WW, Monzack EL, McDougald DS, et al. Gene therapy for sensorineural hearing loss. Ear Hear 2015;36:1–7.

103. Avraham KB. Rescue from hearing loss in Usher's syndrome. N Engl J Med 2013;369:1758–60.

104. Lentz JJ, Jodelka FM, Hinrich AJ, et al. Rescue of hearing and vestibular function by antisense oligonucleotides in a mouse model of human deafness. Nat Med 2013;19:345–50.

105. Muller U, Barr-Gillespie PG. New treatment options for hearing loss. Nat Rev Drug Discov 2015;14(5):346–65.

106. Hu Z, Ulfendahl M. The potential of stem cells for the restoration of auditory function in humans. Regen Med 2013;8:309–18.

107. Rivera T, Sanz L, Camarero G, et al. Drug delivery to the inner ear: strategies and their therapeutic implications for sensorineural hearing loss. Curr Drug Deliv 2012;9:231–42.

108. Stawicki TM, Esterberg R, Hailey DW, et al. Using the zebra fish lateral line to uncover novel mechanisms of action and prevention in drug-induced hair cell death. Front Cell Neurosci 2015;9:46.

109. Xiong W, Wagner T, Yan L, et al. Using injectoporation to deliver genes to mechanosensory hair cells. Nat Protoc 2014;9:2438–49.
110. Behar DM, Davidov B, Brownstein Z, et al. The many faces of sensorineural hearing loss: one founder and two novel mutations affecting one family of mixed Jewish ancestry. Genet Test Mol Biomarkers 2014;18:123–6.

Genetics of Hearing Loss—Nonsyndromic

Kay W. Chang, MD

KEYWORDS

- Nonsyndromic hearing loss • DFNA • DFNB • GJB2 • Next-generation sequencing
- Massively parallel sequencing

KEY POINTS

- Autosomal-recessive (AR) nonsyndromic hearing loss is usually prelingual and frequently results in severe hearing loss, although milder and progressive hearing loss forms also exist. GJB2 and SLC26A4 are the 2 most common AR genes.
- Autosomal-dominant (AD) nonsyndromic hearing loss is often postlingual and progressive. No single gene accounts for any significant proportion of AD hearing loss.
- High-throughput sequencing techniques, also called next-generation sequencing (NGS) or massively parallel sequencing (MPS), now allow comprehensive testing of all known deafness-associated genes in a child presenting with congenital hearing loss.

Hearing loss is the most common congenital sensory impairment, affecting 1 in 500 newborns and 1 in 300 children by the age of 4.[1] Approximately 1 in 1000 newborns has genetically inherited hearing loss. Nonsyndromic etiologies account for 70% of genetic hearing loss, with only 30% being syndromic and demonstrating other clinical findings.[2]

Autosomal-recessive (AR) inheritance accounts for 80% of nonsyndromic genetic hearing loss and is usually prelingual. Autosomal-dominant (AD) inheritance accounts for most of the other 20% and is more often postlingual. AR nonsyndromic hearing loss (designated "DFNB#") most frequently results in severe hearing loss, which presents early, whereas AD nonsyndromic hearing loss (designated "DFNA#") typically results in progressive sensorineural hearing loss (SNHL) with variable severity, which begins at 10 to 40 years.[3] Patients with mitochondrial inheritance tend to develop progressive SNHL, which begins at 5 to 50 years, and the degree of hearing loss is variable.[4] X-linked (designated "DFNX#") and mitochondrial inheritance account for only 1% to 2% of nonsyndromic hearing loss.

Disclosure Statement: The authors have nothing to disclose.
Department of Otolaryngology, Stanford University, 801 Welch Road, Stanford, CA 94305, USA
E-mail address: kchang@ohns.stanford.edu

Otolaryngol Clin N Am 48 (2015) 1063–1072
http://dx.doi.org/10.1016/j.otc.2015.06.005

Nonsyndromic SNHL may be caused by mutations in any one of an increasing number of identified genes. Currently, over 100 genes for SNHL have been mapped, some listed on **Table 1** (a more comprehensive updated list can be found on the Hereditary Hearing Loss Homepage, http://hereditaryhearingloss.org).[5] For AR SNHL, the most frequent causative genes in order of frequency are GJB2, SLC26A4, MYO15A, OTOF, CDH23, and TMC1. Common mutations of AD inheritance include WFS1, TECTA, COCH, and KNCQ4. Several of these genes are also implicated in syndromic hearing loss.

AUTOSOMAL-RECESSIVE GENES

In AR inheritance, there is often no family history of hearing loss. Although AR SNHL is more common in families in which parents are related (consanguinity), they are not exclusive to such families, and most affected individuals have a negative history of consanguinity within the family tree. According to the hereditary hearing loss homepage, 60 genetic mutations have been identified causing nonsyndromic AR hearing loss.[5]

GJB2 (DFNB1A)

GJB2 encodes the gap junction protein Connexin 26, a critical component of the intracellular pathway for potassium cycling between the endolymph and perilymph of the cochlea. Mutations in GJB2 account for up to 50% of patients with nonsyndromic AR SNHL. Hearing loss from GJB2 was first described in 1997,[6] and since then, routine DNA sequencing of the coding region of GJB2 reported across the world has demonstrated interesting patterns of genotypes across populations. Particularly prevalent mutant alleles include 35delG, found in Europe and the Middle East (particularly regions surrounding the Mediterranean); 235delC, found in East Asia, V37I, common in Southeast Asia; and W24X, common in India.[7]

Inactivating truncating mutations in GJB2 (stop codons or frameshift mutations, such as small insertions/deletions) are generally associated with severe-to-profound SNHL. In contrast, noninactivating nontruncating mutations in GJB2 (base changes that result in single amino acid substitutions) are associated with moderate or even mild SNHL.[8] The large, noncoding deletions involving the adjacent GJB6 gene, which encodes for the protein Connexin 30, are thought to cause hearing loss through their effects on GJB2 expression, and not through the effects on GJB6.[9]

Table 2 lists some of the more common truncating and nontruncating GJB2 mutations. The number of discovered mutations continues to increase over time, and a more comprehensive updated list can be found at the Connexin-deafness homepage (http://www.crg.es/deafness).[10] Patients with 2 truncating mutations tend to have severe-to-profound hearing loss, while those with a truncating and nontruncating mutation have more moderate hearing loss, and those with 2 nontruncating mutations tend to have mild hearing loss.[11] However, those with 2 nontruncating mutations, especially those homozygous for V37I, had up to a 39% to 50% rate of progression of hearing loss.[12,13] GJB2 sequencing, along with computed tomography (CT)/MRI of the temporal bone remain 2 of the highest yield diagnostic evaluations for children presenting with SNHL.[14–16]

Although GBJ2 hearing loss is thought to be AR, thus requiring 2 mutations to result in the hearing loss phenotype, meta-analysis of carrier rates between normal hearing and hearing loss populations demonstrates significantly increased rates of truncating mutations in the hearing loss populations, suggesting an unidentified genetic factor contributing to hearing loss in some heterozygote carriers, or alternatively, that there

Table 1
Nonsyndromic SNHL genes

AR genes		AR genes	
DFNB1A	GJB2	DFNB88	ELMOD3
DFNB1B	GJB6	DFNB89	KARS
DFNB2	MYO7A	DFNB91	SERPINB6
DFNB3	MYO15A	DFNB93	CABP2
DFNB4	SLC26A4	DFNB98	TSPEAR
DFNB6	TMIE	DFNB99	TMEM132E
DFNB7/11	TMC1	DFNB101	GRXCR2
DFNB8/10	TMPRSS3	DFNB102	EPS8
DFNB9	OTOF	DFNB103	CLIC5
DFNB12	CDH23		
DFNB15/72/95	GIPC3	**AD genes**	
DFNB16	STRC	DFNA1	DIAPH1
DFNB18	USH1C	DFNA2A	KCNQ4
DFNB21	TECTA	DFNA2B	GJB3
DFNB22	OTOA	DFNA3A	GJB2
DFNB23	PCDH15	DFNA3B	GJB6
DFNB24	RDX	DFNA4	MYH14, CEACAM16
DFNB25	GRXCR1	DFNA5	DFNA5
DFNB28	TRIOBP	DFNA6/14/38	WFS1
DFNB29	CLDN14	DFNA8/12	TECTA
DFNB30	MYO3A	DFNA9	COCH
DFNB31	WHRN	DFNA10	EYA4
DFNB32	GPSM2	DFNA11	MYO7A
DFNB35	ESRRB	DFNA13	COL11A2
DFNB36	ESPN	DFNA15	POU4F3
DFNB37	MYO6	DFNA17	MYH9
DFNB39	HGF	DFNA20/26	ACTG1
DFNB42	ILDR1	DFNA22	MYO6
DFNB44	ADCY1	DFNA23	SIX1
DFNB48	CIB2	DFNA25	SLC17A8
DFNB49	MARVELD2	DFNA28	GRHL2
DFNB49	BDP1	DFNA36	TMC1
DFNB53	COL11A2	DFNA41	P2RX2
DFNB59	PJVK	DFNA44	CCDC50
DFNB61	SLC26A5	DFNA48	MYO1A
DFNB63	LRTOMT (COMT2)	DFNA50	MIRN96
DFNB66/67	LHFPL5	DFNA51	TJP2
DFNB70	PNPT1	DFNA56	TNC
DFNB73	BSND	DFNA64	SMAC (DIABLO)
DFNB74	MSRB3	DFNA65	TBC1D24
DFNB76	SYNE4	DFNA67	OSBPL2
DFNB77	LOXHD1		
DFNB79	TPRN	**X-linked genes**	
DFNB82	GPSM2	DFNX1 (DFN2)	PRPS1
DFNB84	PTPRQ	DFNX2 (DFN3)	POU3F4
DFNB84	OTOGL	DFNX4 (DFN6)	SMPX
DFNB86	TBC1D24		

Table 2
Common truncating and nontruncating GJB2 mutations

	Description	Effect
Truncating mutations		
35delG	del of G at 30–35	Frameshift
235delC	del of C at 233–235	Frameshift
W24X	G to A at 71	Trp at 24 into Stop
E47X	G to T at 139	Glu at 47 into Stop
299–300delAT	del of AT at 299	Frameshift
167delT	del of T at 167	Frameshift
176–191del16	del of 16 nt at 176	Frameshift
Q57X	C to T at 169	Gln at 57 into Stop
269insT	ins of T at 269	Frameshift
290–291insA	Frameshift	Frameshift
Y136X	C to A at 408	Tyr at 136 into Stop
30delG	del of G at 30–35	Frameshift
312del14	del of 14 nt at 312	Frameshift
M1V (p.0)	A to G at 1	No protein production
IVS1 + 1 G to A	G to A at −3172	Splice site
333–334delAA	del of AA at 333–335	Frameshift
E147X	G to T at 439	Glu at 147 into Stop
631delGT	del of GT at 631–632	Frameshift
645–648delTAGA	del of TAGA at 645	Frameshift
W77X	G to A at 231	Trp at 77 into Stop
W44X	G to A at 132	Trp at 44 into Stop
Nontruncating mutations		
V37I	G to A at 109	Val at 37 into Ile
R143W	C to T at 427	Arg at 143 into Trp
V27I + E114G	G to A at 79 + A to G at 341	Val at 27 into Ile and Glu at 114 into Gly
R127H	G to A at 380	Arg at 127 into His
S139N	G to A at 416	Ser at 139 into Gln
G12V	G to T at 35	Gly at 12 into Val
G45E	G to A at 134	Gly at 45 into Glu
H100Y	C to T at 298	His at 100 into Tyr
L90P	T to C at 269	Leu at 90 into Pro
R32L	G to T at 95	Arg at 32 into Leu
V84L	G to C at 250	Val at 84 into Leu
K15T	A to C at 44	Lys at 15 into Thr
V95M	G to A at 283	Val at 95 into Met
K122I	A to T at 365	Lys at 122 into Ile
N206S	A to G at 617	Gln at 206 into Ser
delE120	del of GAG at 360	del of Glu at 119–120
R32C	C to T at 94	Arg at 32 into Cis
R184P	G to C at 551	Arg at 184 into Pro

is a carrier phenotype that is penetrant in a small proportion of carriers.[7] Data from 52,715 normal-hearing controls from 115 studies across 55 countries reveal a worldwide carrier rate of 1.5% for 35delG, ranging from 0% in multiple countries to 5.7% in Belarus. The carrier rate for V37I among 20,866 controls across 72 studies from 26 countries is 2.5%, ranging from 0% to as high as 16.7% in Thailand.[7]

SLC26A4 (DFNB4)

SLC26A4 encodes a chloride and iodide anion transporter and is the second most common nonsyndromic AR SNHL after GJB2.[17,18] Mutations in SLC26A4 may also cause syndromic SNHL, in the form of Pendred syndrome. Because goiter generally does not become apparent until puberty, this form of SNHL characteristically initially presents as nonsyndromic. Not all patients with biallelic SLC26A4 mutations will go on to develop goiter, and thus they will continue to demonstrate true DFNB4 nonsyndromic SNHL.[19]

Many patients with SLC26A4 may demonstrate enlarged vestibular aqueducts (EVA) on CT scan, or enlarged endolymphatic ducts and sacs on MRI. This radiologic finding has important implications for management, because patients with EVA can experience sudden and dramatic hearing loss following minor head trauma.[20] Children with biallelic SLC26A4 mutations are at high risk of developing goiter and hypothyroidism following puberty. Also, about 30% of children with Pendred syndrome have symptomatic vestibular problems, and about another 30% show reduced vestibular function on formal testing.[21]

MYO15A (DFNB3)

Mutations in MYO15A cause congenital severe-to-profound SNHL.[22] Myosin XV is thought to be necessary for actin organization in hair cells and normal stereocilia tip link function.[23,24]

OTOF (DFNB9)

OTOF encodes otoferlin, a protein essential for synaptic vesicle exocytosis, and may act as the major calcium sensor triggering membrane fusion at the inner hair cell ribbon synapse.[25] Mutations in OTOF result in hearing impairment characterized by auditory neuropathy/auditory dissynchrony (AN/AD), which is diagnosed when auditory brainstem responses (ABRs) are absent or severely abnormal, but outer hair cell (OHC) function is normal as indicated by the presence of otoacoustic emissions (OACs) and strong cochlear microphonic. Other nongenetic causes of AN/AD include risk factors such as prematurity, hypoxia, and hyperbilirubinemia.[26] In a Japanese study of AN/AD without environmental risk factors, over 56% of cases had OTOF mutations.[27] Individuals with this disorder can have various degrees of hearing loss by pure tone behavioral audiometry; however they generally have disproportionately poor speech understanding. In contrast to individuals with non-AN/AD SNHL, hearing aids often provide only limited benefit to speech understanding in most individuals with AN/AD.[28] Cochlear implantation has been shown to help the speech understanding in some children with AN/AD from mutations in OTOF.[29]

CDH23 (DFNB12)

Mutations in the gene encoding cadherin-23 (CDH23) result in Usher syndrome type 1D, characterized by SNHL, retinitis pigmentosa, and vestibular dysfunction.[30] The same genetic locus, DFNB12, is the site of a form of nonsyndromic AR SNHL resulting in a moderate-to-profound progressive SNHL.[31]

TMC1 (DFNB7/11)

TMC1 encodes a transmembrane protein that is required for the normal function of cochlear hair cells.[32] TMC1 appears to be a common cause of recessive deafness in consanguineous Indian, Pakistani, Turkish, and Tunisian families. Recessive mutations of TMC1 all result in a prelingual severe-to-profound SNHL.[33–35]

AUTOSOMAL-DOMINANT GENES

AD SNHL is much more easily identified from a multigenerational family history than AR SNHL. However, in contrast to AR SNHL in which 2 genes (GBJ2 and SLC26A4) account for a high proportion of cases, there is no single gene that accounts for any significant proportion of AD SNHL. Most nonsyndromic AD SNHL is postlingual and progressive, and some genes (COCH) may even cause adult-onset SNHL. According to the hereditary hearing loss homepage, 32 genetic mutations have been identified causing nonsyndromic AD hearing loss.[5]

WFS1 (DFNA6/14/38)

Mutations in WFS1 are a common cause of nonsyndromic low-frequency SNHL, predominantly affecting frequencies below 2 kHz. The hearing loss tends to be progressive, ultimately leading to a flattening of the audiogram.[36,37] Some AD missense mutations can cause a syndromic phenotype with congenital profound hearing loss, progressive optic atrophy, and variable penetrance of diabetes mellitus and psychiatric problems. Biallelic mutations in WFS1 cause the AR neurodegenerative condition Wolfram syndrome characterized by the features DIDMOAD (diabetes insipidus, diabetes mellitus, optic atrophy, and deafness).[38]

TECTA (DFNA8/12)

TECTA encodes α tectorin, a component of the tectorial membrane overlying the OHC responsible for transmission and amplification of sound. Nonsense mutations in TECTA may cause DFNB21 AR SNHL, but missense changes result in either high-frequency congenital/early childhood-onset AD hearing loss, or a distinctive midfrequency (U-shaped or cookie-bite) loss.[39,40]

COCH (DFNA9)

COCH mutations typically present as a progressive SNHL with onset in high frequencies. Onset of SNHL in patients with DFNA9 occurs in young adulthood (20–30 years) and displays variable progression to anacusis by 40 to 50 years. A spectrum of clinical vestibular involvement, ranging from lack of symptoms to presence of mild vertigo to complete vestibular hypofunction, has been found.[41]

KNCQ4 (DFNA2A)

KNCQ4 encodes a voltage-gated potassium channel, and is one of the more common genes causing high-frequency AD SNHL.[42,43]

X-LINKED GENES
POU3F4 (DFNX2)

POU3F4 is the most common genetic mutation causing X-linked nonsyndromic hearing loss. It results in a distinct radiological malformation characterized by cochlear hypoplasia and bulbous internal auditory canals. In addition to SNHL, there is often a conductive component to the hearing loss, caused by physiologic stapes fixation, which is not improved by stapes surgery and may cause a gusher of cerebrospinal fluid (CSF) if operated upon.[44,45] Mutations in 4 X-linked genes have been identified causing hearing loss.[5]

MITOCHONDRIAL INHERITANCE
A1555G

Mitochondrial disorders resulting in hearing loss are usually multisystemic and thus syndromic. However, one common nonsyndromic form of mitochondrial deafness is the A1555G mutation in the mitochondrial 12S ribosomal ribonucleic acid (rRNA) gene.[46] The A1555G mutation may be present in up to 1 in 500 Caucasians, and can result in severe hearing loss from exposure to normal therapeutic levels of aminoglycosides.[47] Because of their low cost and high availability, the use of aminoglycosides is widespread in developing countries like China, and this genetic mutation causes an exquisite sensitivity of the cochlea to this class of antibiotic. Up to 22% of all deaf-mutes in one district in China could trace the cause to aminoglycoside use, 28% of them having other relatives with aminoglycoside ototoxicity.[48] It is estimated that up to a third of patients with aminoglycoside ototoxicity in China have the A1555G mutation.[49]

C1494T

C1494T is a different mutation in the 12S rRNA, resulting in aminoglycoside ototoxicity identified in a large Chinese pedigree.[50] Rapid screens for multiple mitochondrial susceptibility mutations (A1555G, C1494T, T1095C, 961delT + C(n), A827G) are becoming more widely available to detect this important etiology of deafness throughout the world.[51]

NEXT-GENERATION OR MASSIVELY PARALLEL SEQUENCING

High-throughput sequencing techniques, also called next-generation sequencing (NGS) or massively parallel sequencing (MPS),[2,52–55] now allow comprehensive testing of all known deafness-associated genes in a child presenting with congenital SNHL. Although complete sequencing of GJB2 could diagnose approximately 25% of all possible genetic hearing losses, utilization of NGS/MPS techniques appears to increase the diagnostic rate to around 50%.[53,56]

The first study using MPS for diagnosis of nonsyndromic SNHL was published in 2010.[52] This platform uses solution-phase custom complementary RNA oligonucleotides for targeted genomic enrichment (TGE), and now includes at least 66 genes and is offered on a clinical basis as OtoSCOPE (http://morl-otoscope.org). An alternative platform using complementary DNA oligonucleotides for array-based TGE[54] is available commercially as OtoGenetics (http://www.otogenetics.com). A third approach uses semiautomated polymerase chain reaction (PCR) amplification paired with MPS to simultaneously sequence 15 deafness genes,[55] and this is available as NXTGNT (http://www.nxtgnt.com). With further advancements in these, as well as future techniques, definitive diagnosis of all possible genetic causes for hearing loss may be a matter of routine in the not-too-distant future.

REFERENCES

1. Morton CC, Nance WE. Newborn hearing screening—a silent revolution. N Engl J Med 2006;354:2151–64.
2. Shearer AE, Smith RJ. Genetics: advances in genetic testing for deafness. Curr Opin Pediatr 2012;24(6):679–86.

3. Liu XZ, Xu LR, Zhang SL, et al. Epidemiological and genetic studies of congenital profound deafness. Am J Med Genet 1994;53:192–5.
4. Liu XZ, Xiaomei KE, Angeli S, et al. Audiological and genetic features of mitDNA deafness. Acta Otolaryngol 2008;128:732–8.
5. Available at: http://hereditaryhearingloss.org. Accessed May 27, 2015.
6. Kelsell DP, Dunlop J, Stevens HP, et al. Connexin 26 mutations in hereditary non-syndromic sensorineural deafness. Nature 1997;387:80–3.
7. Chan DK, Chang KW. GJB2-associated hearing loss: systematic review of world-wide prevalence, genotype, and auditory phenotype. Laryngoscope 2014;124(2):E34–53.
8. Snoeckx RL, Huygen PL, Feldmann D, et al. GJB2 mutations and degree of hearing loss: a multicenter study. Am J Hum Genet 2005;77:945–57.
9. del Castillo I, Villamar M, Moreno-Pelayo MA, et al. A deletion involving the Connexin 30 gene in nonsyndromic hearing impairment. N Engl J Med 2002;346(4):243–9.
10. Ballana E, Ventayol M, Rabionet R, et al. Connexins and deafness homepage. Available at: http://www.crg.es/deafness. Accessed May 27, 2015.
11. Putcha GV, Bejjani BA, Bleoo S, et al. A multicenter study of the frequency and distribution of GJB2 and GJB6 mutations in a large North American cohort. Genet Med 2007;9(7):413–26.
12. Chan DK, Schrijver I, Chang KW. Connexin-26-associated deafness: phenotypic variability and progression of hearing loss. Genet Med 2010;12(3):174–81.
13. Kenna MA, Feldman HA, Neault MW, et al. Audiologic phenotype and progression in GJB2 (Connexin 26) hearing loss. Arch Otolaryngol Head Neck Surg 2010;136(1):81–7.
14. Chan DK, Schrijver I, Chang KW. Diagnostic yield in the workup of congenital sensorineural hearing loss is dependent on patient ethnicity. Otol Neurotol 2011;32(1):81–7.
15. Mafong DD, Shin EJ, Lalwani AK. Use of laboratory evaluation and radiologic imaging in the diagnostic evaluation for children with sensorinueral hearing loss. Laryngoscope 2002;112:1–7.
16. Preciado DA, Lawson L, Madden C, et al. Improved diagnostic effectiveness with a sequential diagnostic paradigm in idiopathic pediatric sensorineural hearing loss. Otol Neurotol 2005;26:610–5.
17. Everett LA, Glaser B, Beck JC, et al. Pendred syndrome is caused by mutations in a putative sulphate transporter gene (PDS). Nat Genet 1997;17:411–22.
18. Scott DA, Wang R, Kreman TM, et al. The Pendred syndrome gene encodes a chloride–iodide transport protein. Nat Genet 1999;21:440–3.
19. Usami S, Abe S, Weston MD, et al. Non-syndromic hearing loss associated with enlarged vestibular aqueduct is caused by PDS mutations. Hum Genet 1999;104:188–92.
20. Colvin IB, Beale T, Harrop-Griffiths K. Long-term follow-up of hearing loss in children and young adults with enlarged vestibular aqueducts: relationship to radiologic findings and Pendred syndrome diagnosis. Laryngoscope 2006;116:2027–36.
21. Luxon LM, Cohen M, Coffey RA, et al. Neuro-otological findings in Pendred syndrome. Int J Audiol 2003;42:82–8.
22. Wang A, Liang Y, Fridell RA, et al. Association of unconventional myosin MYO15 mutations with human non-syndromic deafness DFNB3. Science 1998;280:1447–51.

23. Probst FJ, Fridell RA, Raphael Y, et al. Correction of deafness in shaker-2 mice by an unconventional myosin in a BAC transgene. Science 1998;280:1444–7.
24. Anderson DW, Probst FJ, Belyantseva IA, et al. The motor and tail regions of myosin XV are critical for normal structure and function of auditory and vestibular hair cells. Hum Mol Genet 2000;9:1729–38.
25. Roux I, Safieddine S, Nouvian R, et al. Otoferlin, defective in a human deafness form, is essential for exocytosis at the auditory ribbon synapse. Cell 2006;127:277–89.
26. Norrix LW, Velenovsky DS. Auditory neuropathy spectrum disorder (ANSD): a review. J Speech Lang Hear Res 2014;57:1564–76.
27. Matsunaga T, Mutai H, Kunishima S, et al. A prevalent founder mutation and genotype-phenotype correlations of OTOF in Japanese patients with auditory neuropathy. Clin Genet 2012;82:425–32.
28. Varga R, Avenarius MR, Kelley PM, et al. OTOF mutations revealed by genetic analysis of hearing loss families including a potential temperature sensitive auditory neuropathy allele. J Med Genet 2006;43:576–81.
29. Rouillon I, Marcolla A, Roux I, et al. Results of cochlear implantation in two children with mutations in the OTOF gene. Int J Pediatr Otorhinolaryngol 2006;70:689–96.
30. Yan D, Liu XZ. Genetics and pathological mechanisms of Usher syndrome. J Hum Genet 2010;55:327–35.
31. Schwander M, Xiong W, Tokita J, et al. A mouse model for non-syndromic deafness (DFNB12) links hearing loss to defects in tip links of mechanosensory hair cells. Proc Natl Acad Sci U S A 2009;106:5252–7.
32. Kurima K, Peters LM, Yang Y, et al. Dominant and recessive deafness caused by mutations of a novel gene TMC1 required for cochlear hair-cell function. Nat Genet 2002;30:277–84.
33. Hilgert N, Smith RJ, Van Camp G. Forty-six genes causing nonsyndromic hearing impairment: which ones should be analyzed in DNA diagnostics? Mutat Res 2009;681:189–96.
34. Kalay E, Karaguzel A, Caylan R, et al. Four novel TMC1 (DFNB7/DFNB11) mutations in Turkish patients with congenital autosomal recessive nonsyndromic hearing loss. Hum Mutat 2005;26:591.
35. Sirmaci A, Duman D, Oztürkmen-Akay H, et al. Mutations in TMC1 contribute significantly to nonsyndromic autosomal recessive sensorineural hearing loss a report of five novel mutations. Int J Pediatr Otorhinolaryngol 2009;73:699–705.
36. Despalova IN, Van CG, Born SJ, et al. Mutations in the Wolfram syndrome 1 gene (WFS1) are a common cause of low frequency sensorineural hearing loss. Hum Mol Genet 2001;10:2501–8.
37. Cryns K, Pfister M, Pennings RJ, et al. Mutations in the WFS1 gene that cause low-frequency sensorineural hearing loss are small non-inactivating mutations. Hum Genet 2002;110:389–94.
38. Rendtorff ND, Lodahl M, Boulahbel H, et al. Identification of p.A684V missense mutation in the WFS1 gene as a frequent cause of autosomal dominant optic atrophy and hearing impairment. Am J Med Genet A 2011;155A:1298–313.
39. Verhoeven K, Van Laer L, Kirschhofer K, et al. Mutations in the human alpha-tectorin gene cause autosomal dominant non-syndromic hearing impairment. Nat Genet 1998;19(1):60–2.
40. Hildebrand MS, Morin M, Meyer NC, et al. DFNA8/12 caused by TECTA mutations is the most identified subtype of nonsyndromic autosomal dominant hearing loss. Hum Mutat 2011;32:825–34.

41. Robertson NG, Lu L, Heller S, et al. Mutations in a novel cochlear gene cause DFNA9, a human nonsyndromic deafness with vestibular dysfunction. Nat Genet 1998;20:299–303.
42. Kubisch C, Schroeder BC, Friedrich T, et al. KCNQ4, a novel potassium channel expressed in sensory outer hair cells, is mutated in dominant deafness. Cell 1999;96(3):437–46.
43. Coucke P, Van Camp G, Djoyodiharjo B, et al. Linkage of autosomal dominant hearing loss to the short arm of chromosome 1 in two families. N Engl J Med 1994;331(7):425–31.
44. de Kok YJ, van der Maarel SM, Bitner-Glindzicz M, et al. Association between X-linked mixed deafness and mutations in the POU domain gene POU3F4. Science 1995;267(5198):685–8.
45. Phelps PD, Reardon W, Pembrey M, et al. X-linked deafness, stapes gushers and a distinctive defect of the inner ear. Neuroradiology 1991;33:326–30.
46. Prezant TR, Agapian JV, Bohlman MC, et al. Mitochondrial ribosomal RNA mutation associated with both antibiotic-induced and non-syndromic deafness. Nat Genet 1993;4:289–94.
47. Bitner-Glindzicz M, Pembrey M, Duncan A, et al. Prevalence of mitochondrial 1555A->G mutation in European children. N Engl J Med 2009;360:640–2.
48. Hu DN, Qui WQ, Wu BT, et al. Genetic aspects of antibiotic induced deafness: mitochondrial inheritance. J Med Genet 1991;28:79–83.
49. Fischel-Ghodsian N. Genetic factors in aminoglycoside ototoxicity. In: Roland PS, Rutka JA, editors. Ototoxicity. Hamilton (Canada): BD Decker Inc; 2004. p. 144–52.
50. Zhao H, Li R, Wang Q, et al. Maternally inherited aminoglycoside-induced and nonsyndromic deafness is associated with the novel C1494T mutation in the mitochondrial 12S rRNA gene in a large Chinese family. Am J Hum Genet 2004;74(1):139–52.
51. Bardien S, Human H, Harris T, et al. A rapid method for detection of five known mutations associated with aminoglycoside-induced deafness. BMC Med Genet 2009;10:2.
52. Shearer AE, DeLuca AP, Hildebrand MS, et al. Comprehensive genetic testing for hereditary hearing loss using massively parallel sequencing. Proc Natl Acad Sci U S A 2010;107:21104–9.
53. Brownstein Z, Friedman LM, Shahin H, et al. Targeted genomic capture and massively parallel sequencing to identify genes for hereditary hearing loss in Middle Eastern families. Genome Biol 2011;12:R89.
54. Tang W, Qian D, Ahmad S, et al. A low-cost exon capture method suitable for large-scale screening of genetic deafness by the massively-parallel sequencing approach. Genet Test Mol Biomarkers 2012;16:536–42.
55. De Keulenaer S, Hellemans J, Lefever S, et al. Molecular diagnostics for congenital hearing loss including 15 deafness genes using a next generation sequencing platform. BMC Med Genomics 2012;5:17.
56. Shearer AE, Black-Ziegelbein EA, Hildebrand MS, et al. Advancing genetic testing for deafness with genomic technology. J Med Genet 2013;50:627–34.

Psychosocial Aspects of Hearing Loss in Children

Donna L. Sorkin, MA[a],*, Patricia Gates-Ulanet, PsyD[b], Nancy K. Mellon, MS[b]

KEYWORDS

- Hearing loss • Cochlear implants • Mainstreaming • Inclusive environments
- Self-confidence • Social-emotional learning

KEY POINTS

- The initiation of newborn hearing screening and the resultant opportunity for children with hearing loss to begin early intervention in the first months of life have dramatically changed the landscape of pediatric deafness.
- Federal education and access laws have allowed families to seek and receive the accommodations and services that their children with hearing loss require to attend mainstream schools and excel in the academic realm.
- Despite impressive gains in language development, children with hearing loss are more likely to experience social isolation, feel awkward with peers, and demonstrate immaturity.
- When social-emotional learning programs and approaches are implemented effectively in school settings, children's academic achievement increases, problem behaviors decrease, and the child's relationships with others improve.

EARLY IDENTIFICATION AND INTERVENTION: A NEW PARADIGM

One of the important outcomes of widespread newborn hearing screening in the United States and around the world has been the opportunity early identification affords for children with hearing loss to have access to hearing-assistive technology at a young age, thereby taking advantage of developing brain plasticity and allowing for better language outcomes. Before the initiation of widespread newborn screening, most children born with hearing loss were identified after 20 months of age.[1,2]

It is no longer unusual for children to be fit with hearing aids within the first few months of life,[3–5] which was uncommon even 15 years ago. When parents are given comprehensive, evidence-based information about communication and technology choices during early intervention, children born deaf are able to move through the

The authors have nothing to disclose.
[a] American Cochlear Implant Alliance, PO Box 103, McLean, VA 22101, USA; [b] The River School, 4880 MacArthur Boulevard, Northwest, Washington, DC 20007, USA
* Corresponding author.
E-mail address: dsorkin@acialliance.org

Abbreviations	
CI	Cochlear implant
SEL	Social-emotional learning
ToM	Theory of Mind

hearing evaluation process in a timely way and receive a cochlear implant (CI) at 12 months. In 2015, 12 months was the youngest age under the US Food and Drug Administration guideline for providing the CI intervention to a child with bilateral profound deafness. Providing access to sound through cochlear implantation at the youngest possible age maximizes brain connectivity in the process of hearing and offers crucial opportunities to impact a major childhood disability. With appropriate support, children are now able to achieve the holy grail of pediatric hearing loss; even congenitally deaf children are developing language and reading skills that are close, or equivalent to, that of their hearing peers.[6]

For children with mild to severe hearing loss, technological advances in amplification provide improved outcomes in a range of challenging listening situations. Hearing technology has progressed dramatically, like other consumer electronics, and has also become "cool" in appearance, as exemplified by an incident[7] in which a thief grabbed a CI processor off a child's ear thinking it was a new type of Bluetooth device.

Until recently, typical expectations for a child with a significant hearing loss (and even for many with lesser levels of hearing loss) were that he or she would attend a special school or program with other children with hearing loss. Given late identification, once a child's hearing loss was identified, the hard work ahead was *both* learning language and catching up. Missing the window of language learning meant that many children with hearing loss never did catch up. The median reading level for a child with bilateral deafness graduating from high school was fourth grade.[8] Although there are few recent definitive measures of literacy in children with hearing loss, it is known that early access to language through appropriately fit hearing-assistive technology or early exposure to fluent sign language (via deaf parents who are fluent signers) provides dramatic benefits for language and literacy.[9]

Making full use of federal education and access laws,[1] families are seeking and receiving the accommodations and services that their children require to attend mainstream schools with their siblings and neighborhood friends. The opportunity to go to school, play sports, and pursue cultural activities and other extracurricular activities in inclusive environments allows children the chance to grow up in, and become accustomed to, participation and success in the larger hearing world. Seeking such independence in the mainstream is an important goal for most families.

Federal access laws in the United States have supported and facilitated the shift to a new normal in which it is commonplace for children with hearing loss to grow up and thrive in inclusive environments alongside their siblings and friends.[10,11] Combined with laws that provide children with accommodations and needed support services—regardless of the type of school they attend—this new opportunity has engendered a dramatic change in where children with hearing loss go to school. Society has moved from educating children in special environments to neighborhood school

---

[1] Federal laws such as the Americans with Disabilities Act and Section 504 of the Rehabilitation Act require that public places (including schools) provide accommodations, such as frequency modulation systems, captioning, or sign language, that enable a child with hearing loss access to effective communication.

placements with typically hearing peers. For some, mainstreaming[2] begins before the child enters kindergarten, whereas for others, the process starts later. Regardless, being part of an inclusive classroom setting provides language models with age-appropriate language, content that parallels what other children are learning, and the opportunity for a child with hearing loss to pursue a mainstream journey for growing up.

Mainstream school placement brings with it both challenges and opportunity. Despite impressive performance in one-on-one communication, some children with CIs may struggle to hear peer discussions or teacher directions, depending on class-room acoustics, teaching practices, group size, and classroom dynamics. They may need support to navigate socially in certain learning environments, such as coopera-tive learning groups that require students to discuss, negotiate, and create as a team.[12] These challenges can negatively impact a child's academic and social suc-cess and may be overlooked by professionals. Professionals working to support chil-dren with hearing loss in mainstream placements need to thoughtfully assess and balance both the level of challenge and the needed supports.

THE WHOLE CHILD

Educators and parents tend to focus on the academic elements of childhood develop-ment because that realm has traditionally been so difficult to negotiate given all of the challenges children with hearing loss encountered. Now, there is more attention being given to the psychosocial well-being of these children. Most parents say that they want their child with hearing loss to grow up to be a responsible, independent person able to negotiate his or her own way in life. Developing appropriate psychosocial skills is critical to one's ability to develop a sense of autonomy and self-worth and to develop and maintain successful peer relationships.

Children with hearing loss have historically been more likely to experience social isolation, feel awkward with peers, and demonstrate immaturity[13]; and this was espe-cially true for children attending school in mainstream settings if their language lagged behind hearing peers, and where there may be few opportunities to interact with other students with hearing loss. Self-rated social competence has been found to be higher for children who acquire age-appropriate spoken language skills.[6]

Some children with hearing loss are able to negotiate this aspect of growing up suc-cessfully. It is important for professionals and parents to be aware of factors and stra-tegies that may make a difference in helping children not only develop language and academic skills but also know how to interact effectively with their peers and with a range of people in the larger world. The social-emotional realm of childhood develop-ment cannot be neglected.

SOCIAL COMPETENCY

Psychosocial development is often described in terms of mastering specific stages or progressive steps of social or emotional development. The most commonly refer-enced hierarchy of social development was suggested by Erik Erikson[14] in the 1950s and is still referenced by psychologists and social workers. Erikson suggested

---

[2] Refers to participation of children with disabilities (including hearing loss) side by side with children who do not have disabilities. Support services and access must still be provided to meet the child's communication and educational needs.

that for a young child, the initial developmental stages involve mastering trust, autonomy, and initiative.

All young people go through transitions as they mature and progress from being dependent children to becoming independent adults. Transitions also include moving from primary school to secondary school, and then on to university or out into the working world. At each of these stages, children and young adults must continually develop new skills to mature and eventually self-manage their lives. This process of moving forward with social competency depends on an early framework of comfort and competency in interacting with other people of all ages and all socioeconomic groups.

Irrespective of whether a child has a disability, parents typically watch their children grapple with the challenges of mastering independence. Parents often experience frustration observing their children at various stages of their life journey. One of the most difficult aspects of parenting is judging when to offer help, when to suggest solutions, and when not to intervene. Children and adolescents with hearing loss sometimes have the additional challenge of not being able to consistently understand what is being said to them in various settings, which can create misunderstanding and can also cause the child or young adult to be unsure of themselves in social settings.

The parental role for a family with a child with hearing loss may be complicated because of the number of ways parents must participate in their child's educational program, such as formulating an Individual Education Program (IEP),[3] ensuring that appropriate access services are provided properly, securing therapy or other services outside of school, and arranging opportunities for their child to interact with other children socially outside of school. There is sometimes a tendency for parents to be overprotective of their child with hearing loss; even within the same family, parents often note that they are more involved with their child with hearing loss than they are with their typically hearing children. Prolonged dependency on parents can cause the child to experience delays in developing social skills, overdependence on parents, and low self-confidence. Once a cycle of immaturity develops, it is difficult for the child to know how to overcome what can be very real communication difficulties.

Some of these challenges result because social interactions typically occur in informal settings where there is background noise and distractions. These settings include the lunchroom, hallways, playground, school bus, and athletic events—all listening environments that are often difficult for typically hearing people. Children share information and converse casually in such settings. Because the child with hearing loss will often enter the conversation with no context or knowledge of the topic, he or she can be lost from the start and copes by not participating (for fear of saying the wrong thing), leaving the conversation, or attempting to change the topic. None of these options is a socially positive approach and, over time, can lead other children to view the hearing-impaired child's behavior as odd or negative.

RECENT ADVANCES IN DEVELOPING SOCIAL COMPETENCY

Some early implanted children educated in auditory-oral environments seem to show progress in developing these social skills. Recent findings include the following:

- Most adolescents in a longitudinal cohort study self-reported high self-esteem and well-developed social skills.[15]

---

[3] An Individual Education Program must be developed for a deaf or hard-of-hearing student who requires special education services to receive an education that is appropriate to meet his or her needs.

- Peer ratings and peer nomination of children with deafness in inclusive settings were comparable to hearing peers on measures of peer acceptance and friendship, but lower on social competence.[16]
- Five- and 6-year-old children with CIs showed strong performance on a peer entry task. Better performance was associated with longer duration of implant use and higher self-esteem.[17]

Integrating Social-Emotional Learning Curricula

Although some children with hearing loss are at risk for delays in social development as a consequence of delayed language acquisition,[16] interventions in social-emotional learning (SEL) can be beneficial. Aside from the benefits to their self-esteem and experiences with peers, intervention in the social domain can improve academic performance. Social competence in childhood has been cited as a powerful predictor of academic achievement.[18–20] When SEL programs and approaches are implemented effectively, children's academic achievement increases, problem behaviors decrease, and the child's relationships with others improve.[21] Children who are accepted by their peers and demonstrate prosocial behaviors tend to be high achievers, whereas socially rejected children are at high risk for academic failure.[16,18]

SEL intervention enhances academic achievement; benefits persist over time and positively affect students in multiple areas.[22] After intervention, students demonstrate positive attitudes, more competent social behaviors, fewer problems with conduct, and lower levels of emotional distress. SEL interventions require time during the school day, but they do not detract from students' academic performance. Rather, students in SEL programs show academic improvement of up to 11 percentile points on standardized achievement tests, a significant gain relative to peers not receiving the intervention.[22]

Children with CIs often present with delays in social development, including the quality of reciprocal social interactions, the ability to comprehend the feelings and emotions of others, and the development of Theory of Mind (ToM).[23,24] ToM is typically mastered by hearing children and by deaf children of signing parents by age 5 or 6 but is often delayed in deaf children of hearing parents.[25] Lacking an effective common language, children may miss out on the social mentoring learned from caregiver communications. The child's ability to understand that others have different thoughts, perspectives, and feelings apart from their own is compromised and further compromises the development of specific aspects of social emotional functioning. Early implantation and intervention should lessen this delay in deaf children of hearing parents.

Delays in language acquisition and subsequent delays in exposure to mental state language may cause an atypical developmental sequence of ToM in children with CIs when compared with hearing peers.[26] A child's participation and engagement in pretend play also influence the acquisition of ToM; young children with hearing loss may be more vulnerable to delays due to later acquisition of a common language and less opportunity to engage in social pretend play experiences.[27] Peterson and Wellman[28] documented 2 critical differences between children with and without hearing loss: understanding pretense (imaginary, representational situations) occurs at a later age for children with hearing loss but earlier within the sequence of emergent understanding of the thoughts of others. These findings suggest that cognitive development relating to complexity and executive function may also play a role in ToM development.[29] The differences are attributed to the variability of social interactive experiences between children with hearing loss and those with normal hearing.

THE RIVER SCHOOL: CHILD OUTCOMES IN THE SOCIAL-EMOTIONAL REALM

The River School in Washington, DC was founded in 1999 to provide an inclusive educational environment for young children with hearing loss using CIs or hearing aids. Children from birth to grade 3 with hearing loss learn alongside a classroom of mostly normal-hearing peers, who provide strong language models for them. Classrooms are designed for maximum acoustical access. Each class is taught by a 2-person team, which includes a master's level educator and speech language pathologist. The school provides a challenging academic program with a special focus on language and literacy. There is also a conscious emphasis placed on social outcomes with activities aimed at fostering social cognition including self-esteem, collaboration, critical thinking, and individual responsibility.

Children with CIs at The River School benefit from an intervention program that targets the development of specific skills that can aid social emotional development including social communication, perspective taking, mental state language, and reciprocal social interactions. SEL support includes facilitation during social interactions at school; modeling prosocial behaviors during peer-based social experiences; and direct teaching of social skills. Thoughtful integration of an SEL curriculum can maximize early learning for children with CIs in the context of play and social interactions with hearing peers and lay the foundation for the acquisition of additional skills that enhance a child's emotional intelligence and overall social functioning.

In 2014, The River School began a 3-year longitudinal study entitled "Social Outcomes of Peer Models." As part of the study, all 240 students, 40 of whom have hearing loss, were rated via teacher questionnaires. The Devereux Early Childhood Assessment for Toddlers was used for children ages 18 to 36 months old; the Devereux Early Childhood Assessment for Preschoolers Second Edition was used for children ages 3 through 5, and the Devereux Student Strengths Assessment was used for children in grades K to 3.

Each child was rated by each of their 2 coteachers, an educator and speech pathologist. On initial assessment, no group differences were observed between the 2 groups—children with hearing loss and their hearing peers. All of the participants received scores within normal limits on this standardized, norm-referenced measure. All 240 students were also assessed by a speech-language pathologist using the Pragmatic Judgment subtest of the Comprehensive Assessment of Spoken Language. Although the study is still ongoing and the data have not been comprehensively examined, both groups of students (those with hearing loss and those with normal hearing) demonstrated median scores in the high-average to above-average range. School faculty members hypothesize that having strong language models in the classroom and an intervention program that places priority on SEL is contributing to age-appropriate outcomes among River School students with CIs.

SUMMARY

Infants and children are now identified much earlier with hearing loss. They are more consistently fit at an early age with appropriate hearing technology and are provided with early intervention services. Parents and professionals can begin the process of language development to avoid delays in the academic realm that were so typical in the past. Careful integration of an SEL curriculum can further enhance early learning for children with hearing loss in the context of play and social interactions with hearing peers and lay the foundation for the acquisition of additional skills that enhance a child's emotional intelligence and overall social functioning. Parents should be instructed in how to augment this element of their child's development alongside the day-to-day language learning that occurs outside of school.

REFERENCES

1. Halpin KS, Smith KY, Widen JE, et al. Effects of universal newborn hearing screening on an early intervention program for children with hearing loss, birth to 3 yr of age. J Am Acad Audiol 2010;21(3):169–75.
2. Sininger YS, Martinez A, Eisenberg L, et al. Newborn hearing screening speeds diagnosis and access to intervention by 20–25 months. J Am Acad Audiol 2009; 20(1):49–57.
3. Kerkhofs K, de Smit M. Early hearing aid fitting in children: challenges and results. B-ENT 2013;(Suppl 21):17–25.
4. McCreery RW, Bentler RA, Roush PA. Characteristics of hearing aid fittings in infants and young children. Ear Hear 2013;34(6):701–10.
5. Holte L, Walker E, Oleson J, et al. Factors influencing follow-up to newborn hearing screening for infants who are hard of hearing. Am J Audiol 2012;21:163–74.
6. Geers AE, Hayes H. Reading, writing and phonological processing skills of adolescents with 10 or more years of cochlear implant experience. Ear Hear 2011; 32(1):49S–59S.
7. ABC News. Available at: http://www.deafhh.net/wp/2009/01/04/hearing-aid-mistaken-for-bluetooth-headset-stolen/. Accessed April 1, 2015.
8. Traxler CB. The Stanford Achievement Test, 9th edition: National Norming and Performance Standards for Deaf and Hard-of-Hearing Students. J Deaf Stud Deaf Educ 2000;5(4):337–48.
9. Knorrs H, Marschark M. Language planning for the 21st century: revisiting bilingual policy for deaf children. J Deaf Stud Deaf Educ 2012;17(3):291–305.
10. Sorkin DL. Education and access laws for children with hearing loss. In: Madell J, Flexer C, editors. Pediatric audiology: diagnosis, technology, and management. New York: Thieme; 2014. p. 334–48.
11. Sorkin DL. Disability law and people with hearing loss: we've come a long way (but we're not there yet). Hear Loss 2004;25:13–7.
12. Punch R, Hyde M. Children with cochlear implants in Australia: educational setting, supports, and outcomes. J Deaf Stud Deaf Educ 2010;15(4):405–21.
13. Maxon AB, Bracket D. Psychosocial, familial, and cultural issues. In: Maxon AB, Bracket D, editors. The hearing impaired child: infancy through high school years. Boston: Andover Medical Publishers; 1992. p. 132–6.
14. Erikson EH. Childhood and society. New York: Norton; 1950.
15. Moog JS, Geers AE, Gustus C, et al. Psychosocial adjustment in adolescents who have used cochlear implants since preschool. Ear Hear 2011;32(Suppl 1):75s–83s.
16. Wauters LN, Knoors H. Social integration of deaf children in inclusive settings. J Deaf Stud Deaf Educ 2008;13(1):22–36.
17. Martin D, Bat-Chava Y, Lalwani A, et al. Peer relationships of deaf children with cochlear implants: predictors of peer entry and peer interaction success. J Deaf Stud Deaf Educ 2011;16(1):108–20.
18. Wentzel KR. Motivation and achievement in adolescence: a multiple goal perspective. In: Schunk D, Meece J, editors. Student perceptions in the classroom: causes and consequences. Hillsdale (NJ): Lawrence Earlbaum Assoc; 1992. p. 287–306.
19. Berghout-Austin AM, Draper DC. The relationship among peer acceptance, social impact and academic achievement in middle childhood. Am Educ Res J 1984;21:597–604.

20. Green KD, Forehand R, Beck SJ, et al. An assessment of the relationship among measures of children's social competence and children's academic achievement. Child Dev 1980;51:1149–56.

21. Zins JE, Elias MJ, Greenberg MT. Facilitating success in school and in life through social and emotional learning. Perspectives in education 2003;21(4):59–60.

22. Durlak JA, Weissberg RP, Dymnicki AB, et al. The impact of enhancing students' social and emotional learning: a meta-analysis of school-based universal interventions. Child Dev 2011;82(1):405–32.

23. Peterson CC. Theory of mind development in oral deaf children with cochlear implants or conventional hearing aids. J Child Psychol Psychiatry 2004;45: 1096–106.

24. Peterson CC, Seigal M. Insights into theory of mind from deafness and autism. Mind Lang 2000;15(1):123–45.

25. Peterson CC. Development of social-cognitive and communication skills in children born deaf. Scand J Psychol 2009;50:475–83.

26. Remmel E, Peters K. Theory of min and language in children with cochlear implants. J Deaf Stud Deaf Educ 2000;14(2):218–36.

27. Brown PM, Prescott SJ, Richards FW, et al. Communicating about pretend play: A comparison of the utterances of four-year-old normally hearing and hearing-impaired children in an integrated kindergarten. Volta Review 1997;99:5–17.

28. Peterson CC, Wellman HM. From fancy to reason: Scaling deaf and hearing children's understanding of theory of mind and pretence. Br J Dev Psychol 2009; 27(Pt 2):297–310.

29. Halford GS, Cowan N, Andrews G. Separating cognitive capacity from knowledge: a new hypothesis. Trends Cogn Sci 2007;11(6):236–42.

Communication Assessment and Intervention

Implications for Pediatric Hearing Loss

Lori L. Bobsin, PhD, CCC-SLP, LSLS Cert. AVT[a],*,
K. Todd Houston, PhD, CCC-SLP, LSLS Cert. AVT[b]

KEYWORDS

- Hearing loss • Pediatric • Communication • Assessment • Intervention

KEY POINTS

- Early identification and intervention by qualified professionals is critical to successful outcomes for children with hearing loss.
- Families of children with hearing loss should receive thorough and unbiased information about communication options and guidance to access appropriate local, state, and national resources.
- More families are choosing a listening and spoken language approach for their children with hearing loss, making training of and access to qualified professionals essential.
- Aggressive audiologic management, including communication with all intervention team members, is indispensable in the process of aural (re)habilitation of children.
- Trends in intervention in this field will require reconsideration of the efficiency of current service provision.

DEMOGRAPHICS OF PEDIATRIC HEARING LOSS

Historically, children with hearing loss have fallen well behind their peers with normal hearing in the areas of speech and language development, thus limiting their abilities to participate fully in social, educational, and vocational opportunities.[1–3] However, advances in both the early detection and the identification of hearing loss as well as the technology to improve speech processing through hearing aids, cochlear

Disclosure Statement: The authors have nothing to disclose.
[a] Aural Habilitation Program, University of Virginia Cochlear Implant Program, University of Virginia Health System, 415 Ray C. Hunt Drive, Charlottesville, VA 22903, USA; [b] School of Speech-Language Pathology and Audiology, College of Health Professions, The University of Akron, 184A Polsky Building, Akron, OH 44325-3001, USA
* Corresponding author.
E-mail address: LLP4N@virginia.edu

Otolaryngol Clin N Am 48 (2015) 1081–1095
http://dx.doi.org/10.1016/j.otc.2015.06.003
0030-6665/15/$ – see front matter © 2015 Elsevier Inc. All rights reserved.

implants, and other hearing technology, have provided children with hearing loss unprecedented access to listening and spoken language.[4] In turn, outcome measures for children with hearing loss in the areas of language and literacy have improved significantly in the past 2 decades.[4–8]

According to the most recent Centers for Disease Control and Prevention (CDC) Early Hearing Detection and Intervention (EHDI) Hearing Screening and Follow-Up Survey, the prevalence of congenital hearing loss is 1.6 per 1000 newborns screened in the United States.[9] Each year, 12,000 children in the United States are born with some degree of hearing loss, making it one of the most common birth defects.[10,11] For some children, like the ones included in the CDC survey, hearing loss can be detected soon after birth; other children are older before hearing loss occurs or becomes evident.[12] Hearing loss, regardless of its severity, can interfere with the development of speech and language as well as impede academic success if left undetected or untreated.[13,14] However, when hearing loss is detected early and children are quickly enrolled in appropriate intervention services, most have the ability to progress at age-appropriate rates, to be mainstreamed into regular education classrooms, and to achieve significantly better outcomes than children who receive intervention later.[7,14–17]

EARLY INTERVENTION

Early identification and early intervention are unconditionally critical to the development of listening and spoken language in children with hearing loss. Until the 1990s, the average age of identification for children with permanent hearing loss was 2 $\frac{1}{2}$ to 3 years of age. In the past 20 years, newborn hearing screening has become a standard of care in hospitals and birthing centers nationwide. Today, 98% of newborns in the United States are screened for hearing loss before they leave the hospital.[18] Because of the proliferation of newborn screening programs, the average age of hearing loss identification has decreased to 2 to 3 months of age.[9,19]

Despite these advances, many children with hearing loss still do not receive the follow-up care they need. In 2007, the Joint Commission on Infant Hearing (JCIH) reported that only 54% of babies who are screened subsequently receive the recommended hearing evaluation. The other 46% are "lost to the system." Furthermore, nearly 40% of children identified with hearing loss and their families do not receive a referral to their state's early intervention system and therefore are not aware of the services and funding available to assist with the medical needs of their child.[9] Congress established the Part C (early intervention) program through the Individuals with Disabilities Education Act (IDEA) in 1986 in recognition of "an urgent and substantial need" to

- Enhance the development of infants and toddlers with disabilities;
- Reduce educational costs by minimizing the need for special education through early intervention;
- Minimize the likelihood of institutionalization, and maximize independent living; and
- Enhance the capacity of families to meet their child's needs.

The Part C program was last reauthorized in 2011 and is supported by a federal grant that assists states in operating a comprehensive statewide program of early intervention services for infants and toddlers with disabilities, birth through 3 years of age, and their families.

In 2013, the JCIH updated and expanded on their 2007 position statement to further delineate guiding principles for EHDI systems. In an effort to improve the efficiency of early intervention programs, the JCIH[20] offered a timeline for universal newborn hearing screening, diagnosis, and intervention. As it has been come to be called, the 1:3:6 rule has been adopted by most states as a standard of care for universal newborn hearing screening programs. The 1:3:6 rule states:

- 1 = All infants are screened for hearing loss before discharge from birthing/ neonatal facilities, or within 1 month of birth;
- 3 = All infants referred from the screening process complete diagnostic audiological evaluation by 3 months of age; and
- 6 = All infants with diagnosed hearing loss receive appropriate interventions by 6 months of age, including amplification selection and early intervention services.

Timeliness is vital. These steps provide the greatest opportunities for the child with hearing loss to attain age-appropriate listening and spoken communication skills.[20]

When diagnosis of a hearing loss is confirmed, the audiologist is typically the first professional to inform the parents or caregivers. Receiving the diagnosis can induce a wide range of reactions and emotions in the family. The manner in which this information is imparted is critical to the emotional state of the parents as they begin the process of achieving eventual acceptance. Unlike most parents of children with normal hearing, parents of children with hearing loss must make important decisions about how they and other individuals in their child's life will communicate with their child. Out of necessity, these difficult decisions must occur early in their child's life and are often made during times of uncertainty and sadness. Families must be provided with information, resources, and the opportunity to work through a range of emotions. This process allows for information about hearing loss to be better understood and processed, and for informed decisions about hearing care management and intervention to be made in a timely manner.[21]

The JCIH[10] states that communication-based options need to be presented to parents in a nonbiased manner, and the choice of a communication option needs to be based on the specific needs of the family and the parents' desired communication outcomes. Honest discussions regarding the dedicated effort required from families throughout their child's treatment program must occur. All professionals who provide services to the child need to work in a consistent and collaborative manner in order to maximize the outcomes for each child. In partnership with the family, professionals need to follow the intervention plan for auditory, speech, and language development, monitor growth, and make changes and recommendations based on the progress of the child.[22,23]

COMMUNICATION OPTIONS

Although there are several communication methodologies used with children with hearing loss, communication options generally range on a continuum from mostly visual to mostly auditory in their means of language transmission. Some of the communication options presented to parents and families of children who are deaf or hard of hearing typically include the following: American Sign Language (ASL), Bilingual-Bicultural (Bi-Bi), Total Communication, English-Based Sign Systems, Cued Speech, and Listening and Spoken Language (Auditory-Verbal Therapy [AVT] and Auditory-Verbal Education [AVEd]).[24] Regardless of the communication methodology chosen, all families should receive:

- Thorough information about all communication options;
- Unbiased information about communication options;

- Unconditional support and appropriate resources (local, state, national) and contacts for the methodology the family chooses; and
- Contact information for a local support group or individual parents who have offered support to newly-identified families.

ASL is a visual language with its own unique grammatical structure, morphology, and phonology and is considered the language of Deaf Culture. The Bi-Bi approach emphasizes the use of ASL as the child's first language and is used in academic settings with English taught as a second language through reading and writing. Traditionally, the use of hearing technology is discouraged in these approaches. Both ASL and Bi-Bi focus on integrating the child with hearing loss into the Deaf Culture through a common language.[24]

Other approaches combine auditory- and visually-based communication. Total Communication is not a communication mode as such, but rather an educational philosophy often promoted for children with hearing loss. Its goal is to provide the most appropriate mode of communication for the child's needs at any one time. Children, parents/caregivers, and teachers may use any form of communication, or any combination of communication strategies, to meet the child's communicative and academic needs. English-based sign systems use signs with English grammar and morphologic markers. There are several English-based sign systems, including Signed Exact English, Signed English, Conceptually Accurate Signed English, and Pidgin Signed English. Cued Speech is an approach that uses the movement of hand shapes placed near the mouth to represent the sounds of speech for the purpose of speech-reading, but is not a stand-alone language system.[24]

The Listening and Spoken Language Approaches, namely AVT and AVEd, focus on the development of spoken language through the use of hearing technologies and the engagement of parents as their child's primary language facilitator in the acquisition of spoken communication. AVT, in particular, targets the parents as the main consumer of the approach and provides them with coaching and training to enhance their child's development of spoken conversations primarily though listening.[25,26]

In the past 25 years, there has been a movement toward listening and spoken language approaches for children with severe to profound hearing loss. Likely because approximately 95% of parents of children with hearing loss have normal hearing themselves,[27] trends indicate that many parents are choosing spoken language as the primary mode of communication for their children more than 85% of the time[21]; this is especially true when they realize that spoken language is a viable outcome for their child. Furthermore, these parents typically select listening and spoken language approaches without initiating visual communication systems.[27,28] Although some localities struggle with providing appropriate early intervention services to children with hearing loss and their families, important movements are emerging and a range of communication methodologies and early intervention services are becoming more widely available.

Numerous studies have shown that when children with hearing loss are identified early, use appropriately programmed hearing technology such as digital hearing aids, cochlear implants, and frequency modulation systems from the beginning in conjunction with early auditory-based intervention, they can achieve communication outcomes comparable to their same-age peers with typical hearing[17,25,29] and develop positive speech, language, and social-emotional outcomes.[13,30] More importantly, with early identification and appropriate intervention, these children have the opportunity to enter kindergarten or first grade with age-appropriate language and have been shown to achieve rates of literacy comparable to their peers who have normal hearing.[4–8,31] Communication modes have been shown to have a high statistically significant association with speech and language outcomes of children with cochlear implants.[32] Children exposed to spoken language have a greater probability of scoring higher on speech and language assessments than children exposed to some degree of either sign support or sign language.[33] Children who receive auditory-based intervention score high on speech production and speech recognition measures, and these results improve as the emphasis on audition increases.[34–36]

Improved hearing acuity, as provided by hearing technology, does not, by itself, guarantee the ability to discriminate between sounds nor the ability to develop spoken language. Children with hearing loss require intensive auditory, speech, and language training from professionals who have experience working with children with hearing loss and who possess the specialized training and knowledge to do so.[26,37,38] In addition, parents and caregivers must be active participants in the child's intervention/ rehabilitation. Children's first and most important teacher is their primary caregiver, most often their parents. Therefore, parent training is essential for the linguistic success of the child. Children cannot develop a functional communication system, if the only intervention they receive is in a therapy room. Specific speech, language, and auditory goals should be incorporated daily in the child's home environment.[39]

As discussed previously, children with communication or learning challenges and their families need access to appropriate family-centered early intervention services that are delivered by professionals who are well-trained and experienced in the use of current evidence-based practices; this is particularly true for children with hearing loss.[40] Unfortunately, a lack of qualified practitioners, especially in remote and rural communities, in addition to limited funding, can affect the quality of services that some children receive. The program outlined in Part C of the IDEA of 1997 (PL 105-17) requires the implementation of family-centered intervention in a natural learning environment.[41] Listening and Spoken Language Approaches have always embraced family-centered early intervention as a service delivery model. For children and their families who qualify under this legislation, early intervention services are designed to enhance the quality of their lives by facilitating the parent's capacity to promote the development of skills in their infants and toddlers.[42,43] That is, during family-centered intervention, the professional focuses on enhancing the parent's ability, through coaching, to promote the growth and development of their infant or toddler during daily learning opportunities.[41,44] When parents follow their children's lead by supporting their interests and participation, there is a positive effect on the child's development and learning.[45,46] Families are viewed as having existing capabilities, the ability to make informed decisions, the power to act on their decisions to strengthen family competence and improve family functioning, and the capacity to become increasingly competent.[39,47] These principles serve as the foundation for Auditory-Verbal Practice.

INTERVENTION AND ASSESSMENT

Children with normal hearing thresholds appear to acquire language almost effortlessly by listening to the spoken language that surrounds them daily and by interacting with their environment.[48–50] Borden and colleagues[51(p2)] state: "They (children) are natural language learners, and they develop language by hearing the speech of others. Speech is audible. It can be described in terms of its loudness, its pitch, and its duration. It is meaningful sound strung out in time." For children who have hearing loss, much of the acoustic aspects of speech remain unavailable without appropriate hearing aid amplification or cochlear implantation. These devices can improve access to this information, but are not singly responsible for speech and language development.

Numerous variables have been shown to influence the levels of performance outcomes observed in children with hearing loss. These variables include early diagnosis of the hearing loss, proper audiologic management, familial support, and appropriate aural (re)habilitation. The age of onset of deafness, age of implantation, duration of deafness, chosen communication mode, and duration of implant use also seem to be influential.[32,52] Furthermore, the wear time of hearing technology, the cause of the child's hearing loss, the child's innate cognitive and linguistic abilities, parental motivation and dedication, and quality of therapeutic intervention also seem to influence the ultimate linguistic competence of these children.[1,14,16,46,53] With appropriate medical, therapeutic, and educational management, many children who have hearing loss have the potential to develop language commensurate with their age-matched peers with normal hearing thresholds.[7,15,54] It is clear that achievements of children are guided by both opportunity and ability. Although baseline assessments are completed when services are initiated and periodically thereafter, the professional's mind-set should view each session as diagnostic in nature—an opportunity to observe the child's performance and collect data on the child's and family's progress. With a steadfast commitment to meeting the child's learning needs and assessing when he has the potential to master the content, professionals can ensure that each intervention session is designed to meet the child's skill acquisition for listening, speech, language, cognition, and conversational competence. Similarly, the practitioner should closely monitor the parents' or caregivers' ability to facilitate language and communication and feel comfortable providing the necessary modeling and coaching to finely tune parent-child interactions to maximize learning.[52,55]

Some children meet developmental milestones in a predictable and timely manner, while others may meet some milestones early but then slow down or stop making progress. Other children may make slow but steady gains, and some may make limited progress. Each child with hearing loss presents with individual needs and challenges and follows a unique trajectory in this process. Conservative estimates suggest that approximately 43% of these children present with additional challenges, such as low vision (4.4%), legal blindness (1.2%), developmental delay (8.5%), learning disability (12.4%), orthopedic impairment (4.3%), attention deficit disorder (7.2%), traumatic brain injury (0.3%), intellectual disability (7.7%), emotional disturbance (3.2%), autism (1.9%), Usher syndrome (0.1%), other health impairments (4.1%), and other conditions (8.0%).[56]

By observing the child's behavior during each session and documenting progress on session objectives, the clinician is able to judge if appropriate progress is being made. If expected progress is not occurring, the diagnostic nature of intervention requires a careful review of the factors that may be impeding the child's progress. Some of these factors can be managed fairly easily, while others may require collaboration with other professionals. Once these issues are identified, steps should be taken to reduce their impact on the child's progress.[55]

Although outcomes will differ between children, all therapy should target auditory skills using normal sequences of development and should seek to attain skills at an expected rate. As such, it is necessary for the clinician to have knowledge of the hierarchy of typical development. Concerns about any aspect of the child's development need to be addressed openly and honestly with the parents. Children with additional challenges may require therapy interventions to supplement weekly auditory-verbal sessions or a referral to another therapeutic approach. This process needs to be implemented as quickly as possible to take advantage of the child's critical listening and language-learning years.[26]

AUDIOLOGIC MANAGEMENT

Children need to have complete and consistent access to sound in order to develop listening, speech, and language skills at an acceptable rate. As mentioned previously, an essential precursor to speech and language development is adequate speech perception and the quality of early auditory input; this is especially important for children with significant hearing loss.[57] The deficit in early access to the speech signal can be devastating to the language acquisition process.[58,59]

Attendance at regular appointments, as prescribed by the child's audiologist, is critical to evaluate the functioning of the child's hearing technology and assess progression in speech perception abilities. These appointments are necessary for the optimal functioning of the devices. In addition, parents must maintain extra parts and batteries and become skilled at troubleshooting, in case the hearing aid or cochlear implant becomes unworkable at home.

The Alexander Graham Bell Association (AGBA) for the Deaf and Hard of Hearing has developed a Professional Practice Protocol (2012)[60] for guidance in the audiologic management of children with hearing loss. In addition to the 1:3:6 rule that is explained earlier in this article, this protocol incorporates recommendations for follow-up well after the first 6 months. The following is included as part of the comprehensive protocol:

When hearing loss is diagnosed, routine evaluation should occur ideally at four-to six-week intervals until full audiograms are obtained, and at three-month intervals through age 3 years. Assessment at six-month intervals from age 4 years is appropriate if progress is satisfactory and if there are no concerns about changes in hearing. Immediate evaluation should be undertaken if parent or caretaker concern is expressed or if behavioral observation by parent, therapist or teacher suggests a change in hearing or device function. More frequent evaluation is appropriate when middle ear disease is chronic or recurrent, or when risk factors for progressive hearing loss are present.

One of the goals of thorough audiological management is to assess whether the child's current hearing technology is providing adequate access to sound. If a child is in a listening and spoken language approach, this decision must be made expeditiously. Therefore, communication and collaboration between the child's speech-language pathologist and audiologist are essential. Once it is determined that a child is not getting adequate sound access through his or her current hearing technology, the family should be counseled regarding the potential need for cochlear implantation. According to the US Food and Drug Administration (FDA), as of December 2012, approximately 324,200 people worldwide have received implants. In the United States, roughly 58,000 adults and 38,000 children have received the devices. Since 2000, cochlear implants have been FDA-approved for use in eligible children beginning at 12 months of age. For young children who are deaf or severely hard of hearing, implantation while young exposes them to sounds during an optimal period to develop speech and language skills. Growing evidence has shown that when these children receive a cochlear implant before 18 months of age and participate in an appropriate rehabilitation program, their listening skills, linguistic abilities, and clarity of speech surpass their peers who receive implants when they are older.[32,61,62] Studies have also shown that children who receive a cochlear implant at a young age can develop communication skills at a rate comparable to children with normal hearing and can be successful in mainstream education settings.[4,63] The decision to receive a cochlear implant, like all others, is one that the family of the child needs to make based on the most accurate information available and their goals for their child.

LISTENING AND SPOKEN LANGUAGE AS AN OPTION

For professionals, there is a range of knowledge and skills that support and facilitate positive listening and spoken language outcomes for children with hearing loss and their families. Regardless of the professional preparation, background, or experience, practitioners serving this population should obtain the content, knowledge, and skills for listening and spoken language facilitation, implement family-centered early intervention that incorporates parent engagement and parent coaching as core elements, understand and apply the principles of AVT and AVEd, and possess the experience and skills to carefully plan, evaluate, and deliver their intervention or therapy sessions.

The AGBA for Listening and Spoken Language has a well-established international certification program for Listening and Spoken Language Specialists (LSLS) as Certified Auditory-Verbal Educators (Cert. AVEd) and Certified Auditory-Verbal Therapists (Cert. AVTs). These professionals may be teachers of the deaf and hard of hearing, speech-language pathologists, audiologists, or others from related disciplines who complete this comprehensive certification process.

For the LSLS, the AGBA has defined the foundational knowledge that the practitioner should possess before certification. These domains of knowledge span a range of disciplines including but not limited to medical intervention, psychology, social sciences, linguistics, audiology, speech-language pathology, early intervention, early childhood education, and education of the deaf and hard of hearing. More specifically, the practicing LSLS must integrate these knowledge domains into intervention when working with children with hearing loss and their families:

- Hearing and hearing technology (ie, digital hearing aids, cochlear implants, and assistive listening devices);
- Auditory functioning;
- Spoken language communication;
- Child development;
- Parent guidance, education, and support;
- Strategies for listening and spoken language development;
- Education (ie, supporting the child with hearing loss in the general education curriculum); and
- Emergent literacy.

The knowledge domains on which the certification is based continue to evolve and be refined as new research, public policy, and clinical outcomes shape the practice of LSLS professionals and their delivery of services.

Auditory-verbal practice is defined as the application and management of hearing technology, in conjunction with specific strategies, techniques, and conditions, which promote optimal acquisition of spoken language primarily through listening for children who are deaf and hard of hearing. The principles of LSLS Auditory-Verbal practice are well established[60] and have been defined for the both the Cert. AVT and the Cert. AVEd. These principles are presented in **Boxes 1** and **2**. In addition to following these principles in their practice and mastering the auditory-verbal techniques and strategies[26,37,64] that facilitate listening and spoken language, professionals must maintain the skills to carefully plan, evaluate, and deliver their intervention services.

Box 1

Principles of listening and spoken language educator auditory-verbal therapy (LSLS Cert. AVT)

1. Promote early diagnosis of hearing loss in newborns, infants, toddlers, and young children, followed by immediate audiologic management and AVT.

2. Recommend immediate assessment and use of appropriate, state-of-the-art hearing technology to obtain maximum benefits of auditory stimulation.

3. Guide and coach parents to help their child use hearing as the primary sensory modality in developing listening and spoken language.

4. Guide and coach parents to become the primary facilitators of their child's listening and spoken language development through active consistent participation in individualized AVT.

5. Guide and coach parents to create environments that support listening for the acquisition of spoken language throughout the child's daily activities.

6. Guide and coach parents to help their child integrate listening and spoken language into all aspects of the child's life.

7. Guide and coach parents to use natural developmental patterns of audition, speech, language, cognition, and communication.

8. Guide and coach parents to help their child self-monitor spoken language through listening.

9. Administer ongoing formal and informal diagnostic assessments to develop individualized Auditory-Verbal treatment plans, to monitor progress, and to evaluate the effectiveness of the plans for the child and family.

10. Promote education in regular schools with peers who have typical hearing and with appropriate services from early childhood onwards.

An Auditory-Verbal Practice requires all 10 principles.
Reprinted with permission of the Alexander Graham Bell Association for the Deaf and Hard of Hearing. http://www.listeningandspokenlanguage.org/uploadedFiles/Get_Certified/Getting_Certified/Final%202012%20Handbook.pdf.

Box 2

Principles of listening and spoken language educator auditory-verbal education (LSLS Cert. AVEd)

A listening and spoken language educator (LSLS Cert. AVEd) teaches children with hearing loss to listen and talk exclusively though listening and spoken language instruction.

1. Promote early diagnosis of hearing loss in infants, toddlers, and young children, followed by immediate audiologic assessment and use of appropriate state-of-the-art hearing technology to ensure maximum benefits of auditory stimulation.

2. Promote immediate audiologic management and development of listening and spoken language for children as their primary mode of communication.

3. Create and maintain acoustically controlled environments that support listening and talking for the acquisition of spoken language throughout the child's daily activities.

4. Guide and coach parents to become effective facilitators of their child's listening and spoken language development in all aspects of the child's life.

5. Provide effective teaching with families and children in settings such as homes, classrooms, therapy rooms, hospitals, or clinics.

6. Provide focused and individualized instruction to the child through lesson plans and classroom activities while maximizing listening and spoken language.

7. Collaborate with parents and professionals to develop goals, objectives, and strategies for achieving the natural developmental patterns of audition, speech, language, cognition, and communication.

8. Promote each child's ability to self-monitor spoken language through listening.

9. Use diagnostic assessments to develop individualized objectives, to monitor progress, and to evaluate the effectiveness of the teaching activities.

10. Promote education in regular classrooms with peers who have typical hearing, as early as possible, when the child has the skills to do so successfully.

Reprinted with permission of the Alexander Graham Bell Association for the Deaf and Hard of Hearing.   http://www.listeningandspokenlanguage.org/uploadedFiles/Get_Certified/Getting_Certified/Final%202012%20Handbook.pdf.

SUMMARY

Hearing technologies will continue to evolve, providing greater access to sound and the potential for even greater spoken language outcomes for children with hearing loss. Early intervention professionals, speech-language pathologists, audiologists, pediatricians, otolaryngologists, and other allied health care professionals share a responsibility to ensure that children with hearing loss and their families have access to appropriate, coordinated, and consistent intervention, therapy, and rehabilitation services. If the family selects listening and spoken language as the mode of communication for their child, they should seek out a professional with the specialized knowledge and experience to facilitate this approach. LSLS-trained professionals have the capacity to guide listening and spoken language through use of natural hierarchies of development and by following specific principles of the approach as outlined by the AGBA for the Deaf and Hard of Hearing.

However, with all of the technology and information available, some children do not have these opportunities for success. The provision of services to these children needs to be met through additional training opportunities for professionals seeking LSLS certification as well as the evolution of new service delivery models. Telepractice is quickly becoming an accepted mode of service provision.[65] Children with hearing loss and their families can access high-quality AVT and education, individualized auditory skills training, and programming of cochlear implants and other hearing devices through the use of telepractice.[65–68] In addition, social-emotional support for cochlear implant users of all ages and their family members can be found online through social networks, blogs, or Web sites of cochlear implant companies. With the coordinated efforts of families and professionals coupled with the remarkable advances in both hearing and communication technology, listening and spoken language outcomes for children with hearing loss will be obtainable for all.

RESOURCES
Alexander Graham Bell Association for the Deaf and Hard of Hearing (www.agbell.org)

International nonprofit membership organization, support network, and resource center on pediatric hearing loss and spoken language approaches and related issues.

Address: 3417 Volta Place, NW, Washington, DC 20007
(202) 337–5220 (Voice)

(202) 337–5221 (TTY)
(202) 337–8314 (Fax)

American Academy of Audiology (AAA) (www.audiology.org)

Dedicated to providing quality hearing care to the public and providing consumer and professional resources related to hearing care.

Address: 11730 Plaza America Drive, Suite 300, Reston, VA 20190
(800) AAA-2336 (Voice, Toll-free)
(703) 790–8466 (Voice)
(703) 790–8631 (Fax)

American Speech-Language-Hearing Association (ASHA) (www.asha.org/public/hearing/testing/)

Provides information on newborn hearing screening guidelines and current legislation.

Address: 10801 Rockville Pike, Rockville, MD 20852
E-mail: actioncenter@asha.org
(800) 638–8255 (Voice, TTY)

Centers for Disease Control and Prevention; National Center on Birth Defects and Developmental Disabilities; Early Hearing Detection and Intervention Program (www.cdc.gov/ncbddd/ehdi/default.htm) (Federal Web Site)

Provides information about children and hearing loss and answers some commonly asked questions. Information about state EHDI programs is also available.

Address: MS E-88, 1600 Clifton Road, Atlanta, GA 30333
E-mail: ehdi@cdc.gov
1–800-CDC-INFO (1–800–232–4636)

National Center for Hearing Assessment and Management (NCHAM) (www.infanthearing.org/screening/index.html)

Provides information on newborn hearing screening programs, legislation, equipment, and other related issues.

Utah State University
Address: 2880 Old Main Hill, Logan, UT 84322
E-mail: mail@infanthearing.org
(435) 797–3584 (Voice)

National Institutes of Health; National Institute on Deafness and Other Communication Disorders (www.nidcd.nih.gov/[Federal Web Site])

Federal government's focal point for biomedical and behavioral research in human communication. Web site provides information about hearing, ear infections, and deafness.

Address: 31 Center Drive, MSC 2320, Bethesda, MD 20892–2320
E-mail: nidcdinfo@nidcd.nih.gov
(800) 241–1044 (Toll-free, Voice)
(800) 241–1055 (Toll-free, TTY)

Office of Special Education and Rehabilitation Services (OSERS), US Department of Education (www.ed.gov/about/offices/list/osers/aboutus.html [Federal Web Site])

OSERS supports programs that help educate children and youth with disabilities, provides for the rehabilitation of youth and adults with disabilities, and supports research to improve the lives of individuals with disabilities.

Address: 400 Maryland Avenue, S.W. Washington, DC 20202-7100
(800) 872–5327 (Toll-free)
(202) 245–7468 (Voice)
(800) 437–0833 (TTY)

ZERO TO THREE: National Center for Infants, Toddlers, and Families (www. zerotothree.org)

A national nonprofit organization that promotes the healthy development of infants and toddlers by supporting and strengthening families, communities, and those who work on their behalf. Dedicated to advancing current knowledge; promoting beneficial policies and practices; communicating research and best practices to a wide variety of audiences; and providing training, technical assistance, and leadership development.

Address: 2000 M Street, NW, Suite 200, Washington, DC 20036
(202) 638–1144 (Voice)

REFERENCES

1. Geers AE. Factors affecting the development of speech, language, and literacy in children with early cochlear implantation. Lang Speech Hear Serv Sch 2002; 33(3):172–83.
2. United States Preventative Services Task Force. Summary of recommendations: newborn hearing screening. Rockville (MD): U.S. Preventative Services Task Force Guide to Clinical Preventative Services; 2001.
3. Wake M, Hughes EK, Poulakis Z, et al. Outcomes of children with mild-profound congenital hearing loss at 7-8 years: a population study. Ear Hear 2004;1(25):1–8.
4. Cole EB, Flexer C. Children with hearing loss: developing listening and talking, birth to six. 2nd edition. San Diego (CA): Plural Publishing; 2011.
5. Desjardin JL, Ambrose SE. The importance of the home literacy environment for developing literacy skills in young children who are deaf or hard of hearing. Young Except Child 2010;13:28–44.
6. Flexer C. Technology and listening. In: Robertson L, editor. Literacy and deafness, listening and spoken language. San Diego (CA): Plural Publishing; 2009. p. 43–63.
7. Fulcher A, Purcell AA, Baker E, et al. Listen up: children with early identified hearing loss achieve age-appropriate speech/language outcomes by 3-years-of-age. Int J Pediatr Otorhinolaryngol 2012;76(12):1785–94.
8. Robertson L. Literacy and deafness: listening and spoken language. 2nd edition. San Diego (CA): Plural Publishing; 2009.
9. Centers for Disease Control and Prevention. Annual data for the early hearing detection and intervention program. 2013. Available at: www.cdc.gov/ncbddd/ ehdi/data.htm. Accessed March 17, 2015.
10. Joint Committee on Infant Hearing of the American Academy of Pediatrics, Muse C, Harrison J, et al. Supplement to the JCIH 2007 position statement:

principles and guidelines for early intervention after confirmation that a child is deaf or hard of hearing. Pediatrics 2013;131(4):e1324–49.

11. Ross D, Holstrum WJ, Gaffney M, et al. Hearing screening and diagnostic evaluation of children with unilateral and mild bilateral hearing loss. Trends Amplif 2008;12(1):27.

12. Shargorodsky J, Curhan SG, Curhan GC, et al. Change in prevalence of hearing loss in US adolescents. JAMA 2010;304(7):772–8.

13. Fitzpatrick EM, Crawford L, Ni A, et al. A descriptive analysis of language and speech skills in 4- and 5-yr-old children with hearing loss. Ear Hear 2011;32(5): 605–16.

14. Yoshinaga-Itano C. Principles and guidelines for early intervention after confirmation that a child is deaf or hard of hearing. J Deaf Stud Deaf Educ 2014;19(2):143–75.

15. Geers A, Moog J, Biedenstein J, et al. Spoken language scores of children using cochlear implants compared to hearing age-mates at school entry. J Deaf Stud Deaf Educ 2009;14(3):371–85.

16. Moeller MP. Early intervention and language development in children who are deaf or hard of hearing. Pediatrics 2000;106:e43.

17. Yoshinaga-Itano C, Sedey AL, Coulter DK, et al. Language of early- and later-identified children with hearing loss. Pediatrics 1998;102:1161–71.

18. National Institute on Deafness and Other Communication Disorders. Infographic: 20 years of newborn hearing screenings. Bethesda (MD): US. Department of Health and Human Services; 2015. Available at: http://www.nidcd.nih.gov/Pages/Infographic-20-Years-of-Newborn-Screenings. Accessed March 17, 2015.

19. White KR. The current status of EHDI programs in the United States. Ment Retard Dev Disabil Res Rev 2008;9(2):70–88.

20. Joint Committee on Infant Hearing. Year 2007 position statement: principles and guidelines for early hearing detection and intervention programs. Pediatrics 2007;120(4):898–921.

21. Anderson K, Madell J. Improving hearing and hearing aid retention for infants and young children. Hearing Review 2014;21(2):16–20.

22. Brown C. Early intervention: strategies for public and private sector collaboration. 2006 Convention of the Alexander Graham Bell Association for the Deaf and Hard of Hearing, Pittsburgh (PA), June 23–27, 2006.

23. Moeller MP, Carr G, Seaver L, et al. Best practices in family-centered early intervention for children who are deaf or hard of hearing: an international consensus statement. J Deaf Stud Deaf Educ 2013;18(4):429–45.

24. Houston KT. Ensuring access to communication for young children with hearing loss: auditory learning and spoken language;2010. Available online at: http://www.speechpathology.com. Accessed March 3, 2015.

25. Dornan D, Hickson L, Murdoch B, et al. Is auditory-verbal therapy effective for children with hearing loss? Volta Rev 2010;110(3):361–87.

26. Estabrooks W, editor. 101 FAQs about auditory-verbal practice. Washington, DC: Alexander Graham Bell Association for the Deaf and Hard of Hearing; 2012.

27. Mitchell RE, Karchmer MA. Chasing the mythical ten percent: parental hearing status of deaf and hard of hearing students in the United States. Sign Lang Stud 2004;4:138–63.

28. Alberg J, Wilson K, Roush J. Statewide collaboration in the delivery of EDHI services. Volta Rev 2006;106(3):259–74.

29. Dornan D, Hickson L, Murdoch B, et al. Speech and language outcomes for children with hearing loss in AVT programs: A review of the evidence. Communicative Disorders Review 2008;2(3–4):157–72.

30. Percy-Smith L, Jensen JH, Caye-Themasen P, et al. Factors that affect the social well-being of children with cochlear implants. Cochlear Implants Int 2008;9(4):199–214.

31. Yoshinaga-Itano C. Early intervention after universal neonatal hearing screening: impact on outcomes. Ment Retard Dev Disabil Res Rev 2003;9:252–66.

32. Dettman S, Wall E, Constantinescu G, et al. Communication outcomes for groups of children using cochlear implants enrolled in auditory-verbal, auditory-oral, and bilingual-bicultural early intervention programs. Otol Neurotol 2013;34(3):451–9.

33. Percy-Smith L, Cayé-Thomasen P, Breinegaard N, et al. Parental mode of communication is essential for speech and language outcomes in cochlear implanted children. Acta Otolaryngol 2010;130(6):708–15.

34. Peterson NR, Pisoni DB, Miyamoto RT. Cochlear implants and spoken language processing abilities: review and assessment of the literature. Restor Neurol Neurosci 2010;28(2):237–50.

35. Wie OB, Falkenberg ES, Tvete O, et al. Children with a cochlear implant: characteristics and determinants of speech recognition, speech-recognition growth rate, and speech production. Int J Audiol 2007;46(5):232–43.

36. Yanbay E, Hickson L, Scarinci N, et al. Language outcomes for children with cochlear implants enrolled in different communication programs. Cochlear Implants Int 2014;15(3):121–35.

37. Estabrooks W, Houston KT, MacIver-Lux K. Therapeutic approaches following cochlear implantation. In: Waltzman SB, Roland JT, editors. Cochlear implants. 3rd edition. New York: Thieme Medical Publishers; 2014.

38. Houston KT, Perigoe C. Future directions in professional preparation and development. Volta Rev 2010;110(2):339–40.

39. Holzinger D, Fellinger J, Beitel C. Early onset of family centered intervention predicts language outcomes in children with hearing loss. Int J Pediatr Otorhinolaryngol 2011;75(2):256–60.

40. Hoffman J, Beauchaine K. Babies with hearing loss: steps for effective intervention. ASHA Lead 2007;12(2):8–9, 22–3.

41. Rush D, Sheldon M. The early childhood coaching handbook. Baltimore (MD): Brookes; 2011.

42. Cason J. Telerehabilitation: an adjunct service delivery model for early intervention services. Int J Telerehabil 2011;3(1):19–28.

43. Leffel K, Suskind D. Parent-directed approaches to enrich the early language environments of children living in poverty. Semin Speech Lang 2013;34(4):267–78.

44. McWilliam RA. Working with families of young children with special needs. New York: Guilford Press; 2010.

45. Dunst CJ, Bruder MB, Trivette CM, et al. Everyday activity settings, natural learning environments, and early intervention practices. J Policy Pract Intellect Disabil 2006;3:3–10.

46. Vohr B, Pierre LS, Topol D, et al. Association of maternal communicative behavior with child vocabulary at 18-24 months for children with congenital hearing loss. Early Hum Dev 2010;86(4):255–60.

47. Hintermeir M. Parental resources, parental stress, and socioemotional development of deaf and hard of hearing children. J Deaf Stud Deaf Educ 2006;11(4):493–513.

48. Saffron JR, Werker JF, Werner LA. The infant's auditory world: hearing, speech, and the beginnings of language. In: Kuhn D, Siegler M, editors. The handbook of child psychology. 6th edition. Hoboken (NJ): John Wiley & Sons, Inc; 2006. p. 58–108.

49. Soderstrom M, Seidl A, Kemler Nelson D, et al. The prosodic bootstrapping of phrases: evidence from prelinguistic infants. J Mem Lang 2003;49:249–67.
50. Werker JF, Yeung HH. Infant speech perception bootstraps word learning. Trends Cogn Sci 2005;9(11):519–27.
51. Borden GJ, Harris KS, Raphael LJ. Speech science primer: physiology, acoustics, and perception of speech. 3rd edition. Baltimore (MD): Williams & Wilkins; 1994.
52. Niparko JK, Tobey EA, Thal DJ, et al. Spoken language development in children following cochlear implantation. JAMA 2010;303(15):1498–506.
53. Indiana University School of Medicine. Word learning better in deaf children who receive cochlear implants by age 13 months. Science Daily. 2010. Available online at: http://www.sciencedaily.com/releases/2010/02/100221143158.htm. Accessed March 10, 2011.
54. Hayes H, Geers A, Treiman R, et al. Receptive vocabulary development in deaf children with cochlear implants: achievement in an intensive auditory-oral educational setting. Ear Hear 2009;30:128–35.
55. Bradham T, Houston KT, editors. Assessing listening and spoken language in children with hearing loss. San Diego (CA): Plural Publishing; 2014.
56. Gallaudet Research Institute. Regional and national summary report of data from the 2009-2010 annual survey of deaf and hard of hearing children and youth. Washington, DC: Gallaudet University; 2011.
57. Kushalnagar P, Mathur G, Moreland CJ, et al. Infants and children with hearing loss need early language access. J Clin Ethics 2010;21(2):143–54.
58. Sharma A, Dorman M. Central auditory development in children with cochlear implants: clinical impressions. Adv Otorhinolaryngol 2006;64:66–8.
59. Sharma A, Dorman M, Kral A. The influence of a sensitive period on central auditory development in children with bilateral and unilateral cochlear implants. Hear Res 2005;203:134–43.
60. AGBell Academy for Listening and Spoken Language. 2012 Certification Handbook. Available at: www.agbellacademy.org. Accessed June 11, 2015.
61. Ganek H, McConkey Robbins A, Niparko JK. Language outcomes after cochlear implantation. Otolaryngol Clin North Am 2012;45(1):173–85.
62. Sharma A, Dorman MF, Spahr AJ. A sensitive period for the development of the central auditory system in children with cochlear implants: implications for age of implantation. Ear Hear 2002;23(6):532–9.
63. Kirk KI, Miyamoto RT, Lento CL, et al. Effects of age at implantation in young children. Ann Otol Rhinol Laryngol Suppl 2002;189:69–73.
64. Pollack CA, Goldberg D, Caleffe-Schenck N. Educational audiology for the limited-hearing infant and preschooler: an auditory-verbal program. 3rd edition. Springfield (IL): Charles C. Thomas; 1997.
65. Houston KT, editor. Telepractice in speech-language pathology. San Diego (CA): Plural Publishing; 2014.
66. Brown J. The state of telepractice in 2014. ASHA Lead 2014;19:54–7.
67. Coleman M. Telemedicine making its way to cochlear implants. Hear J 2011; 64(11).
68. McElveen JT, Blackburn EL, Green JD, et al. Remote programming of cochlear implants: a telecommunications model. Otol Neurotol 2010;7:1035–40.

On the Horizon
Cochlear Implant Technology

Joseph P. Roche, MD[a], Marlan R. Hansen, MD[a,b],*

KEYWORDS

- Cochlear implant • Future designs • Optogenetics • Intraneural electrodes
- Intracochlear drug delivery

KEY POINTS

- Cochlear device implantation (CDI) remains the only reliable option for auditory communication rehabilitation in cases of severe and profound sensorineural hearing loss (SNHL) where the site of lesion is outside the central auditory processing stream.
- Cochlear implants (CIs) sample the acoustic environment, process the input signal into discrete frequency bands, compress the amplitude into an electrically useable range, and then stimulate the residual neural elements in a tonotopic manner to reproduce the frequency- and amplitude-analyzing capability of the cochlea.
- CIs represent the most successful neural prosthesis in clinical use and have a long and interesting history that has led to the modern devices that are currently available. Further refinements of the existing current iteration of these devices and the development of novel technology hold promise to continue to improve and benefit patient experience.

INTRODUCTION

Most patients with hearing loss significant enough to result in social dysfunction can be treated with nonsurgical interventions. In many instances, environmental manipulations are sufficient to improve auditory communication, typically by way of improving the signal-to-noise ratio or relative amplification. Examples include minimizing ambient noise such as avoiding crowded or noisy listening situations, selective seating such as sitting closer or with the better ear near important sound sources, or the use of frequency-modulated or infrared (IR) devices. When these manipulations are insufficient, amplification of the acoustic environment can be used. This amplification may

[a] Department of Otolaryngology – Head and Neck Surgery, The University of Iowa Carver College of Medicine, 21151 Pomerantz Family Pavilion, 200 Hawkins Drive, Iowa City, IA 52242-1089, USA; [b] Department of Neurosurgery, The University of Iowa Carver College of Medicine, 200 Hawkins Drive, Iowa City, IA 52242-1089, USA
* Corresponding author. Department of Otolaryngology – Head and Neck Surgery, The University of Iowa Carver College of Medicine, 21151 Pomerantz Family Pavilion, 200 Hawkins Drive, Iowa City, IA 52242-1089.
E-mail address: marlan-hansen@uiowa.edu

Otolaryngol Clin N Am 48 (2015) 1097–1116
http://dx.doi.org/10.1016/j.otc.2015.07.009
0030-6665/15/$ – see front matter © 2015 Elsevier Inc. All rights reserved.

take many forms including personal listening devices or conventional hearing aids. In those with conductive hearing loss that is not amenable to conventional amplification that uses air conduction mechanisms, bone conductive solutions are available including osseointegrated and active middle ear implants.

CDI remains the only reliable option for auditory communication rehabilitation in cases of severe and profound SNHL where the site of lesion is outside the central auditory processing stream. CIs sample the acoustic environment, process the input signal into discrete frequency bands, compress the amplitude into an electrically useable range, and then stimulate the residual neural elements in a tonotopic manner to reproduce the frequency- and amplitude-analyzing capability of the cochlea. CIs represent the most successful neural prosthesis in clinical use and have a long and interesting history that has led to the modern devices that are currently available. Further refinements of the existing devices and the development of novel technology hold promise to continue to improve and benefit patient experience.

HISTORY OF COCHLEAR IMPLANT DEVELOPMENT

The history of CDI spans over 60 years and has seen multiple iterations of the devices and speech processing strategies utilized, although the initial use of electrical audition preceded CDI by almost 200 years. Alessandro Volta performed the first documented electrical stimulation of the auditory system in 1790 when he applied a large voltage across his own ears and was able to generate auditory percepts he described as crackling or bubbling.[1–4] Later experiments applied alternating currents (Duchenne of Boulogne) as well as various charges, polarities, and intensities (Brenner).[2,4] Weaver and colleagues[5] (1930) described electrical signals from the feline cochlea that closely resembled the input stimulus waveform with the implication that it might be possible to replicate this result with electrical signals.[4]

Djourno and colleagues[6] (1957) implanted an electrode coupled with a receiver coil into a patient having undergone resection of the distal cochlear nerve during the treatment of an extensive cholesteatoma and were able to stimulate the apparatus with an external coil for several months. Amazingly, this patient was able to develop sound awareness and simple word recognition.[1,2,4,6–8] William House began his pioneering work in the early 1960s, inspired by the work of Djourno and Eyries, starting with the implantation of either simple wires, wires with ball electrodes, and even simple arrays into the scala tympani.[1,2,9] This early work in partnership with Jack Urban eventually resulted in the development of a commercially available implantable device in 1972 with clinical trials beginning the following year.[1,9]

Although met with considerable skepticism and resistance from the basic science community including leading neurophysiologists and otologists,[1,2,4,10] the validity of direct electrical stimulation of auditory nerve fibers as a rehabilitative strategy was confirmed in 1977 by a team commissioned by the National Institutes of Health that evaluated the outcomes from patients implanted with single-channel devices.[1,4,11] In a major advancement, Clark[12] developed a multichannel CI, which was able to produce open-set word recognition.[12] Following the Food and Drug Administration (FDA) approval of the single-channel CI, multichannel devices soon replaced the single-channel device because of better frequency spectrum percepts and open-set word recognition.[1,4] Based on these developments, multiple multichannel CI devices are available with varying numbers of electrode contacts, electrode lengths, electrode widths, and electrode positioning technologies from 3 device manufactures (Advanced Bionics, Cochlear, and MED-EL).

Environmental speech formant processing and electrode activation strategies developed in parallel to that of CI design over the past several decades.[1] The initial single-channel CIs used simple sinusoidal currents to drive neural responses, whereas multichannel CIs used simultaneous stimulation of discrete locations of the modiolus in a tonotopic manner, this being termed compressed analog strategy.[1,2] Although this latter stimulation paradigm allowed for limited open-set word recognition, the spread of the temporally synchronous current resulted in issues of channel interaction. Other early speech processing strategies included feature extraction (called the PEAK strategy) and the use of multiple filter banks (Spectral Peak Extraction or SPEAK).[2] In 1991, Wilson and colleagues[13] introduced the continuous interleaved sampling (CIS) strategy, which demonstrated significantly improved open-set word recognition when compared with previous analog strategies. Today, all commercially available pulsatile strategies are based on CIS.[1]

CONTEMPORARY COCHLEAR IMPLANTS AND TARGETS FOR INNOVATION

Successful auditory system stimulation resulting in meaningful perceptions requires several technological and biological components, all of which are targets for continued innovations. Acoustic stimuli must be detected and captured (microphone), processed (speech processing software and circuitry), turned into electrical signals (coil, receiver/stimulator) that are delivered to the spiral ganglion neurons (SGNs) (electrode array), transduced into action potentials, and delivered to the central auditory processing stream. Carlson and colleagues[1] (2012) provide a review of the components of the modern CI. Briefly, most CIs consist of an external device worn as a behind-the-ear device incorporating one or more microphones that convert acoustic energy into an analog signal. This signal is then typically digitized, compressed, filtered, and encoded into a signal that is used to drive SGN stimulation. This code is transmitted through the skin using radiofrequency signals to a completely subcutaneous signal receiver that drives intracochlear electrode activation. A variable number of electrodes are encased within a carrier (commonly referred to as the electrode or electrode array), the length of which varies according to the specific device. SGNs are directly driven with electrical voltage delivered by the electrode array to generate action potentials, which are conducted to more central locations in the auditory system. Most CIs also have a return/inactive (ground) electrode that is either part of the body of the receiver/stimulator or a separate lead implanted in the soft tissues around the ear, typically deep to the temporalis muscle. The active electrodes (intracochlear) can be activated in 2 main configurations: monopolar and bipolar. In monopolar stimulation, each intracochlear active electrode uses the extracochlear inactive electrode as the current return. In the bipolar mode, 2 neighboring electrodes form an active/inactive pair. Each mode has its advantages and disadvantages, which are beyond the scope of this review.

The premise of CDI is simple: patterned electrical stimulation of cochlear afferent fibers. Thus both the processing of the acoustic signal (electrical stimulation code) and the neural responses are critical. Unfavorable electrical stimulation or neural response characteristics results in poor perceptual outcomes. The residual neural elements and their health as well as the ability of the CI to deliver high-fidelity electrical stimulation are the basic substrates of contemporary cochlear implantation. Neuronal health has received considerable attention in recent years with several works demonstrating that reduced intracochlear damage with device placement, presumably resulting in improved neuronal survival, is associated with improved speech perceptual abilities.[1,14]

Remote CI programming, totally implanted devices, improved neural health and survival through targeted drug therapy and delivery, intraneural electrode placement, electroacoustical stimulation and hybrid CIs, and methods to enhance the neural-prosthesis interface are evolving areas of innovation reviewed in this article.

TOTALLY IMPLANTABLE COCHLEAR IMPLANTS

Totally implanted cochlear implants (TICIs) may have advantages when compared with current commercially available devices,[1,15] which require an external device that couples to the implanted receiver/stimulator. External devices are exposed to the environment, which may render them more vulnerable to damage from extremes of temperature, moisture, and dislodgement. In addition, implantees typically remove the external device when water exposure is likely (eg, bathing, swimming) or when perspiration is great (vigorous exercise) and thus are off-line during these activities.[15,16] Although the size and profile of current external devices are smaller and less conspicuous than those of earlier-generation devices, they are visible (more so than modern behind-the-ear hearing aids), which may not be desirable to many potential candidates for social reasons.[1] There are several technical barriers to implantation of a TICI including power source management, environmental sound detection, and management of component breakdown.[1,15] Contemporary CIs are powered via electromagnetic induction using radiofrequency signals via the coil of the external device and antenna of the receiver/stimulator. Any TICI would need to be powered internally, likely with the use of a rechargeable battery. Batteries need to be able to recharge quickly, hold enough charge to power the CI for about a day, not generate significant heat, and have a very low chance of leaking potentially dangerous battery chemicals even in the event of battery failure.[1,15,16] At this time, all rechargeable batteries eventually fail to hold significant charge and need to be replaced (a strategy used with pacemakers). In addition, current CIs use an external device worn behind the ear that houses one or more microphones and provides a largely unfettered access to the acoustic environment and takes advantage of the filtering properties of the head. A TICI needs to overcome the more limited direct access to sound sources. Options include microphone placement subcutaneously in the external auditory canal or behind the ear or using the tympanic membrane and/or ossicular chain as a microphone directly.[1,15,17–19] The speech processor and related electrical components also needs to be implanted. It is likely that with the increased number of components implanted, an explantation strategy will need to be devised because component failure becomes more likely. It is also probable that TICI will need some type of external hardware for battery recharging, programming, and switching between programs. It may also be desirable to allow the TICI to be powered and stimulated using a conventional external device.[15,16] Briggs and colleagues[16] (2008) published the first report using a TICI system in 3 subjects. The investigators termed the use of the TICI alone as invisible hearing. The devices used a subcutaneous microphone near the radiofrequency coil, lithium ion battery, and the ESPrit 3G (Cochlear Corporation, New South Wales, Australia) external sound processor for use in a conventional mode. Results indicated that the devices can be safely implanted and all 3 subjects reported benefit when using the devices in the invisible hearing mode. However, the subjects scored higher in measures of consonant-nucleus-consonant word testing in quiet and City University of New York sentence scores in noise when using the devices in conventional mode with the external speech processor. With continued improvement, it is likely that TICI will become a viable and common device option for patients.

TELEMEDICINE AND REMOTE PROGRAMMING OF COCHLEAR IMPLANTS

After CDI, the brain learns to use the encoded electrical stimulation to extract information about the acoustic environment; this is a dynamic process with continued improvements being seen years after the initial device activation. Each electrode in the array must be tuned to the response properties of the region that it stimulates, which typically involves determining the psychophysical threshold and the maximum comfortable level of stimulation (also known as T and C levels, respectively). Over time, changes in T and/or C levels, individual electrode failures or extrusions, and nonauditory stimulations (eg, facial nerve stimulation) require reprogramming the speech processor. CI programming has traditionally been performed in the clinical setting by an implant audiologist using proprietary equipment and software. This programming has required health care encounters at dedicated CI program centers, often necessitating a travel requirement for patients and their families. Modern telecommunication technologies may offer an approach to programming where patients and their CI team can work together to maximize each user's performance without a physical visit to the implant center. This approach can offer specific benefit to patients with limited access to transportation or who live in remote areas. Several recent reports document the safety and efficacy of remote programming.[20–22] Ramos and colleagues[20] (2009) describe a fairly simple setup for remote programming based on software for video conferencing, computer operating systems, and standard CI programming software and hardware. In their experimental setup, a remote unit equipped with all required programming equipment and attended by a local representative interacted with a remote location equipped with similar computing equipment and programs. The remote computer was able to control the local computer and thus run the programming software. In their study of 5 subjects who were programmed both with standard and remote programming sessions, they found that remote programming was safe and was not statistically different from standard programming. McElveen and colleagues[21] (2010) also demonstrated the safety and noninferiority of remote programming in 7 patients compared with 7 matched controls using a setup similar to that of Ramos and colleagues[20] (2009). Wesarg and colleagues[22] (2010) evaluated 70 subjects over several different implant centers using a variety of technology and found no significant difference in map characteristics between remote and local programming sessions. One common finding in these 3 studies is the presence of monitoring personnel to ensure the safety of the subject being programmed by watching for signs of painful stimulation and ensuring that there are no communication issues between the remote programming audiologist and the subject.[20–22] Patient and health care professional satisfaction with remote CI programming in these and other studies has been quite high, with one recent study reporting that greater than 96% of respondents were satisfied with remote programming sessions and 100% reporting that they would use remote programming in the future.[20–23] These studies demonstrate that remote programming is safe and feasible and may offer an opportunity for better access and possibly improved outcomes for patients undergoing CDI who live at a considerable distance from their implant center.

OPTICAL NEURAL STIMULATION AND OPTICAL COCHLEAR IMPLANTS

Contemporary hearing rehabilitation currently relies on 2 main modalities: acoustic stimulation to the cochlea and electrical stimulation of remaining cochlear nerve afferents.[24] Both strategies have advantages and limitations. Acoustic stimulation relies on the presence of mechanoacoustic stimulation of the cochlea, typically with amplified and filtered signals (eg, conventional hearing aids) and necessarily relies on cochlear functions including the biomechanics of the basilar membrane and organ of Corti as well as the physiology of the inner and outer hair cells. In the case of conventional hearing aids, this requires a patent external auditory canal that can tolerate the placement of the hearing aid. In severe cases of SNHL, these biomechanical and physiologic properties are deranged to the point where mechanoacoustical stimulation does not provide the subject with a hearing benefit. In many of these patients, a reduced but viable population of SGNs remain that can be driven with nearby electrical voltage changes and this provides the neural basis for electrical hearing via CDI. With modern CI electrode arrays and stimulation paradigms, CI users are commonly performing at perfect or near-perfect levels on word recognition tests including hearing in noise situations.[25] However, despite these results, many patients continue to report difficulty hearing in noisy environments and with music perception.[24,26,27] As reviewed by Richter and colleagues[28] (2013), although there are at most 22 electrodes, only 4 to 7 channels are truly independent versus the estimated 30 to 50 channels in subjects with normal hearing. The main problem is thought to be the spread of current (spread of excitation) away from active electrodes.[29] This spread of excitation may degrade the specificity of the neural elements being stimulated through channel interaction or cross talk.[30,31] Channel interaction is an example of how the spread of the excitatory currents degrade the neural percepts with CIs. It is likely that increasing the number of independent channels will improve listening in noise or music appreciation.[28,29] Virtual channels, created by steering current between 2 electrodes, and bipolar electrode stimulation[32] have been used to decrease channel interaction but have yet to result in significant improvement over more traditional stimulation methods.[28]

The use of photons as the energy source for neural stimulation has been proposed as one mechanism to more specifically stimulate neural elements (reviewed in Richter and colleagues,[28] 2013; Eshraghi and colleagues,[4] 2012; Jeschke and Moser 2015[27]; and Moser,[24] 2015). **Fig. 1** provides a demonstration of how optical stimulation may provide more precise stimulation when compared to current cochlear implant devices. The precision that light stimulation may offer could allow for the creation of more focal stimulation and thus more independent channels of information flow.[27] Light energy has been found to excite many different types of tissues including peripheral nerve, cortical cells, cardiomyocytes, and isolated neurons.[27,28] In addition, the light energy could be delivered via local light sources such as miniature light-emitting diodes or could be transported via special wave guides.[27] There are several proposed mechanisms for how light can stimulate neural tissues: (1) photoactivation of light-gated ion channels (optogenetics), (2) thermal stimulation of heat-gated ion channels (thermogenetics), (3) direct activation through alterations in local plasma membrane electrical properties, (4) uncaging of neurostimulatory compounds, and (5) modulation of intracellular calcium metabolism.[4,24,27,28] Optical stimulation mechanisms, specifically optogenetic and IR light stimulation, have received the most attention.

Optogenetics and thermogenetics require the expression of ion channels in the tissue to be excited, which in the case of hearing loss and CIs in particular, are the SGNs.[27,28] Since the discovery of channelrhodopsin (ChR) 1 and 2, the expression of these channels has become a popular method for neural stimulation throughout the neurosciences.[24,27,33,34] The molecules function as transmembrane light-gated ionotropic channels. Several ChRs have been developed with a variety of kinetic properties,[27] which with creative expression including specific subcellular compartmental localization could allow for a variety of light wavelengths and channels to precisely tune neural responses. Although cation channels and anion pumps have been expressed and used to drive neuronal activity in rodent auditory brainstem neurons and auditory neocortex, the expression of these channels requires either the

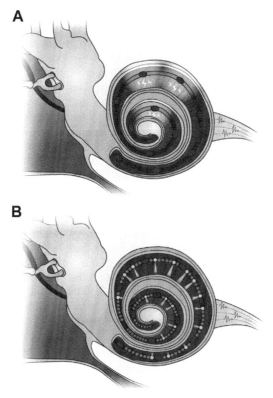

Fig. 1. Schematic representation of cochlear implant devices using either electrical (*A*) or optical (*B*) stimulation. Devices that are in clinical use at present use electrical stimulation and contain variable numbers of electrode channels depending on the specific design of the electrode array; electrical currents spread outward from the electrodes to depolarize the remaining spiral ganglion cells. Overlapping electrical fields result in channel interactions and degradation of the spectral and temporal resolution that is possible from the stimulating signal pattern. Optical stimulation, such as focused light delivered through microscale light-emitting diodes, may allow for more focused stimulation of spiral ganglion cells. Thus it should be possible to generate more independent channels of information, which could result in better spectral and temporal percepts of the acoustic environment. (*From Jeschke M, Moser T. Considering optogenetic stimulation for cochlear implants. Hearing Res 2015;322:224–34; with permission.*)

postfertilization transfer of the genetic material, typically using a viral vector, or transgenic techniques, neither of which is used in humans at this time.[24,27,28,35,36] In addition, the channel kinetics of the available channels limit the rate of stimulation to around 50 to 60 Hz, much lower than the several hundred Hertz spiking that can been seen in SGNs as they follow the envelope of a sound stimulus.[24,37]

Similar to optogenetics, thermogenetics uses a thermosensitive ion channel that has recently been described, which has been shown to allow for depolarization of neurons with the focal application of heat, such as IR light.[28,38] Similar limitations to the expression of these channels as for optogenetic stimulation exist.

In addition to excitation of exogenously expressed thermosensitive channels, IR light has been shown to directly stimulate neurons.[28,39] The mechanism underlying this is thought to be focal thermal changes in the plasma membrane capacitance, which results in depolarization. Shapiro and colleagues[35] (2012) demonstrated that this excitation is due to a focal, reversible increase in temperature because of IR energy absorption by water. This increase in temperature results in a change in the local capacitance of the plasma membrane and leads to membrane depolarization. When compared with optogenetic and thermogenetic techniques, IR stimulation has the advantage of not requiring the expression of special ion channels or the infusion of special compounds. In a series of reports, Richter and colleagues[40] demonstrated neural excitation with IR energy and defined the amount of energy required for this excitation, the temporal fidelity, and the spread of excitation from focal IR pulse, which was better than that of electrical stimulation.[39,41–43] Littlefield and colleagues[39] (2010) demonstrated that IR light could activate auditory nerve fibers by using IR light directed through the round window. However, several recent studies have challenged the underlying assumptions of how IR energy stimulates the auditory system. The rapid rise in temperature could result in pressure wave formation (up to about 60 dB sound pressure level equivalent), which could then stimulate remaining hair cells and drive an auditory response (optoacoustic effect).[37,44] In addition, Verma and colleagues[37] (2014) demonstrated that in a completely deafened cochlea, IR stimulation was unable to drive cochlear nucleus responses. There are numerous challenges to implementing these strategies. However, as water is the main molecule that absorbs IR energy, the light source needs to be very close to the target neuron because the surrounding fluids cause a significant decrement in the amount of energy available to drive neural responses.[28] When compared with existing CI technology, the energy requirement for IR stimulation was far in excess.[24,40] Further work needs to be performed to clarify the mechanisms of how IR energy directly stimulates central auditory pathways.

IR light can also be used to free caged compounds that can drive neural excitation.[4] One example of this would be the use of light to break a photosensitive bond between glutamate and an inactivating caging compound.

With continued refinement, focused optical stimulation of the SGNs holds promise to overcome many of the technical and perceptual challenges currently present with modern CIs; this may take several forms but is mainly geared toward the creation of more functionally independent channels of information flow. It is also likely that novel coding and stimulation strategies will be needed for optical CIs to take advantage of the increased information channels and channel independence.[24]

INTRANEURAL COCHLEAR IMPLANTATION

Contemporary intrascalar CI electrode arrays are arguably the most successful neurosensory rehabilitation prosthesis, although as reviewed above, significant perceptual challenges remain including listening in noise, music perception, impaired pitch perception, and poor sound localization even with bilateral CIs.[45] These deficits may be a result of the spread of excitation due to the high levels of current required to overcome the distance between the electrodes in the array and the excitable neural elements, the shunting of current away from these neural elements by the electroconductive perilymph, and the shielding effects of the modiolar bone covering the neural elements.[8,45] Optical stimulation, as outlined above, is one mechanism that holds promise to refine the ability to precisely stimulate neural elements and thus reduce the spread of excitation and channel interaction. Another strategy is direct stimulation of the neural elements in the modiolus with intraneural electrodes. Intraneural implantation may offer several advantages over intrascalar electrode arrays including lower threshold currents because of direct interaction of the electrode and the neural elements (possibly allowing for an increased number of independent channels), the ability to access more apical fibers resulting in better stimulation of lower-characteristic-frequency neural elements, lower risk of facial nerve stimulation due to the electrode being farther from the facial nerve, and less anatomic limitations to implantation for dysplastic or ossified cochleas.[8] Increased potential for neural injury because of insertional trauma represents a significant hurdle for stimulation with intraneural electrodes.

Djourno and colleagues[6] (1957) were the first to chronically implant an electrical auditory prosthesis as described above. From 1964 through the middle of the 1980s, Simmons and colleagues[46–54] published a series of reports investigating the direct intraoperative stimulation of the auditory nerve, implantation of an intraneural device into the auditory nerve, subsequent work in animal models, and a return to human direct nerve implantation.[8] Amazingly, the initial human experiments resulted in auditory perceptions.[46,48] Subsequent work in cats and then humans demonstrated that chronically implanted intraneural electrodes yield stable long-term thresholds and were well tolerated, although evidence of partial SGN loss and insertional neural trauma was found.[49–51,53,54] As reviewed and cited in Arts and colleagues'[8] article (2003), the next development was that of the Michigan array, a series of electrodes on one or more thin shanks. In a series of experiments, these arrays were found to be well tolerated in both stimulating and nonstimulating conditions of the cochlear nerve and cochlear nuclei in animal models. When implanted in the modiolus, there was comparatively less cochlear and neural damage reported by Arts and colleagues[8] than that reported by Simmons (1979).[54] Both modiolar and intracanalicular auditory nerve implantations have been used. Investigators at the University of Utah have developed a multielectrode implant, termed the Utah electrode array (UEA) that uses a series of needle electrodes arranged in a square configuration that could be implanted into the modiolar nerve after a facial recess surgical approach.[55] Badi and colleagues[55–57] demonstrated that in cats implantation with variations of the UEA into the auditory nerve is feasible, seems to result in minimal histologic trauma to implanted nerves, and can elicit auditory responses. Lastly, Middlebrooks and Snyder[45] (2007) implanted straight electrode arrays into the modiolar nerve and found that these electrodes could produce low current threshold, frequency-specific responses in the inferior colliculus central nucleus with less electrode interaction, and spread of excitation when compared with intrascalar electrodes. The studies by Simmons,[54] those with the Michigan array by Arts and colleagues,[8] those with the UEA by Badi and colleagues,[56] and the work by Middlebrooks and Snyder (2007)[45] all demonstrate that intraneural electrodes evoke auditory neural responses with less current levels than intrascalar electrodes.[8,45,54,56] These studies demonstrate the feasibility of chronic intraneural implantation and stimulation and the possibility of increased numbers of independent channels with reduced channel interaction compared with current intrascalar electrode arrays. Furthermore, intraneural implants, if proven to be safe and at least not inferior to conventional intrascalar CIs, may offer a more reliable option for patients with malformed, brittle, or ossified cochleae.

HEARING PRESERVATION AND ELECTROACOUSTICAL STIMULATION

The benefits of CDI and electrical hearing are well established, and CDI can now be considered the standard of care for patients with severe-to-profound SNHL and no meaningful benefit from conventional amplification. However, many patients with severe-to-profound high-frequency hearing loss and limited word discrimination retain substantial residual hearing in the low frequencies. This residual hearing often provides significant benefit; however, the profound SNHL in the high frequencies results in poor speech and language abilities.[58] These patients are able to gain information about the low-frequency components of speech (vocal fold vibratory patterns) but are not able to process high-frequency components of speech such as fricative phonemes.[59] Conventional amplification is of limited benefit in these situations.[60] Such patients are left in a therapeutic bind: they do not benefit significantly from amplification but conventional cochlear implantation with standard electrode arrays and carriers typically results in complete loss of the residual hearing.

Considerable recent work has focused on preserving the residual low-frequency hearing after CDI, such that the implanted ear is simultaneously stimulated with electrical signals with higher-frequency information (where many formants of English language speech are found) and acoustic signals, which will convey low-frequency information. Two main hearing preservation strategies have been used: incomplete insertion of standard electrodes and design of shorter-electrode carriers. Preservation of low-frequency hearing with standard-length electrode arrays is typically accomplished by terminating electrode advancement at the level of the basal turn,[58,61–65] thereby reducing the risk of the electrode traversing the basilar membrane and damaging the organ of Corti and neural elements. Shorter-electrode carrier designs include the Hybrid S, Hybrid S10, and L24 by Cochlear Corporation (Cochlear Americas, Boulder, CO) and the M or Flex-EAS electrodes by MED-EL Corporation (Durham, NC). As reviewed in Mowry and colleagues[58] (2012), results from studies of speech and language outcomes and preservation of hearing have been favorable with shorter-electrode carriers (from both companies) and standard electrode carriers with shorter insertion angles. Controversy exists as to whether a standard or short-electrode carrier is the best. Standard electrode carriers have higher rates of loss of residual hearing including anacusis. However, if residual hearing is lost, longer electrodes have the potential to offer more independent channels of information, depending on insertion depth, because of the higher number of electrodes in the array and wider spacing, which can reduce channel interaction. **Fig. 2** provides a graphical representation of current implant criteria for both conventional and hearing preserving

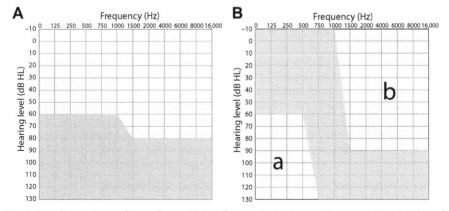

Fig. 2. Audiometric profiles of candidates for implantation with conventional (A) and hybrid (B) devices. The blue shaded area represents where pure-tone thresholds should lie. Candidates for hybrid cochlear implant devices must not have pure-tone thresholds in the gray regions representing thresholds that are either too poor (a) to use acoustic stimulation or good (b) to benefit from electrical stimulation of high-frequency regions.

cochlear implants that allow for both electrical and acoustic stimulation (so called hybrid CI).

The initial short-electrode device, the Hybrid S (Cochlear Corporation) had 6 electrodes in the array in a carrier that was 6 mm in length.[58] Results from the first 6 patients, 3 implanted with a 6-mm carrier and 3 with a 10-mm carrier, demonstrated that all 6 subjects preserved their hearing and all demonstrated benefit; the 3 subjects implanted with the 10-mm carrier performed considerably better than those implanted with the 6-mm carrier.[66] Based on these successful results, a phase 1 FDA trial using the Hybrid S 10-mm carrier enrolled 87 patients with severe-to-profound high frequency SNHL and the preliminary results again demonstrated favorable results.[67] The vast majority of subjects demonstrated initial and long-term hearing preservation after surgery (98% and 91%, respectively). About 30% of subjects had a 30 dB HL or greater loss in the low frequencies. Most patients performed better than preoperative measures; 18% did not show any improvement or performed worse.[67] The L24 carrier (Cochlear) is 16 mm in length but has 22 electrodes in the array. Results from a multicenter trial in Europe demonstrated that subjects maintained low-frequency hearing within 30 dB HL (96%) and 15 dB HL (68%) of preoperative thresholds and this was stable over time.[68] Both the Hybrid S and L24 trials found that habituation periods were significant with continued improvement occurring after 12 months of use.[58] In a study of 18 patients undergoing implantation with the M electrode (MED-EL Corporation), 12 patients had residual hearing that could be amplified, although only 6 consistently used their CI in the hybrid mode on a routine basis.[69] Numerous studies have reported preservation of hearing after subtotal insertion of various full-length standard carriers.[58] Patients implanted with short-electrode carriers (Hybrid S/L24 or M/Flex-EAS) achieve significant improvements in speech discrimination in quiet as well as in noisy listening conditions.[58,67,68] Similar results have been found in subjects implanted with standard electrode arrays with subtotal insertion.[58] Electrical and acoustic stimulation with residual hearing preservation seems to be a viable option for patients with significant levels of preoperative low-frequency hearing (**Fig. 1**).

NEUROPROTECTION

Most patients with severe-to-profound hearing loss have a reduced population of SGNs presumably as a result of gradual neural degeneration following injury to the cochlear epithelium and hair cell loss. While the residual neurons in these patients suffice to perform well on standard speech perception testing using previous versions of electrode arrays and stimulation strategies,[70,71] it is likely that emerging devices and stimulation strategies will depend more on a healthy complement of neurons to achieve optimal results.[72] Furthermore, insertion of the electrode array itself into the scala tympani can result in trauma to the neurosensory elements through violation of the basilar membrane, entry into the scala media, disruption of the organ of Corti, injury to the stria vascularis, and/or fracture of the modiolus.[1,9] As reviewed in Carlson and colleagues[1] (2012), damage to the residual neural elements is thought to underlie some of the variability in CI outcomes. These findings have led to the development and refinement of less-traumatic surgical techniques (so-called soft surgery).[4,9,73–76] As reviewed in Eshraghi and colleagues[9,73] (2012 and 2013, respectively), even in situations in which no identifiable macroscopic trauma can be found in animal cochleae undergoing implantation, molecular and cellular evidence for damage can be found and may explain the losses of residual hearing seen in several hearing preservation trials using specialized electrodes and techniques (see above).[58,67,68] Molecular events that could contribute to cell death include the generation of reactive oxygen species and proinflammatory cytokines that lead to the activation of proapoptotic signals such as c-Jun-N-terminal kinase (JNK), a member of the mitogen-activated protein kinase family.[9,73] Various drugs that target the aforementioned molecular signals and various delivery systems to deliver these drugs are currently being investigated. The glucocorticoid, dexamethasone, and JNK pathway inhibitors are the most well-studied pharmaceutical therapeutics. Targeted delivery systems have included transtympanic injections (such as transtympanic corticosteroids for sudden hearing loss), miniosmotic pumps, and biodegradable gels that elute the compound of interest over time. Targeted delivery is preferable to systemic administration because this can reduce the side effects and other nondesirable effects of the medications,[9,73] which in turn may allow for higher local doses and longer treatment durations. For example, in the setting of sudden hearing loss, intratympanic corticosteroids can be used instead of systemic therapy in cases in which the biochemical side effects are difficult to tolerate (eg, diabetes).

Dexamethasone has been used by numerous investigators to reduce inflammation induced by CDI and has demonstrated a protective effect in animal models. Eshraghi and colleagues[77] (2007) and Vivero and colleagues[78] (2008) found that infusion of the dexamethasone via miniosmotic pumps protected the operated ears in guinea pigs from trauma-induced hearing loss with electrode insertion. Likewise, Ye and colleagues[79] (2007) found that triamcinolone, another glucocorticoid compound, reduced hearing loss caused from surgical trauma (cochleostomy). James and colleagues[80] (2008) used dexamethasone in a hyaluronic acid/carboxymethylcellulose bead placed near the round window, and this was found to protect against hearing loss from electrode trauma.

The JNK pathway mediates apoptosis signaling, and pathway inhibitors have been used in various organ systems as neuroprotectants (eg, retinal ganglion cells and cortical neurons).[73] Ex vivo studies of murine cochleae found that treatment with D-JNKI-1, a peptide JNK inhibitor, prevented hair cell apoptosis induced with acoustic or aminoglycoside trauma.[81] Eshraghi and colleagues[82,83] performed a series of experiments in guinea pigs that demonstrated the protective effects of D-JNK-1 from hearing loss induced by trauma due to electrode insertion, both acute and delayed components. Both these studies used minipumps to infuse the JNK inhibitor. Eshraghi and colleagues[73] (2013) used D-JNK-1 mixed with a hyaluronate gel applied to the round window membrane half an hour before electrode insertion and again demonstrated physiologic and histologic protection from the damaging effects of electrode insertion. Furthermore, inhibition of JNK using genetic and molecular approaches and pharmacologic compounds rescues cultured SGN from apoptosis.[84] However, general JNK inhibitors, such as D-JNK-1, inhibit SGN neurite regeneration. To the extent that neural regeneration (see below) becomes a therapeutic goal in addition to prevention of neuron apoptosis, it will be important to consider the effects of specific molecular targets on neurite growth in addition to neuronal survival. Other examples of stimuli and signaling molecules that promote SGN survival yet inhibit neurite regeneration include membrane depolarization, protein kinase A, calcium-calmodulin-dependent kinase II, and members of the Bcl-2 family of proteins.[85–89] Meanwhile, other factors, in particular, the neurotrophins (NTs) NT-3 and brain-derived neurotrophic factor (BDNF), promote both SGN survival and neurite regeneration (see below).[90]

Typically, pharmacologic compounds must diffuse through the round window to gain access to the scalar contents. As reviewed in Salt and Plontke[91] (2009), a variety of substances (local anesthetics, ototoxic medications, neurotransmitters, and monoclonal antibodies) have been placed into the middle ear with the goal of intralabyrinthine distribution. Recently, measurements from the scala tympani have demonstrated that drug distribution is accomplished mainly with passive diffusion movement and that a concentration gradient is found between the basal and apical ends of the scala; thus to achieve high apical drug concentrations, prolonged exposure to the round window is required.[9,91] The drug of interest must be able to liberate from the carrier substance, be absorbed into the perilymph (typically through the round window membrane), and distribute throughout the inner ear tissue via diffusion.[91] Carrier compounds that allow for the sustained release of drug over time include liposomes, drug-loaded biodegradable microspheres, and drug-polymer congregates.[91] Alternatively, microcatheters and pumps can be used to infuse the drug to the round window membrane.[73,82,91] With specific regard to the CI, several investigators have discussed strategies for drug delivery using the CI device including bathing the implant in a drug or gel before implantation, drug liberation from the electrode array carrier, drug release from a reservoir within the carrier, infusion through a separate channel in the carrier, and coating the carrier with a sustained-release formulation.[91–94] Richardson and colleagues[93] (2009) demonstrated that polymer electrodes that elute NTs with electrical stimulation resulted in lower brainstem response thresholds and higher SGN counts when compared with controls (nonelectrically stimulated).

In summary, targeted drug therapy to help improve hair cell and neuronal survival, as well as innovative drug delivery mechanisms, hold significant promise for improving performance with current devices and preserve residual structures.

IMPROVING THE ELECTRODE AND COCHLEAR NERVE INTERACTIONS

As reviewed above, CDI allows for the perception of the acoustic environment by selective stimulation of the remaining modiolar neural elements in a frequency-specific manner. However, the distance between the stimulating electrodes and the neural elements that they activate fails to recapitulate the intimate, precise innervation pattern of the cochlea. Improvements in how the electrode and neural elements interact may allow for enhanced specificity in the coupling of specific electrodes and nerve fibers, resulting in lower stimulation current requirements and thus potentially less channel interaction.[1] Direct nerve implantation (reviewed above) is one mechanism being studied that results in physical contact of the electrodes in the array with cochlear nerve afferent fibers. Two other strategies are currently being studied: electrode carrier positioning techniques that result in a perimodiolar position of the electrode array and neural stimulation to induce neural growth to the electrode. It is possible that a combination of all 3 strategies will be used in some combination in the future to take selective advantage of benefits that each strategy may offer.

Perimodiolar positioning strategies have been used clinically in the past decade. Early designs used ridged positioning elements that resulted in significant intracochlear trauma and were associated with a significantly elevated risk of meningitis and were subsequently withdrawn from the market.[1,95,96] Animal models have corroborated the clinical findings that cochlear trauma increases the risk of otogenic meningitis.[97] Recently, precurved electrode carriers (Cochlear Corporation [Cochlear Americas, Boulder, CO] Contour Advance electrode array) have been used with great success. Roland[98] (2005) demonstrated that with the advance of stylet (AOS) technique there were low levels of cochlear trauma through a reduction in the forces imparted to the lateral cochlear wall. This device uses a rigid stylet that is contained within the electrode carrier that holds the carrier in a nearly straight alignment for the initial insertion. Once the electrode carrier is at the first turn of the cochlea, the stylet is grasped and the electrode is advanced further allowing the carrier to return to its nascent, curved shaped in a tight spiral around the modular wall. This device is now routinely used in many institutions. Midscalar positioning (electrode carrier array located in the middle of the scala tympani without contact to either the modiolus or lateral wall) can also be used. An advantage of this intrascalar position is that it may avoid some of the trauma that is seen with electrode carrier interactions with either the lateral or modular walls while bringing the electrodes closer to the remaining neural elements than traditional lateral wall configurations.[99,100] Histologic studies have demonstrated that the midscalar electrode carrier (HiFocus Mid-scala, Advanced Bionics [Valencia, CA]) does allow for low insertional trauma when inserted off of a stylet.

CIs require the presence of type I afferent fibers to work as evidenced by the profound lack of benefit seen in children with cochlear nerve aplasia who have undergone CDI. Progressive loss of these auditory fibers or other neuropathologic changes has been postulated to result in reduced performance with CIs.[101] One explanation for the loss of SGNs with hearing loss is the resulting loss of neurotrophic factors produced in the cochlear epithelium.[101] NTs are implicated in the development of SGNs and their long-term survival in both ex vivo and in vivo animal models when exogenously administered.[101,102] In addition to their neuroprotective effects, NTs have also been demonstrated to enhance resprouting of auditory nerve peripheral processes.[102] Wise and colleagues[103] (2005) demonstrated that the application of BDNF and NT3 enhanced sprouting from neural elements near the site of drug application. Viral vectors have been used to force expression of BDNF in a murine model and found enhanced neural regrowth.[104] Thus it appears possible that exogenously administered or endogenously expressed neurotrophic factors may have a role in preserving the neural substrate for CIs and possibly inducing neural sprouting to further enhance the prosthesis-nerve interface. However, for such axon regeneration to be useful, it must be precisely guided to faithfully recapitulate the precise tonotopic arrangement of the afferent auditory innervation. Thus, additional work has been performed to look at neurite guidance cues in an effort to understand and potentially modulate and control neurite growth patterns with the idea that it might be possible to guide neurite growth in an advantageous way. Patterning of biochemical guidance clues have been shown to direct SGN growth cone pathfinding and neurite growth. For example, stripes of EphA4, a chemorepulsive peptide, guide neurite growth because the neurites avoid the EphA-coated stripes.[105] In addition to biochemical factors, physical surface features have recently been shown to precisely direct SGN neurite growth.[106,107] The ability of these surface features to guide SGN neurite growth depends on channel amplitude and periodicity, mechanical and surface properties (eg, polarity), and pattern complexity.[108–110] Advantages of such surface features compared with patterning of bioactive molecules include ease and cost of production, reproducibility, and shelf-life stability.[108,110] Taken together, neurotrophic-enhanced neural sprouting and the use of directional neurite growth strategies including physical surface and biochemical cues may allow for a more intimate interface of the CI electrode array and the neural elements it stimulates.

SUMMARY

Cochlear implantation and CIs have a long history filled with innovations that have resulted in the high-performing device's currently available. Several promising technologies have been reviewed in this article, which hold the promise to drive performance even higher.

REFERENCES

1. Carlson ML, Driscoll CL, Gifford RH, et al. Cochlear implantation: current and future device options. Otolaryngol Clin North Am 2012;45(1):221–48.
2. Ramsden RT. History of cochlear implantation. Cochlear Implants Int 2013; 14(Suppl 4):S3–5.
3. Volta A. On electricity excited by the mere contact of conducting substances of different kinds. Phil. Trans. R. Soc. Lond 1800;90:403–31.
4. Eshraghi AA, Nazarian R, Telischi FF, et al. The cochlear implant: historical aspects and future prospects. Anat Rec (Hoboken) 2012;295(11):1967–80.
5. Weaver E, Bray C, Wever EG, et al. The nature of the acoustic response: the relation between sound frequency of impulses in the auditory nerve. J Exp Psychol 1930;13:373–87.
6. Djourno A, Eyries C, Vallancien B. Electric excitation of the cochlear nerve in man by induction at a distance with the aid of micro-coil included in the fixture. C R Seances Soc Biol Fil 1957;151(3):423–5 [in French].
7. Eisen MD. Djourno, Eyries, and the first implanted electrical neural stimulator to restore hearing. Otol Neurotol 2003;24(3):500–6.
8. Arts HA, Jones DA, Anderson DJ. Prosthetic stimulation of the auditory system with intraneural electrodes. Ann Otol Rhinol Laryngol Suppl 2003;191:20–5.
9. Eshraghi AA, Gupta C, Ozdamar O, et al. Biomedical engineering principles of modern cochlear implants and recent surgical innovations. Anat Rec (Hoboken) 2012;295(11):1957–66.
10. Kiang NY, Moxon EC. Physiological considerations in artificial stimulation of the inner ear. Ann Otol Rhinol Laryngol 1972;81(5):714–30.
11. Bilger RC, Black FO. Auditory prostheses in perspective. Ann Otol Rhinol Laryngol Suppl 1977;86(3 Pt 2 Suppl 38):3–10.
12. Clark GM, Tong YC, Martin LF. A multiple-channel cochlear implant: an evaluation using open-set CID sentences. Laryngoscope 1981;91(4):628–34.
13. Wilson BS, Finley CC, Lawson DT, et al. Better speech recognition with cochlear implants. Nature 1991;352(6332):236–8.
14. Carlson ML, Driscoll CL, Gifford RH, et al. Implications of minimizing trauma during conventional cochlear implantation. Otol Neurotol 2011;32(6):962–8.
15. Cohen N. The totally implantable cochlear implant. Ear Hear 2007;28(2 Suppl): 100s–1s.
16. Briggs RJ, Eder HC, Seligman PM, et al. Initial clinical experience with a totally implantable cochlear implant research device. Otol Neurotol 2008;20(2):114–9.
17. Huttenbrink KB, Zahnert TH, Bornitz M, et al. Biomechanical aspects in implantable microphones and hearing aids and development of a concept with a hydroacoustical transmission. Acta Otolaryngol 2001;121(2):185–9.
18. Maniglia AJ, Abbass H, Azar T, et al. The middle ear bioelectronic microphone for a totally implantable cochlear hearing device for profound and total hearing loss. Am J Otol 1999;20(5):602–11.
19. Zenner HP, Leysieffer H, Maassen M, et al. Human studies of a piezoelectric transducer and a microphone for a totally implantable electronic hearing device. Am J Otol 2000;21(2):196–204.
20. Ramos A, Rodriguez C, Martinez-Beneyto P, et al. Use of telemedicine in the remote programming of cochlear implants. Acta Otolaryngol 2009;129(5):533–40.
21. McElveen JT Jr, Blackburn EL, Green JD Jr, et al. Remote programming of cochlear implants: a telecommunications model. Otol Neurotol 2010;31(7): 1035–40.

22. Wesarg T, Wasowski A, Skarzynski H, et al. Remote fitting in nucleus cochlear implant recipients. Acta Otolaryngol 2010;130(12):1379–88.

23. Kuzovkov V, Yanov Y, Levin S, et al. Remote programming of MED-EL cochlear implants: users' and professionals' evaluation of the remote programming experience. Acta Otolaryngol 2014;134(7):709–16.

24. Moser T. Optogenetic stimulation of the auditory pathway for research and future prosthetics. Curr Opin Neurobiol 2015;34C:29–36.

25. Gifford RH, Shallop JK, Peterson AM. Speech recognition materials and ceiling effects: considerations for cochlear implant programs. Audiol Neurootol 2008; 13(3):193–205.

26. Kohlberg G, Spitzer JB, Mancuso D, et al. Does cochlear implantation restore music appreciation? Laryngoscope 2014;124(3):587–8.

27. Jeschke M, Moser T. Considering optogenetic stimulation for cochlear implants. Hear Res 2015;322:224–34.

28. Richter CP, Rajguru S, Bendett M. Infrared neural stimulation in the cochlea. Proc SPIE Int Soc Opt Eng 2013;8565:85651Y.

29. Friesen LM, Shannon RV, Baskent D, et al. Speech recognition in noise as a function of the number of spectral channels: comparison of acoustic hearing and cochlear implants. J Acoust Soc Am 2001;110(2):1150–63.

30. Kral A, Hartmann R, Mortazavi D, et al. Spatial resolution of cochlear implants: the electrical field and excitation of auditory afferents. Hear Res 1998;121(1–2): 11–28.

31. Shannon RV. Multichannel electrical stimulation of the auditory nerve in man. I. Basic psychophysics. Hear Res 1983;11(2):157–89.

32. Donaldson GS, Kreft HA, Litvak L. Place-pitch discrimination of single- versus dual-electrode stimuli by cochlear implant users (L). J Acoust Soc Am 2005; 118(2):623–6.

33. Nagel G, Ollig D, Fuhrmann M, et al. Channelrhodopsin-1: a light-gated proton channel in green algae. Science 2002;296(5577):2395–8.

34. Nagel G, Szellas T, Huhn W, et al. Channelrhodopsin-2, a directly light-gated cation-selective membrane channel. Proc Natl Acad Sci U S A 2003;100(24): 13940–5.

35. Shapiro MG, Homma K, Villarreal S, et al. Infrared light excites cells by changing their electrical capacitance. Nat Commun 2012;3:736.

36. Shimano T, Fyk-Kolodziej B, Mirza N, et al. Assessment of the AAV-mediated expression of channelrhodopsin-2 and halorhodopsin in brainstem neurons mediating auditory signaling. Brain Res 2013;1511:138–52.

37. Verma RU, Guex AA, Hancock KE, et al. Auditory responses to electric and infrared neural stimulation of the rat cochlear nucleus. Hear Res 2014;310: 69–75.

38. Albert ES, Bec JM, Desmadryl G, et al. TRPV4 channels mediate the infrared laser-evoked response in sensory neurons. J Neurophysiol 2012;107(12):3227–34.

39. Littlefield PD, Vujanovic I, Mundi J, et al. Laser stimulation of single auditory nerve fibers. Laryngoscope 2010;120(10):2071–82.

40. Richter CP, Rajguru SM, Matic AI, et al. Spread of cochlear excitation during stimulation with pulsed infrared radiation: inferior colliculus measurements. J Neural Eng 2011;8(5):056006.

41. Izzo AD, Richter CP, Jansen ED, et al. Laser stimulation of the auditory nerve. Lasers Surg Med 2006;38(8):745–53.

42. Izzo AD, Walsh JT Jr, Ralph H, et al. Laser stimulation of auditory neurons: effect of shorter pulse duration and penetration depth. Biophys J 2008;94(8):3159–66.

43. Izzo AD, Suh E, Pathria J, et al. Selectivity of neural stimulation in the auditory system: a comparison of optic and electric stimuli. J Biomed Opt 2007;12(2):021008.
44. Teudt IU, Maier H, Richter CP, et al. Acoustic events and "optophonic" cochlear responses induced by pulsed near-infrared laser. IEEE Trans Biomed Eng 2011;58(6):1648–55.
45. Middlebrooks JC, Snyder RL. Auditory prosthesis with a penetrating nerve array. J Assoc Res Otolaryngol 2007;8(2):258–79.
46. Simmons FB, Mongeon CJ, Lewis WR, et al. Electrical stimulation of acoustical nerve and inferior colliculus. Arch Otolaryngol 1964;79:559–68.
47. Simmons FB, Epley JM, Lummis RC, et al. Auditory nerve: electrical stimulation in man. Science 1965;148(3666):104–6.
48. Simmons FB. Electrical stimulation of the auditory nerve in man. Arch Otolaryngol 1966;84(1):2–54.
49. Simmons FB. Permanent intracochlear electrodes in cats, tissue tolerance and cochlear microphonics. Laryngoscope 1967;77(2):171–86.
50. Simmons FB, Glattke TJ. Comparison of electrical and acoustical stimulation of the cat ear. Ann Otol Rhinol Laryngol 1972;81(5):731–7.
51. Simmons FB, Mathews RG, Walker MG, et al. A functioning multichannel auditory nerve stimulator. A preliminary report on two human volunteers. Acta Otolaryngol 1979;87(3–4):170–5.
52. Simmons FB. Percepts from modiolar (eighth nerve) stimulation. Ann N Y Acad Sci 1983;405:259–63.
53. Simmons FB, Schuknecht HF, Smith L. Histopathology of an ear after 5 years of electrical stimulation. Ann Otol Rhinol Laryngol 1986;95(2 Pt 1):132–6.
54. Simmons FB. Electrical stimulation of the auditory nerve in cats. Long term electrophysiological and histological results. Ann Otol Rhinol Laryngol 1979;88(4 Pt 1):533–9.
55. Badi AN, Hillman T, Shelton C, et al. A technique for implantation of a 3-dimensional penetrating electrode array in the modiolar nerve of cats and humans. Arch Otolaryngol Head Neck Surg 2002;128(9):1019–25.
56. Badi AN, Kertesz TR, Gurgel RK, et al. Development of a novel eighth-nerve intraneural auditory neuroprosthesis. Laryngoscope 2003;113(5):833–42.
57. Badi AN, Owa AO, Shelton C, et al. Electrode independence in intraneural cochlear nerve stimulation. Otol Neurotol 2007;28(1):16–24.
58. Mowry SE, Woodson E, Gantz BJ. New frontiers in cochlear implantation: acoustic plus electric hearing, hearing preservation, and more. Otolaryngol Clin North Am 2012;45(1):187–203.
59. Turner CW, Gantz BJ, Karsten S, et al. Impact of hair cell preservation in cochlear implantation: combined electric and acoustic hearing. Otol Neurotol 2010;31(8):1227–32.
60. Hogan CA, Turner CW. High-frequency audibility: benefits for hearing-impaired listeners. J Acoust Soc Am 1998;104(1):432–41.
61. Rizer FM, Arkis PN, Lippy WH, et al. A postoperative audiometric evaluation of cochlear implant patients. Otolaryngol Head Neck Surg 1988;98(3):203–6.
62. Kiefer J, Gstoettner W, Baumgartner W, et al. Conservation of low-frequency hearing in cochlear implantation. Acta Otolaryngol 2004;124(3):272–80.
63. Hodges AV, Schloffman J, Balkany T. Conservation of residual hearing with cochlear implantation. Am J Otol 1997;18(2):179–83.
64. Balkany TJ, Connell SS, Hodges AV, et al. Conservation of residual acoustic hearing after cochlear implantation. Otol Neurotol 2006;27(8):1083–8.

65. von Ilberg C, Kiefer J, Tillein J, et al. Electric-acoustic stimulation of the auditory system. New technology for severe hearing loss. ORL J Otorhinolaryngol Relat Spec 1999;61(6):334–40.

66. Gantz BJ, Turner CW. Combining acoustic and electrical hearing. Laryngoscope 2003;113(10):1726–30.

67. Gantz BJ, Hansen MR, Turner CW, et al. Hybrid 10 clinical trial: preliminary results. Audiol Neurootol 2009;14(Suppl 1):32–8.

68. Lenarz T, Stover T, Buechner A, et al. Hearing conservation surgery using the Hybrid-L electrode. Results from the first clinical trial at the Medical University of Hannover. Audiol Neurootol 2009;14(Suppl 1):22–31.

69. Gstoettner WK, Van De Heyning P, O'Connor AF, et al. Electric acoustic stimulation of the auditory system: results of a multi-centre investigation. Acta Otolaryngol 2008;128:1–8.

70. Fayad J, Linthicum FH Jr, Otto SR, et al. Cochlear implants: histopathologic findings related to performance in 16 human temporal bones. Ann Otol Rhinol Laryngol 1991;100(10):807–11.

71. Khan AM, Handzel O, Burgess BJ, et al. Is word recognition correlated with the number of surviving spiral ganglion cells and electrode insertion depth in human subjects with cochlear implants? Laryngoscope 2005;115(4):672–7.

72. Roehm PC, Hansen MR. Strategies to preserve or regenerate spiral ganglion neurons. Curr Opin Otolaryngol Head Neck Surg 2005;13(5):294–300.

73. Eshraghi AA, Gupta C, Van De Water TR, et al. Molecular mechanisms involved in cochlear implantation trauma and the protection of hearing and auditory sensory cells by inhibition of c-Jun-N-terminal kinase signaling. Laryngoscope 2013;123(Suppl 1):S1–14.

74. Adunka O, Kiefer J, Unkelbach MH, et al. Development and evaluation of an improved cochlear implant electrode design for electric acoustic stimulation. Laryngoscope 2004;114(7):1237–41.

75. Eshraghi AA, Yang NW, Balkany TJ. Comparative study of cochlear damage with three perimodiolar electrode designs. Laryngoscope 2003;113(3):415–9.

76. Adunka OF, Pillsbury HC, Buchman CA. Minimizing intracochlear trauma during cochlear implantation. Adv Otorhinolaryngol 2010;67:96–107.

77. Eshraghi AA, Adil E, He J, et al. Local dexamethasone therapy conserves hearing in an animal model of electrode insertion trauma-induced hearing loss. Otol Neurotol 2007;28(6):842–9.

78. Vivero RJ, Joseph DE, Angeli S, et al. Dexamethasone base conserves hearing from electrode trauma-induced hearing loss. Laryngoscope 2008;118(11):2028–35.

79. Ye Q, Tillein J, Hartmann R, et al. Application of a corticosteroid (triamcinolone) protects inner ear function after surgical intervention. Ear Hear 2007;28(3):361–9.

80. James DP, Eastwood H, Richardson RT, et al. Effects of round window dexamethasone on residual hearing in a Guinea pig model of cochlear implantation. Audiol Neurootol 2008;13(2):86–96.

81. Wang J, Van De Water TR, Bonny C, et al. A peptide inhibitor of c-Jun N-terminal kinase protects against both aminoglycoside and acoustic trauma-induced auditory hair cell death and hearing loss. J Neurosci 2003;23(24):8596–607.

82. Eshraghi AA, He J, Mou CH, et al. D-JNKI-1 treatment prevents the progression of hearing loss in a model of cochlear implantation trauma. Otol Neurotol 2006;27(4):504–11.

83. Eshraghi AA, Wang J, Adil E, et al. Blocking c-Jun-N-terminal kinase signaling can prevent hearing loss induced by both electrode insertion trauma and neomycin ototoxicity. Hear Res 2007;226(1–2):168–77.

84. Atkinson PJ, Cho CH, Hansen MR, et al. Activity of all JNK isoforms contributes to neurite growth in spiral ganglion neurons. Hear Res 2011;278(1–2):77–85.

85. Roehm PC, Xu N, Woodson EA, et al. Membrane depolarization inhibits spiral ganglion neurite growth via activation of multiple types of voltage sensitive calcium channels and calpain. Mol Cell Neurosci 2008;37(2):376–87.

86. Renton JP, Xu N, Clark JJ, et al. Interaction of neurotrophin signaling with Bcl-2 localized to the mitochondria and endoplasmic reticulum on spiral ganglion neuron survival and neurite growth. J Neurosci Res 2010;88(10):2239–51.

87. Hansen MR, Roehm PC, Xu N, et al. Overexpression of Bcl-2 or Bcl-xL prevents spiral ganglion neuron death and inhibits neurite growth. Dev Neurobiol 2007; 67(3):316–25.

88. Hansen MR, Bok J, Devaiah AK, et al. Ca2+/calmodulin-dependent protein kinases II and IV both promote survival but differ in their effects on axon growth in spiral ganglion neurons. J Neurosci Res 2003;72(2):169–84.

89. Xu N, Engbers J, Khaja S, et al. Influence of cAMP and protein kinase A on neurite length from spiral ganglion neurons. Hear Res 2012;283(1–2):33–44.

90. Green SH, Bailey E, Wang Q, et al. The Trk A, B, C's of neurotrophins in the cochlea. Anat Rec (Hoboken) 2012;295(11):1877–95.

91. Salt AN, Plontke SK. Principles of local drug delivery to the inner ear. Audiol Neurootol 2009;14(6):350–60.

92. Garnham C, Reetz G, Jolly C, et al. Drug delivery to the cochlea after implantation: consideration of the risk factors. Cochlear Implants Int 2005;6(Suppl 1): 12–4.

93. Richardson RT, Wise AK, Thompson BC, et al. Polypyrrole-coated electrodes for the delivery of charge and neurotrophins to cochlear neurons. Biomaterials 2009;30(13):2614–24.

94. Hochmair I, Nopp P, Jolly C, et al. MED-EL Cochlear implants: state of the art and a glimpse into the future. Trends Amplif 2006;10(4):201–19.

95. Aschendorff A, Klenzner T, Richter B, et al. Evaluation of the HiFocus electrode array with positioner in human temporal bones. J Laryngol Otol 2003;117(7): 527–31.

96. Reefhuis J, Honein MA, Whitney CG, et al. Risk of bacterial meningitis in children with cochlear implants. N Engl J Med 2003;349(5):435–45.

97. Wei BP, Shepherd RK, Robins-Browne RM, et al. Effects of inner ear trauma on the risk of pneumococcal meningitis. Arch Otolaryngol Head Neck Surg 2007; 133(3):250–9.

98. Roland JT Jr. A model for cochlear implant electrode insertion and force evaluation: results with a new electrode design and insertion technique. Laryngoscope 2005;115(8):1325–39.

99. Hassepass F, Bulla S, Maier W, et al. The new mid-scala electrode array: a radiologic and histologic study in human temporal bones. Otol Neurotol 2014;35(8): 1415–20.

100. Wanna GB, Noble JH, Carlson ML, et al. Impact of electrode design and surgical approach on scalar location and cochlear implant outcomes. Laryngoscope 2014;124(Suppl 6):S1–7.

101. Pettingill LN, Richardson RT, Wise AK, et al. Neurotrophic factors and neural prostheses: potential clinical applications based upon findings in the auditory system. IEEE Trans Biomed Eng 2007;54(6 Pt 1):1138–48.

102. Budenz CL, Pfingst BE, Raphael Y. The use of neurotrophin therapy in the inner ear to augment cochlear implantation outcomes. Anat Rec (Hoboken) 2012; 295(11):1896–908.

103. Wise AK, Richardson R, Hardman J, et al. Resprouting and survival of guinea pig cochlear neurons in response to the administration of the neurotrophins brain-derived neurotrophic factor and neurotrophin-3. J Comp Neurol 2005; 487(2):147–65.

104. Shibata SB, Cortez SR, Beyer LA, et al. Transgenic BDNF induces nerve fiber regrowth into the auditory epithelium in deaf cochleae. Exp Neurol 2010; 223(2):464–72.

105. Brors D, Bodmer D, Pak K, et al. EphA4 provides repulsive signals to developing cochlear ganglion neurites mediated through ephrin-B2 and -B3. J Comp Neurol 2003;462(1):90–100.

106. Reich U, Mueller PP, Fadeeva E, et al. Differential fine-tuning of cochlear implant material-cell interactions by femtosecond laser microstructuring. J Biomed Mater Res B Appl Biomater 2008;87(1):146–53.

107. Clarke JC, Tuft BW, Clinger JD, et al. Micropatterned methacrylate polymers direct spiral ganglion neurite and Schwann cell growth. Hear Res 2011; 278(1–2):96–105.

108. Tuft BW, Li S, Xu L, et al. Photopolymerized microfeatures for directed spiral ganglion neurite and Schwann cell growth. Biomaterials 2013;34(1):42–54.

109. Tuft BW, Zhang L, Xu L, et al. Material stiffness effects on neurite alignment to photopolymerized micropatterns. Biomacromolecules 2014;15(10):3717–27.

110. Tuft BW, Xu L, White SP, et al. Neural pathfinding on uni- and multidirectional photopolymerized micropatterns. ACS Appl Mater Interfaces 2014;6(14): 11265–76.

Pediatric Auditory Brainstem Implant Surgery

Sidharth V. Puram, MD, PhD[a,b], Daniel J. Lee, MD[a,b],*

KEYWORDS

- Auditory brainstem implant (ABI) • Pediatric • Congenital hearing loss
- Cochlear nerve hypoplasia or aplasia • Cochlear hypoplasia or aplasia
- Retrosigmoid craniotomy

KEY POINTS

- Evaluation for pediatric auditory brainstem implant (ABI) candidacy includes a thorough neurotologic and neurosurgical consultation, audiologic evaluation including both behavioral and electrophysiologic testing, speech and language consultation, high-resolution temporal bone computed tomography and MRI imaging, and neuropsychological assessment of developmental milestones.
- Indications for an ABI in infants and children include bilateral cochlea aplasia/hypoplasia, cochlear nerve hypoplasia/aplasia, cochlear ossification, cochlear nerve fracture or cochlear nerve injury from bilateral temporal bone fractures, failed cochlear implantation caused by anatomic constraints or auditory neuropathy. Older children and teenagers with neurofibromatosis type 2 (NF2) are also candidates for the ABI.
- The retrosigmoid craniotomy approach is recommended for pediatric ABI because of the relative small size of the temporal bone in young children that would make a translabyrinthine craniotomy more difficult.
- Most complications following ABI surgery are minor in the hands of an experienced neurotology/neurosurgery team. The most common complication is a cerebrospinal fluid leak after surgery.
- Outcomes are generally modest among most pediatric ABI users, with most achieving sound awareness that enhances lip reading, but some realize closed-set or open-set speech recognition. Patients who do not have NF2 as the cause of deafness have better audiologic outcomes than those with NF2.
- Standardized outcome reporting across a growing number of pediatric ABI centers worldwide will be important in order to identify the factors that predict safe and effective ABI surgery in children.

Disclosures/conflict of interest: The authors have nothing to disclose.
[a] Department of Otolaryngology, Massachusetts Eye and Ear Infirmary, 243 Charles Street, Boston, MA 02114, USA; [b] Department of Otology and Laryngology, Harvard Medical School, 25 Shattuck St, Boston, MA 02115, USA
* Corresponding author. Massachusetts Eye and Ear Infirmary, 243 Charles Street, Boston, MA 02114.
E-mail address: Daniel_lee@meei.harvard.edu

Abbreviations

ABI	Auditory brainstem implant
CAP	Category of auditory performance
ChR	Channel rhodopsin
CI	Cochlear implant
CN	Cochlear nucleus
CNS	Central nervous system
CSF	Cerebrospinal fluid
DCN	Dorsal cochlear nucleus
EMG	Electromyographic
FDA	Food and Drug Administration
IAC	Internal auditory canal
IC	Inferior colliculus
NF2	Neurofibromatosis type II
PABI	Penetrating auditory brainstem implant
VCN	Ventral cochlear nucleus

 Videos of typical operating room setup for pediatric ABI surgery and key steps in pediatric ABI surgery accompany this article at http://www.oto.theclinics. com/

INTRODUCTION

Providing meaningful sound perception to pediatric and adult patients with profound hearing loss has been the subject of intense research efforts for decades. Beginning with Djourno and Eyriès more than 50 years ago, the idea of an auditory prosthesis has undergone a dramatic evolution. These pioneers provided a detailed description for artificially transducing sound with an implantable induction coil that created auditory sensations via transcutaneous electric stimulation. Since then, technological advancements have facilitated the development of both cochlear implants (CIs) and auditory brainstem implants (ABIs). In parallel with improved microphone and battery technology, more advanced algorithms for speech processing as well as postoperative auditory rehabilitation and training on device use has further advanced the audiologic gains with implantable prostheses, offering the possibility of open-set speech recognition in most patients with severe to profound sensorineural deafness.

Although the CI implant has gained widespread acceptance and use, this technology has limitations. In cases whereby the cochlea and cochlear nerve are fully developed or are only mildly malformed (eg, Mondini or incomplete partition type 2 deformity), the CI is a reasonable option for hearing habilitation (in congenitally deaf children) or rehabilitation (in patients with postlingual deafness). The CI bypasses the inner hair cells of the cochlea to directly stimulate spiral ganglion cells, the first-order neurons of the auditory pathway. However, there is a subset of patients who are not candidates for a CI because of abnormal anatomy, such as an absent, scarred, or small cochlea or cochlear nerve. A CI is likely to provide modest benefits in these patients, with some exceptions.[1] The ABI is an alternative approach to the CI and bypasses the cochlea, cochlear nerve, and any associated peripheral disease to electrically stimulate the second-order auditory neurons found in the cochlear nucleus (CN). The ABI is a modified CI whose surface electrode array is placed on or near the brainstem CN via the lateral recess of the fourth ventricle. The CN is the primary brainstem hub for type 1 auditory afferents originating in the cochlea and is the first center of auditory processing in the brain. Electrical stimulation of the electrode array crudely approximates the input that normally arises from the cochlear nerve by leveraging the tonotopic distribution of second-order auditory neurons within the CN. Most ABI users have neurofibromatosis type II (NF2) and receive sound detection that aids in lip reading.

In 1979, William Hitselberger and William House performed the first successful ABI surgery for an adult woman with NF2 following removal of her second vestibular schwannoma via a translabyrinthine craniotomy. This prototype implant had a single glass ball electrode that was placed via the lateral recess of the fourth ventricle in proximity to the dorsal CN (DCN) to provide auditory sensations. Eventually, technology developed to include a multiple electrode array and receiver stimulator that is forward compatible with modern receiver stimulators used with the CI. In 2000, Cochlear Corporation (Engelwood, CO) received approval from the Food and Drug Administration (FDA) for the 21 electrode Nucleus 24 ABI system for patients with NF2 aged 12 years and older. There are no audiologic candidacy criteria for the ABI in patients with NF2. Today, more than 1000 patients have received ABI surgery worldwide.

As of May 2015, the Nucleus 24 ABI system (**Fig. 1**) was phased out; Cochlear Corporation will be introducing a new ABI system pending regulatory approval in the United States that until then may be used under FDA compassionate use exemption. The MED-EL (Durham, NC) also manufactures an ABI device (**Fig. 2**) that has been used internationally for pediatric ABI surgery. Although it has not been submitted for formal FDA approval in the United States, it has been used under the FDA compassionate use exemption.

Patients with NF2 are the most common cohort of ABI candidates with deficits of the cochlear nerve related to tumor growth and compression that are not typically amenable to CI. Patients with NF2 have an autosomal dominant mutation that triggers the formation of vestibular schwannomas bilaterally along with a myriad of synchronous central nervous system (CNS) tumors. Growth of these vestibular schwannomas as well as resection with surgery and/or treatment with radiation often damages the cochlear nerve, resulting in bilateral retrocochlear hearing loss not helped with hearing aids or CIs.

Over the past decade, there has been growing interest in the ABI to provide hearing sensations to non-NF2 patients with cochlear or cochlear nerve pathology. Professor Vittorio Colletti's work at the University of Verona and more recently in Milan has propelled enthusiasm for ABI surgery in non-NF2–related deafness. Colletti and colleagues[2,3] demonstrated that open-set sentence recognition is possible with the ABI

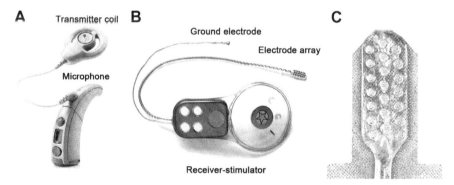

Fig. 1. The Nucleus 24 ABI system includes (*A*) the externally worn device, including a behind-the-ear microphone, speech processor, and transmitter coil, and (*B*) the internal receiver-stimulator, electrode array, and ground electrode. The array consists of 21 active platinum electrodes on a polyethylene terephthalate mesh backing as shown in (*C*). (*Courtesy of* Cochlear Corporation, Englewood, CO; with permission.)

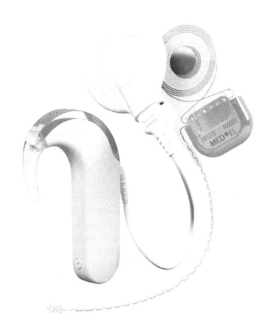

Fig. 2. The MED-EL SYNCRONY ABI implant and SONNET audio processor. The SYNCRHONY system features a unique self-aligning magnet that greatly reduces torque during MRI scanning when the magnet is left in place. The magnet is optionally removable if necessary. The array consists of 12 active electrodes on a mesh backing as shown. (*Courtesy of* MED-EL Corporation North America, Durham, NC; with permission.)

in adult non-NF2 users compared with NF2 users. Since those initial studies in adult patients, Colletti's group[4] expanded the indications for ABI surgery to children and infants who are not CI candidates. Colletti performed the first pediatric ABI surgery for auditory nerve aplasia in 2001 and has performed approximately 100 non-NF2 pediatric ABI surgeries since that time, including surgery on an 8 month old, the youngest infant to date. Much like Colletti, Professor Levent Sennaroglu[5] from the University of Hacettepe, Turkey has driven international experience in Ankara with more than 70 non-NF2 pediatric ABIs. Remarkably, the combined experience of these two groups has been associated with relatively low morbidity. There have been a small number of transient facial nerve palsies and cerebrospinal fluid (CSF) leaks, which have been managed conservatively.[6] More strikingly, a significant number of these children who were implanted at a young age and had no significant developmental issues have subsequently achieved either closed or open-set speech recognition following ABI surgery. Pediatric ABI surgery in non-NF2 children in the United States began initially in 2012, with the first child implanted in 2012 at New York University. There are now 4 investigational device exemption clinical trials in the United States: University of North Carolina-Chapel Hill, Massachusetts Eye and Ear Infirmary-Harvard Medical School, the Los Angeles Pediatric ABI team, and New York University.

In this article, we summarize the preoperative assessment of pediatric ABI candidates, the surgical approach, postoperative management issues, complications, and review published outcomes in this unique cohort. Based on findings from Italy and Turkey and our early experience in the U.S., we believe that ABI surgery is a safe and effective option for auditory habilitation in deaf children who are not candidates for the CI.

TREATMENT GOALS AND OUTCOMES

The treatment goals for pediatric ABI surgery are (1) safe and successful placement of ABI electrode array through the foramen of Luschka (to bring electrode in close proximity to cochlear nucleus), (2) measurable electrically-evoked auditory brainstem responses (EABR) seen intraoperatively, (3) minimizing surgical complications such as CSF leak and facial nerve injury, (4) habilitation/rehabilitation of deafness with meaningful sound detection on behavioral testing, and (5) avoidance of side effects caused by stimulation of non-auditory pathways (e.g. facial nerve, glossopharyngeal nerve). As the range of clinical outcomes varies widely (see Outcomes), the stated goals should include a substantial conversation with families and patients regarding both the risks of craniotomy surgery in a young child as well as the reasonable expectation of audiologic outcomes. A team based tertiary care setting is the ideal environment where pediatric ABI candidates and their families can be carefully evaluated for possible surgery. At the Wilson ABI Program at Massachusetts Eye and Ear Infirmary and Massachusetts General Hospital, all candidates participate in a formal consultation with pediatric neurotology, neurosurgery, audiology, speech therapy, and neuropsychology to ensure adequate communication regarding the treatment goals, frank discussion of surgical risks, and review of outcomes.

PREOPERATIVE PLANNING AND PREPARATION
Implant Systems

The ABI system is modular, with both external and internal components that capture, transduce, process, and propagate auditory stimuli into electrical signals to the electrode array, similar to that of the CI. The external components include a microphone, battery, speech processor, and transmitter coil. Acoustic stimuli are processed and transmitted as electronic signals to a receiver-stimulator via an induction coil. The surgically implanted receiver-stimulator then carries these signals to the CN via a rigid surface multi-electrode array that consists of 12 (MED-EL) to 21 (Cochlear) electrode contacts (see **Figs. 1** and **2**). These platinum alloy electrode contacts trigger neuronal signaling in the CN, thereby stimulating upstream auditory pathways and providing sound perception.

The ABI continues to leverage sound-processing algorithms originally developed for CIs. However, because the tonotopic arrangement of the DCN is orthogonal to the surface of the brainstem, capturing a specific spectral frequency with each electrode is more challenging. This organization is in contrast to the CI electrode whose position in the scala tympani follows the tonotopic organization of the cochlea. Indeed, some studies suggest that there is limited benefit to an ABI electrode array beyond 7 leads,[7] providing a rationale for exploring penetrating electrodes that can better stimulate multiple tonotopic layers of the DCN. However, the initial experience using a novel penetrating ABI (PABI) array developed in Los Angeles in adult patients with NF2 was not associated with improved outcomes.[8] This PABI system also includes surface contacts, and overall auditory performance was not enhanced in the PABI-only condition. Side effects were also seen in patients even with the ABI turned off.[8] Finally, stimulation one level higher at the inferior colliculus (IC) has been proposed, with the hypothesis that patients with NF2 may have damage to the CN that limits the utility of an ABI.[9] However, outcomes in a small cohort of patients with IC electrode placement (either penetrating or surface) have not demonstrated improved outcomes compared with traditional electrode placement near the CN.

In the United States, Cochlear Corporation previously offered the multichannel Nucleus 24 ABI system, which was approved by the FDA in 2000 for patients with NF2 aged 12 years and older (see **Fig. 1**). The Nucleus 24 ABI consists of 21 electrode contacts measuring 0.7 mm in diameter arranged along a polymeric silicon (Silastic) paddle with polyethylene terephthalate (Dacron) mesh backing. This ABI has been used for the approximately 20 pediatric ABI surgeries performed in the United States. The Cochlear system uses the SPEAK coding strategy, originally developed for the Nucleus CI. Although the Nucleus 24 ABI is technically capable of more sophisticated speech-processing algorithms, including continuous interleaved sampling (CIS) and advanced combination encoding, the FDA has not approved these other sound-processing strategies.

However, as of May 2015, the Nucleus 24 ABI has been phased out. In late 2015 or 2016, Cochlear Corporation will be introducing a new ABI system pending US regulatory approval of their new profile platform. Until then, their new ABI may only be used in the United States after securing approval through an FDA compassionate use exemption.

The magnet within the polymeric silicon pocket of the surgically implanted ABI receiver stimulator is retained to improve close contact between the external speech processor and the internal components. This retention is possible because most non-NF2 pediatric ABI candidates do not require routine MRI surveillance in comparison with all patients with NF2. Ideally, future ABI designs that reach regulatory approval for use in the United States should include magnet designs that allow for MRI scans, as a young non-NF2 child who receives an ABI may need imaging done in their lifetime for unrelated reasons. As one example, MED-EL has a SYNCHRONY ABI (not approved for the United States) that allows for 1.5-T MRI scans without the need for magnet removal or even a pressure dressing.

In contrast, patients with NF2 require serial MRIs to monitor the growth of multiple CNS tumors; therefore, most centers will replace the ABI magnet during craniotomy surgery with a nonmagnetic metallic spacer provided by the company's prior electrode placement. The scalp is tattooed in the region of the receiver-stimulator telecoil after the ABI is inserted into the subperiosteal pocket. The tattoo provides a visual guide for patients to place an adhesive magnetic disk on the scalp, facilitating head-piece retention. At Massachusetts Eye and Ear, we also offer focal laser hair removal of the scalp in the region of the telecoil (especially important in patients with thick or coarse hair) to improve retention of the adhesive magnetic disk.

A 1.5-T MRI can be obtained in the United States with the magnet surgically removed from the FDA-approved ABI. Some international centers will retain the magnet in the ABI in patients with NF2 to improve device retention and patient use. In these cases, a 1.5-T MRI scan is performed with a tight mastoid dressing and a custom mold or plastic card placed over the scalp flap in the location of the receiver-stimulator.

MED-EL offers an ABI, but this device is only available in the United States through compassionate use exemption from FDA. The MED-EL ABI has mirrored advancements in the MED-EL CI over the last two decades, with the current iteration being the SYNCRHONY ABI, and has been used internationally for both NF2 and non-NF2 applications. It consists of an internal receiver-stimulator and external microphone speech processor with attached transmission coil. The MED-EL ABI has 12 platinum electrode contacts (.55 mm diameter) and uses a simplified placing electrode to identify the optimal location for EABRs. This placing electrode is smaller than the actual ABI paddle and can help localize the CN before committing to the actual ABI. This system includes the SONNET audio processor which offers the High Definition Continuous Interleaved Sampling (HDCIS) coding strategy. Finally, the SYNCRHONY ABI has approval in Europe for MRI at 0.2, 1.0 and 1.5T without the need to remove the magnet, although the magnet is optionally removable in the event that the area to be imaged is in the vicinity of the implant itself.

The Advanced Bionics (Valencia, CA) ABI was based on the Clarion 1.2 CI; however, after a brief period of use in Europe, Advanced Bionics discontinued the Clarion ABI. This device consisted of a polymeric silicone electrode array with 16 platinum-iridium electrodes (1.0 mm diameter). This implant was manufactured without a magnet and used a special headset to hold the external headpiece in position.

Evaluation

Evaluation of a child for possible ABI surgery is a multidisciplinary effort requiring evaluation of several specialists in addition to the neurotologist and neurosurgeon. All patients undergo a preoperative history and examination and complete surgical assessment, behavioral and electrophysiologic measurement of hearing, formal speech therapy evaluation, and neuropsychological consultation. In prelingually deafened patients, both behavioral thresholds and acoustically evoked auditory brainstem responses (ABRs) are carefully analyzed and repeated as needed to ensure that there is no residual hearing that might support a CI trial before consideration of an ABI. Pediatric patients receive a comprehensive evaluation of their language skills by a speech and language pathologist as well as a formal neuropsychological evaluation to assess overall progress with cognitive, motor, and language development. Sign language is encouraged in order to provide a basis for language development in prelingually deafened pediatric ABI candidates as overall outcomes with the ABI still lag behind the CI. In addition, neurodevelopmental delay is more commonly found among pediatric ABI candidates compared with CI candidates. Finally, a crucial component of the preoperative evaluation is determining whether there is an appropriate level of family support and realistic expectations to facilitate success with an ABI in a congenitally deafened child.

Radiographic Assessment

Imaging with high-resolution computed tomography (CT) and MRI followed by interpretation by a tertiary center neuroradiologist is essential to assess the anatomic details of the internal auditory canal (IAC), lateral recess, and brainstem. Typically this imaging consists of a temporal bone CT as well as MRI with T2-weighted fast imaging employing steady-state acquisition (FIESTA)/constructive interference into steady state sequences. At Massachusetts Eye and Ear, we rely on T2-weighted 3-dimensional turbo spin echo with *direct* driven equilibrium radio frequency reset pulse parasagittal imaging of the IAC. Reconstructions of the IAC on MRI to image the cross section of the auditory nerve are often not sufficient to rule out auditory nerve hypoplasia compared with direct parasagittal imaging.[10] The Massachusetts Eye and Ear imaging protocol for pediatric ABI candidates offers enhanced visualization of the IAC and neural anatomy (**Fig. 3**), with a direct impact on clinical decision making.[10] The surgical team should also carefully evaluate the pontomedullary junction, taking note of the lower cranial nerves and lateral recess of the fourth ventricle. The presence of vascularity, scar tissue, or anomalous lower nerves may influence the surgical approach with the ABI electrode. Because the CN is not easily distinguishable on MRI, the surgeon is limited to a gross evaluation of the brainstem and cranial nerve rootlets.

Selection Criteria and Candidacy

In the United States, the FDA has approved ABI surgery in patients with NF2 fulfilling several specific criteria (**Box 1**). There are no audiologic criteria for this cohort because of (1) the history of ABI surgery with early cases performed in patients who were

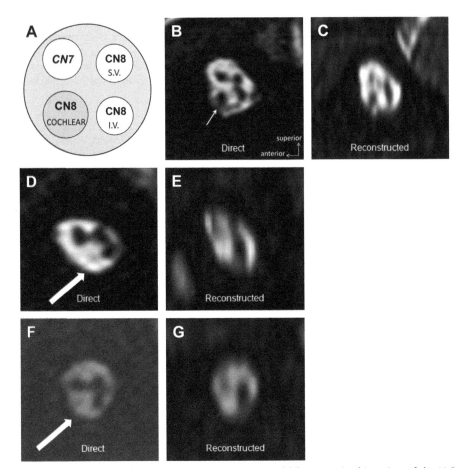

Fig. 3. (*A*) The IAC. (*B, C*) Direct (*B*) versus reconstructed (*C*) parasagittal imaging of the IAC in a healthy pediatric patient. The cochlear nerve is identified with a white arrow, with images demonstrating the clear difference in quality between the direct and reconstructed images. (*D–G*) Direct (*D, F*) versus reconstructed (*E, G*) parasagittal imaging of the IAC in 2 patients with hypoplastic cochlea. In the second case (*F, G*), although the cochlear nerve is visible on direct imaging (*F*), it is not appreciated on the reconstructed image (*G*). CN, cranial nerve; I.V., inferior vestibular nerve; S.V., superior vestibular nerve. (*Adapted from* Noij KS, Remenschneider AK, Kozin ED, et al. Direct parasagittal magnetic resonance imaging of the internal auditory canal to determine cochlear or auditory brainstem implant candidacy in children. Laryngoscope. 2015 Mar 16. [Epub ahead of print]; with permission.)

Box 1
US FDA criteria for auditory brainstem implantation

- Diagnosis of NF2
- 12 years old or older
- High degree of motivation to comply with rehabilitation
- Reasonable patient and family expectations

Notably, there are no audiologic criteria.

undergoing removal of a second vestibular schwannoma and left with no hearing after tumor resection and (2) the natural history of NF2 resulting in profound hearing loss in virtually all affected patients. Clinical studies have shown that about 8% of patients will fail to gain any useful hearing with the ABI.[11] Hence, some centers have placed the ABI even when there is residual hearing in the contralateral ear in order to maximize the chances of providing sound awareness in at least one ear. With the advent of chemotherapeutic options for NF2 including bevacizumab, a monoclonal antibody against the ecto-domain of vascular endothelial growth factor, early ABI placement has been increasingly deferred in favor of maximizing the duration of acoustic hearing before tumor resection and ABI surgery.[12] At the Massachusetts Eye and Ear, all patients with NF2 with tumor burden and progressive hearing loss are first evaluated at the Neurofibromatosis Clinic at Massachusetts General Hospital for a multidisciplinary evaluation and possible chemotherapy trial before consideration for tumor and/or ABI surgery.

Although most adult ABI users have NF2, only a small percentage of pediatric patients are implanted because of NF2. Most pediatric ABI users are younger children with anatomic limitations that preclude successful CI surgery. Several studies from Europe have suggested improved outcomes in nontumor adult and pediatric patients compared with patients with NF2. Accordingly, a European ABI consensus group concluded that indications for pediatric ABI surgery should include the following (**Box 2**)[13]:

- Prelingually deafened children with inner ear malformation and cochlear nerve hypoplasia/aplasia
- Postlingually deafened children with cochlear ossification from meningitis, cochlear nerve avulsion from bilateral temporal bone fractures, gross cochlear ossification caused by otosclerosis, or intractable facial nerve stimulation with CI.

In pediatric patients with cochlear and cochlear nerve aplasia, consideration of an ABI without a CI trial is reasonable. In contrast, a CI could be offered as a first option for a child with profound hearing loss and cochlear nerve hypoplasia or partial cochlear ossification, provided that the inner ear anatomy supports reasonable electrode insertion with a standard array. The decision to pursue CI surgery should also be influenced by any detectable behavioral thresholds that may be associated with auditory neuronal viability. Ultimately, comprehensive psychophysical and electrophysiologic measurements obtained by an experienced pediatric audiologist is critical to determine whether a congenitally deafened child with poor neural anatomy would benefit from a CI trial before ABI surgery. In some centers, EABRs generated by cochlear promontory electrical stimulation can help discern whether a functional neural connection exists between the cochlea and central auditory pathways. Patients with inconsistent or absent EABR responses are unlikely to derive substantial benefit from the CI.[14]

The ABI research team at Massachusetts Eye and Ear recently reviewed auditory implant candidacy in the United States to determine the relative need for ABI surgery.[15] Based on documented rates of cochlear and cochlear nerve aplasia/hypoplasia and population-level sensorineural hearing loss data, we estimated that 2.1% of potential implant candidates (1266 children) meet absolute indications for an ABI in the United States, with another 3.2% of potential implant candidates (1928 children) meeting relative indications for an ABI. The actual number may be smaller after imaging, as most children who undergo MRI scans to evaluate the auditory nerve rely on reformatted parasagittal images that do not provide adequate resolution of detailed neural anatomy. Pediatric ABI candidates are rare, but there is a legitimate need for

---

Box 2
Pediatric ABI patient indications based on European consensus statement

Well-defined congenital indications

1. Complete labyrinthine aplasia (Michel aplasia)

2. Cochlear aplasia

3. Cochlear nerve aplasia

4. Cochlear aperture aplasia

Possible congenital indications

1. Hypoplastic cochleae with cochlear aperture hypoplasia

2. Common cavity and incomplete partition type I cases if the cochlear nerve is not present.

3. Common cavity and incomplete partition type I cases if the cochlear nerve is present. If the nerve is present, the distribution of the neural tissue in the abnormal cochlea is unpredictable and an ABI is indicated if CI fails to elicit an auditory sensation.

4. Unbranched cochleovestibular nerve is a challenge. If there is a doubt, a CI can be used first, and ABI can be reserved for the patients with an insufficient response.

5. Hypoplastic cochlear nerves (<50% of usual size of cochlear nerve or less than diameter of the facial nerve) present a dilemma. If a sufficient amount of neural tissue cannot be followed into the cochlear space, an ABI may be indicated.

Acquired indications

1. Postlingual deafness caused by meningitis with severe ossification of the cochlea (white cochleae on CT with no cochlear duct signal on MRI) should undergo ABI surgery. If the cochlea appears patent on T2 MRI, CI should be the first option.

2. Bilateral temporal bone transverse fractures with cochlear nerve avulsion.

3. Cochlear otosclerosis with gross destruction of the cochlea; in addition, some otosclerosis patients have abnormal facial nerve stimulation, which may limit CI use.

4. Unmanageable facial nerve stimulation with CI.

Data from Sennaroglu L, Colletti V, Manrique M, et al. Auditory brainstem implantation in children and non-neurofibromatosis type 2 patients: a consensus statement. Otol Neurotol 2011;32:187–91.

---

dedicated ABI centers of excellence to gather the experience and expertise required to offer safe surgery and ABI mapping for this specialized cohort of deaf children who are not candidates for the CI.

The European consensus group on ABI surgery in children has explored the optimal time for ABI surgery in children. At earlier ages, children demonstrate increased plasticity and are likely to accrue greater benefit from early auditory sensations; however, infants less than 1 year of age have less blood and CSF volume with a smaller window of access to the lateral recess, potentially increasing the risks of craniotomy and ABI surgery. Based on these factors, there is consensus that implanting pediatric patients between 18 months and 3 years of age may provide a compromise between these physiologic and surgical considerations.[13] To date, almost 200 children have received ABIs internationally, with approximately 20 non-NF2 pediatric ABIs placed in the United States as of June 2015.

Our pediatric ABI candidacy algorithm at Massachusetts Eye and Ear includes a formal multidisciplinary preoperative evaluation, retrosigmoid craniotomy and ABI placement, and postoperative care as outlined in **Box 3**.

Box 3
Pediatric ABI surgery algorithm including preoperative assessment, ABI surgery, and postoperative care

Preoperative evaluation

  History and physical

  Formal speech, language, developmental testing

  Audiology and speech evaluation

  Radiographic assessment with direct IAC imaging

  Genetic testing (if indicated)

Formal multidisciplinary evaluation by auditory implant board

Surgical planning with coordination of multidisciplinary team (neurotology, neurosurgery, audiology, anesthesia)

ABI surgery using retrosigmoid approach

  CN monitoring: CN V and VII via needle electrode, VIII via EABRs, X via NIM tube or modified firefly monitored endotracheal tube intraoperative EABRs

  Multilayered dural closure around the electrode array to prevent CSF leak

  Postoperative CT/skull films to confirm device proximity to the brainstem and to check for hemorrhage

  Intensive care unit monitoring with sedation for first 24 hours followed by routine postoperative care

  Mastoid dressing in place for 5 to 7 days postoperatively to avoid CSF hygroma

Device activation and programming

  Initial activation 4 to 6 weeks postoperatively under anesthesia with dexmedetomidine

  Awake activation with physician monitoring the following day if activation is well tolerated

  Device programming using pitch ranking with age-appropriate testing

Routine neurotology and audiologic follow-up

  Routine wound checks by neurotology

  Scheduled audiologic testing and device reprogramming

SURGICAL APPROACH

Choosing which side to implant is primarily based on anatomic considerations and evidence of any detectable thresholds on behavioral or electrophysiologic testing. If both ears demonstrate no functional hearing, then the side with the most accessible lateral recess and radiographic evidence of a cochlear nerve should be implanted. If both sides are similar audiologically and on radiology, the right ear is chosen based on the hypothesis that speech perception abilities rely more on left-brain activity in response to input from the right auditory periphery.[16] If detectable thresholds are found in one ear based on behavioral or ABR testing, and the child is otherwise not a CI candidate or has failed CI surgery, that side should be selected as there may be a chance that central auditory neuronal pathways may be better developed.

Traditionally, most ABIs in adults have been placed via translabyrinthine craniotomy; but increasingly the retrosigmoid approach has been favored in some centers to reduce operating room time and avoid destroying the vestibular labyrinth.[17] In the pediatric population, the retrosigmoid craniotomy is preferred in order to avoid a space-constrained transmastoid approach as well as preserve any residual inner ear bony and neural anatomy.

Translabyrinthine Craniotomy

The translabyrinthine approach to ABI surgery is commonly used for adult patients with NF2 and offers access to the lateral recess of the fourth ventricle with a wide-angle view brainstem and adjacent structures. Using this approach for patients with NF2, complete tumor resection from the fundus can be accomplished with early identification of the facial nerve and minimal cerebellar retraction. The facial nerve is routinely monitored (and occasionally the glossopharyngeal) to avoid traction injury during tumor resection and minimize the risk of inadvertent stimulation of these nerves during tumor dissection, electrode positioning, and intraoperative electrical testing of the ABI paddle. Detailed and careful planning of the operating room setup ensures a smooth operative workflow between surgeons, anesthesiologists, audiologists, and scrub technicians (Video 1; available online at http://www.oto.theclinics.com).

In patients with NF2, the initial surgical procedure often involves tumor resection. After this is completed, ABI placement can proceed. A bony well is drilled in the calvarium superior and posterior to the pinna for placement of the receiver-stimulator and electrode paddle. A polymeric silicone device template is used to confirm adequate shape and positioning of the bony well. The lateral recess is identified, and access to the region near the DCN is obtained using the glossopharyngeal nerve and choroid plexus as landmarks. CN VII and VIII superiorly and CN IX inferiorly border the foramen of Luschka, and a Valsalva maneuver can be helpful for identifying the egress of CSF and the location of the foramen. These landmarks guide the placement of the ABI electrode, as the human CN is not directly visualized using the surgical microscope. The CN is found along the dorsolateral brainstem at the pontomedullary junction, with only a small portion (1.0–1.28 cm^2) of the DCN theoretically accessible for contact with a surface electrode.[18] In the future, as demonstrated by Friedland and colleagues,[19] endoscopic approaches may provide more direct visualization to facilitate insertion of the ABI electrode while minimizing cerebellar retraction. An ABI mimics signals from the cochlear nerve, creating sound perception by electrically stimulating the bushy cells of the ventral CN (VCN); however, the relative inaccessibility and small size of the VCN necessitates electrode stimulation of the DCN. Current spread extends the reach of ABI stimulation to the underlying VCN.

The ABI electrode array is blindly placed within the lateral recess adjacent to the presumptive location of the CN. At some centers, gentle retraction may be used to place the array under direct visualization. The polyethylene terephthalate mesh wings are trimmed off in pediatric ABI surgery because of the smaller dimensions of the lateral recess in children and the theoretic advantage of removing the electrode more easily (as the mesh will adhere to the surrounding brainstem) for any future revision surgery. After electrode positioning, intraoperative EABRs are measured to determine if the appropriate waveform morphology is generated with activation of the array. Bipolar stimulation is used with pairs of electrodes that represent different regions of the paddle to understand the relative location of the electrode to the CN. A multi-peaked response within the first 2 to 3 milliseconds of the onset of stimulus using the ABI is generally associated with an auditory response (**Fig. 4B**). In addition, this step is critical to check for unintended stimulation of adjacent cranial nerves. Larger broad-based waveforms with longer amplitudes are often nonauditory. If stimulation does not generate an appropriate EABR or is associated with nonauditory responses, the array can be repositioned. Once the array is optimally placed, a small piece of fat,

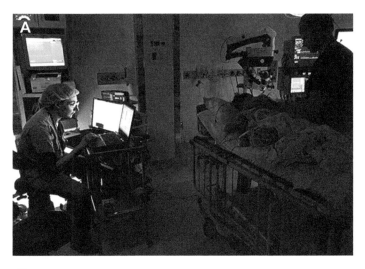

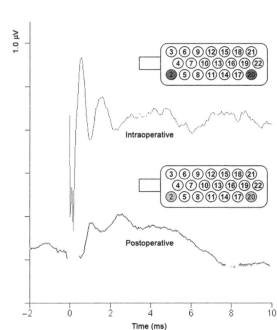

Fig. 4. (*A*) Typical setup for activation under anesthesia, which is completed with a multidisciplinary team consisting of audiology, pediatric anesthesia, and neurotology. (*B*) Representative EABR waveforms elicited from an ABI user during electrode positioning. Evoked responses were generated by stimulating bipolar electrode pair E2 and E20 with single biphasic pulses (pulse width = 150 microseconds). The top trace was recorded intraoperatively during ABI placement, and the bottom trace was recorded 3 months following ABI activation.

muscle, polytetrafluoroethylene felt, or a combination is used to secure its position. The receiver stimulator is placed in the bony well of the skull and anchored. Redundant coils of the electrode array are curled into the mastoid cavity, while taking great care to avoid any tugging on the device or the array seated in the brainstem. The ground electrode, if applicable, is placed underneath the temporalis muscle, and the mastoid cavity is packed with abdominal fat. The craniotomy site is closed with a titanium mesh and the incision sutured with a watertight closure, followed by a pressure dressing.

Retrosigmoid Craniotomy

The retrosigmoid approach for the ABI offers advantages of a shorter surgical time, decreased risk of intracranial contamination with flora of the tympanomastoid cavity, and preservation of inner ear structures compared with a translabyrinthine craniotomy. Some argue that the retrosigmoid approach offers a more en face view of larger tumors in the cistern, greater access to the lateral recess, and improved visualization of lower cranial nerves. Although retrosigmoid craniotomy for ABI placement has been used commonly outside the United States, it has only recently gained interest within the United States. At our institution, all non-NF2 pediatric ABIs are performed using a retrosigmoid craniotomy (Video 2; available online at http://www.oto.theclinics.com).

With this approach, older children or adults are placed in a lateral decubitus position with appropriate bolsters to support the upper torso and extremities. Infants can be placed supine with a head turn. The surgeon begins with a curvilinear postauricular incision with elevation of a skin flap along the temporoparietal fascia (**Fig. 5**A). A plane is maintained superficial to the periosteum of the mastoid and occipital bones as well as the temporalis fascia. The periosteum is then elevated and suboccipital muscle attachments are removed. Like the translabyrinthine approach, a subperiosteal pocket is made for the device above the craniotomy site (see **Fig. 5**B, C). The craniotomy itself is usually 3 × 3 cm, bounded by the sigmoid sinus anteriorly and transverse sinus superiorly (see **Fig. 5**D). It is important to partially decompress the sigmoid sinus anteriorly in order to provide as much exposure in front of the cerebellum and avoid excessive brain retraction in order to visualize the lateral recess. After drilling the craniotomy, the dura is incised and dural flaps are retracted. The cerebellum is decompressed by draining CSF, and gentle retraction is used to identify the lateral recess and adjacent cranial nerves (**Fig. 6**A).

The device is opened and inspected. The receiver-stimulator is anchored; the grounding electrode is positioned (see **Fig. 6**B); the array is placed in the CN as described with the translabyrinthine approach (see **Fig. 6**C; **Fig. 7**). After confirming proper placement of the array, the dura, craniotomy site, and incision are closed as previously described (see **Fig. 5**E). Meticulous, watertight, multilayer closure of the dural defect with both autologous tissue and a bovine collagen dural graft around the electrode array reduces the risk of a CSF leak as does a secure mastoid dressing to be worn for at least 5 to 7 days (see **Fig. 5**F).

Intraoperative EABRs

Intraoperative EABRs are critical for validating placement of the electrode array (see **Fig. 4**B). If EABRs are inadequate, the device is repositioned until appropriate waveforms are obtained in order to increase the probability of auditory perception with the ABI. In the case of NF2, tumor growth and resection can distort landmarks. Nevertheless, even in nontumor cases, the complexity of the brainstem anatomy and the blind electrode placement into the CN makes positioning a challenge. Intraoperative EABRs are generated in the bipolar condition using pairs of electrodes (as shown in **Fig. 4**B) to maximize the chance of useful auditory sensations postoperatively and to reduce nonauditory stimulation. EABR surface electrodes are placed at the vertex (positive electrode), seventh cervical vertebrae (reference electrode), and base of the neck

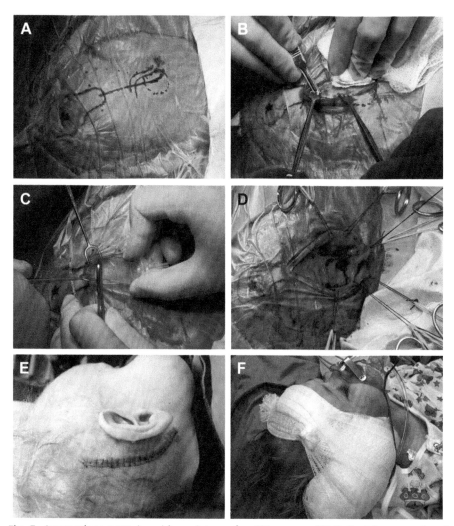

Fig. 5. Approach to retrosigmoid craniotomy for ABI surgery. (*A*) Patient is prepped and draped with a plan for a postauricular incision and a periosteal pocket for device implantation superior to the incision. (*B*) After making an incision, anterior and posterior flaps are raised and a pocket is created for the implanted receiver-stimulator. (*C*) A plastic dummy device is used to confirm an adequately sized periosteal pocket for the implanted receiver-stimulator. (*D*) An inferiorly based periosteal flap approximately 3 cm in width is created, exposing the underlying calvarium to allow an approximately 3 × 3 cm retrosigmoid craniotomy. (*E*) The periosteal flap and skin are closed in layers to ensure a watertight closure over the dura and craniotomy site. (*F*) A firm pressure dressing is maintained in place for 5 to 7 days postoperatively to reduce the risk of CSF leak. (*Adapted from* Puram SV, Tward AD, Jung DH, et al. Auditory brainstem implantation in a 16-month-old boy with cochlear hypoplasia. Otol Neurotol 2015;36(4):621; with permission.)

(ground electrode). By stimulating distinct electrode pairs in the bipolar condition, the relative location of the CN can be inferred. With any EABR, inadvertent stimulation of vasoactive centers and cranial nerves is possible; thus, the surgeon should alert anesthesia before any intraoperative stimulation.

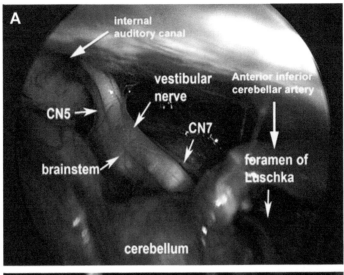

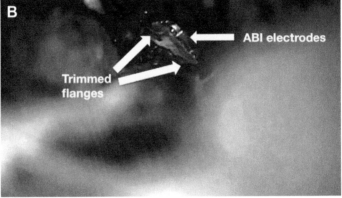

Fig. 6. (*A*) A 0°, 4 mm diameter, rigid endoscopic view of the posterior fossa as seen via retro-sigmoid craniotomy, highlight aberrant neural anatomy. The facial nerve is hypoplastic, the IAC is rotated more superiorly than in the normal posterior fossa and the vestibular nerve runs with trigeminal nerve before entering the IAC. The cochlear nerve as the Imaging suggested was absent. (*B*) Magnified microscope view of the electrode array positioned in the CN. Note that the electrodes are placed facing away from the surgeon and towards the surface of the brainstem. The Dacron mesh as shown is also fully trimmed off to provide passage through a typically smaller foramen of Luschka in children as well as to reduce scarring to surround neural tissues in the event that revision surgery is needed in the future. See also Video 2.

Because the cochlea and auditory nerves are bypassed, an EABR from an ABI will lack waves I and II with amplitude and latency characteristics that differ from acoustic or electrically evoked ABRs generated at the level of the cochlea. Multi-peaked waveforms generated in the first 2 to 3 milliseconds of the onset of the stimulus are thought to be auditory responses, whereas larger waveforms that have longer amplitudes are generally nonauditory. Awake ABI users (in the monopolar stimulation condition) that have a stable electrode position can exhibit similar waveform morphology to those seen intraoperatively, but latencies may be slightly longer because of the lower current used when patients are awake.

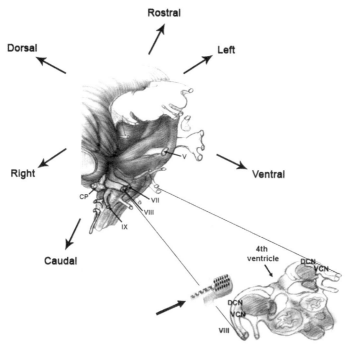

Fig. 7. Three-dimensional illustration of the human pontomedullary junction demonstrating the relationships among the anatomic landmarks used during ABI placement (*upper left*). The choroid plexus (CP) and glossopharyngeal nerve (IX) are used to identify the foramen of Luschka (lateral recess of the fourth ventricle). Magnified section through the brainstem at the level of CN (*lower right*) showing placement of the electrode paddle of the ABI in close proximity to the right DCN and VCN. As shown in this magnified section, neurons of the DCN are closer to the surface electrodes than the VCN. V, trigeminal nerve; VII, facial nerve; VIII, vestibulocochlear nerve. (*Adapted from* Schwartz MS, Otto SR, Shannon RV, et al. Auditory brainstem implants. Neurotherapeutics 2008;5(1):130; with permission.)

Cranial Nerve Monitoring: Cranial Nerve VII and Cranial Nerve X

Intraoperative monitoring of cranial nerves near the foramen of Luschka and the CN is essential to avoid inadvertent injury to these structures as well as to minimize stimulation of nonauditory cranial nerve centers with the ABI. At our institution, facial nerve electromyographic (EMG) responses are monitored with needle electrodes placed in the orbicularis oculi and orbicularis oris on the same side as the craniotomy as well as a high-definition infrared video camera on the ipsilateral face. During EABR testing, in addition to confirming an adequate multiphasic peak waveform, monitoring of CNVII will detect inadvertent stimulation of the facial nerve, necessitating shifting of the electrode paddle.

Similarly, CNX is followed intraoperatively through an EMG monitoring system. An electrode is placed along the side of an appropriately sized endotracheal tube before intubation (**Fig. 8**). The neural integrity monitor (NIM) electrode is placed lateral to the endotracheal tube (and proximal to the cuff) in close apposition to one of the true vocal folds. Video laryngoscopy is used to confirm the position of the electrode. Anesthesia is briefly lightened to trigger vocal fold movement and electrophysiologically confirm

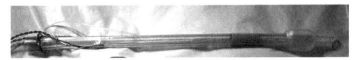

Fig. 8. NIM monitored endotracheal tube with lateral electrodes placed against the vocal folds to detect possible injury or stimulation of CNX during ABI surgery.

the adequacy of monitoring. As an alternative, a premodified firefly monitored endotracheal tube can be used. Monitoring of laryngeal EMGs prevents caudal placement of the electrode array and reduces the risk of hemodynamic instability at ABI activation caused by stimulation of the vagus nerve.

POSTOPERATIVE MANAGEMENT

All pediatric patients are monitored in a dedicated pediatric surgical intensive care unit after ABI surgery with hourly neurologic checks for the first 24 hours. A head CT is ordered on the evening of surgery to confirm stable electrode placement and absence of intracranial bleed or midline shift. Perioperative steroids can reduce edema and can be tapered over the patients' inpatient admission. In our initial experience with 5 retrosigmoid craniotomies for ABI placement in children, the hospital stay ranged from 2 to 4 days. Follow-up occurs at 7 to 10 days. We typically activate the ABI device approximately 4 to 6 weeks after surgery, first under anesthesia and the following day in the awake condition (see *Rehabilitation and Recovery*).

COMPLICATIONS ASSOCIATED WITH PEDIATRIC ABI SURGERY

Most of the studies looking at complication rates in ABI surgery have been completed in adults and in the context of vestibular schwannoma excision. Thus, we review these data here as dedicated studies of complications following pediatric surgery are limited. The translabyrinthine approach has been the primary approach for ABI surgery historically. Among 258 patients who underwent vestibular schwannoma resection over a 14-year period, perioperative complications included CSF leak (7.8%), bacterial meningitis (1.6%), incomplete tumor resection (1.6%), neurovascular compromise (1.1%), and facial nerve palsy (House-Brackmann V or VI) (6.0%).[20] Occlusion of the eustachian tube with bone wax or muscle and obliteration of the mastoid cavity with abdominal fat reduce rates of CSF leak. At many centers, patients are immunized preoperatively with the pneumococcal vaccine to reduce the risk of meningitis.

Compared with the translabyrinthine approach, the retrosigmoid approach has been associated with higher rates of CSF leak (2%–30%), meningitis (up to 2.9%), and postoperative headache (up to 54%).[21] Notably, this analysis does not account for technical modifications to the retrosigmoid approach that have likely improved complication rates. In contrast, the retrosigmoid approach has better reported rates of postoperative facial nerve function compared with a middle fossa craniotomy or translabyrinthine approaches for tumor resection.[22]

The overall rates of complications with the addition of ABI surgery do not vary significantly from those with vestibular schwannoma resection. Colletti and colleagues[6] have reported on their experience at the University of Verona. In their retrospective study of 114 adult and pediatric ABI cases (83 adults, 31 children) over an 11-year period, they found that complications could be divided into major complications (14%), minor complications (65%), and nonauditory side effects (45%). Among the major complications, 3 patients died of unrelated causes, whereas the other patients had complications, such as pseudomeningoceles, cranial nerve palsy, hydrocephalus, and meningitis. Minor complications, such as wound seroma, resolved with conservative care or minor interventions, such as oral antibiotics, whereas issues with transient balance resolved without intervention. Nonauditory sensations included ipsilateral body tingling, facial nerve stimulation, dizziness, and throat irritation following ABI activation. Complication rates did not vary significantly from CI based on their analyses, but there was a statistically significant decrease in complications for nontumor patients compared with the NF2 cohort.

Similar to the University of Verona, Otto and colleagues[23] at the House Ear Institute described 61 patients who had undergone vestibular schwannoma resection and ABI surgery via the translabyrinthine approach. CSF leak occurred in 3.3% of patients, with meningitis rates of 1.6%. Implant-specific complications included failure to provide useful auditory sensations (9.8%) and electrode displacement/migration (1.6%). Twenty-four percent of individual electrodes on ABI arrays could not be used because of nonauditory sensations including dizziness, tingling, and visual jitter. Indeed, as many as 69% of ABI users have reported these nonauditory side effects. These nonauditory side effects are caused by unintended stimulation of nearby cranial nerves, such as VII (facial twitching), IX (tingling and throat constriction), X (nausea), and XI (shoulder contraction), as well as the cerebellar flocculus (jittering of the visual field). Usually, these are associated with the array being positioned too high or low in the brainstem leading to off-target effects. Side effects can be reduced by turning problematic electrodes down or completely off, increasing the duration of the electrical pulse, or changing the reference electrodes. Off-target symptoms become less prominent over time, often allowing the affected electrodes to be reactivated at a later date. At our institution, we have found that the retrosigmoid approach is a safe and effective means of placing the ABI in patients with NF2, offering reliable electrode placement and audiologic benefits with no cases of CSF leak.[17]

More recently, our own experience with 5 cases of pediatric ABI surgery has been favorable with a 2- to 4-day postoperative stay for all patients and no CSF leaks, electrode migration, or other adverse events.[24] However, one of our patients did have total device failure requiring revision surgery after mild blunt head trauma during attempted ambulation. He underwent successful replacement of his device on the same side via revision retrosigmoid craniotomy, with robust postoperative EABRs and behavioral sound detection. Further evaluation of long-term outcomes in this group is ongoing.

RECOVERY AND AUDITORY HABILITATION

As CSF leak is the most common complication seen following retrosigmoid craniotomy for ABI in children, a meticulous multilayer closure and use of firm pressure dressing for 5 to 7 days are crucial. Soft splints over the upper extremities are used to reduce displacement of the pressure dressing in the vigorous child. A formal face-lift wrap can be used to provide durable and stable placement of the mastoid dressing. Hospital stay following ABI surgery has ranged from 2 to 4 days for our first pediatric ABI recipients and we ask all families to remain in the Boston metropolitan area with their child for at least 10 days before flying home.

The first step in auditory habilitation involves device activation and programming (see **Fig. 4**), which typically occurs 4 to 6 weeks after surgery. ABI position is variable between patients, and we have not identified a clear correlation between electrode position and the spatial organization of the CN or psychophysical responses. As a result, empirical testing and activation of electrodes must be performed by an experienced audiologist/electrophysiologist to optimize auditory sensations while minimizing nonauditory stimulation. By analyzing 33 bipolar pairs in a series of adult ABI patients with NF2 , we recently identified an association between auditory perceptual sensations and bipolar ABI electrical stimulation that elicits an evoked response with a P3 wave or middle-latency wave.[25] Thus, as our understanding of ABI electrophysiology improves, it may be possible to better predict the electrophysiologic correlates of perceived auditory responses.

In pediatric patients, we perform initial activation under sedation, typically using dexmedetomidine managed by a dedicated pediatric anesthesia team and overseen by a surgeon (see **Fig. 4**A). This approach allows safe assessment of whether the ABI triggers off-target effects on nearby cranial nerves, such as facial stimulation, gag reflex, or bradycardia. During initial activation under anesthesia (and in the awake condition), the monopolar current is used to stimulate the CN and obtain physiologic feedback from patients. If initial testing is favorable, patients return the following day for testing while awake. If patients are very young, electrical stimulation is paired with visual cues to assess the efficacy of stimulation, whereas, if older, the audiologist can directly solicit feedback from patients regarding quality, level, and pitch of auditory sensation, the extent of nonauditory side effects (if any), and the identification of maximum current levels based on patient comfort. Stimulation parameters are adjusted to optimize audiologic outcomes while minimizing off-target stimulation. Vasoactive centers may be inadvertently stimulated; thus, emergency equipment should be available during activation and testing.

After identifying the specific electrodes that contribute meaningful electrophysiologic and behavioral responses, patients go through a programming process known as pitch ranking, providing detailed feedback on the pitch associated with each electrode: Two electrodes are successively activated and patients note which electrode has a higher perceived pitch. In pediatric patients, this process is simplified. Over time, the audiologist attempts to rank all of the electrodes and generate a tonotopic map that can be downloaded to the speech processor. At follow-up appointments, various speech perception testing is completed with frequent reassessment of electrode sensation and reprogramming. Initially, follow-up appointments are more frequent, but follow-up intervals lengthen with time. We typically see ABI patients 1 week after activation, monthly for 3 months, every 3 months until the first year, and then every 6 months thereafter. Neurotology and neurosurgery follow-up continues at regular intervals ranging from every 3 to 6 months.

Methods for audiologic testing are highly variable. At our institution, early behavioral testing has been limited by the young age of implanted patients (average implant age of 14 months). In this setting, audiologic assessments are performed using the Infant-Toddler Meaningful Auditory Integration of Sound (IT-MAIS) scale, a parental questionnaire used when a child cannot participate in dedicated audiologic testing. As these children progress, formal testing will be completed with LING 6 sounds and eventually Early Speech Perception testing (closed-set format) and Consonant-Nucleus-Consonant (open-set format) may be used. In pediatric patients younger than 3 years, standard audiometric techniques are used with visual reinforcement audiometry to determine sound field thresholds. Although we have not yet completed speech and language assessments in our cohort because of the short follow-up period and young age of their pediatric ABI recipients, we will soon be relying on standard clinical tests, including the MacArthur-Bates

Communicative Development Inventories, Preschool Language Scale, Clinical Evaluation of Language Fundamentals, and Goldman-Fristoe Test of Articulation, to gauge progress.

After activation, families frequently require counseling to help with expectation management. Families and patients may be disappointed with the level of auditory sensation and need to be reminded that sound quality as well as nonauditory sensation usually improves over several years. Given that some patients will not achieve significant speech perception, it is emotionally easier for patients and families to begin with simpler audiologic tasks. With this approach, audiologic testing can be scaled down, allowing a child to master basic tests while avoiding failure on tasks that might be too difficult and result in frustration.

OUTCOMES AND CLINICAL RESULTS IN THE LITERATURE

Dedicated pediatric ABI outcomes are not well described in the literature. Thus, we focus on ABI outcomes in both adults and children, which includes a summary of the few pediatric studies completed to date. ABI outcomes vary depending on the patient population, with nontumor patients typically achieving better outcomes than patients with NF2. ABI users with NF2 can expect auditory sensation, environmental sound awareness, and, occasionally, closed-set word recognition. Rarely, these patients can achieve open-set word recognition. Nevertheless, environmental sound awareness combined with lip reading does improve speech perception abilities in ABI users.[26,27]

Otto and colleagues[23] reported that most adult ABI users with NF2 achieved sound awareness. In these studies, 84% of patients performed greater than chance on closed-set word recognition tests. Although few patients achieve sound-only sentence recognition, when ABI-mediated inputs were combined with lip reading, there was a significant overall gain in comprehension. Importantly, there was continued improvement in test scores and audiologic performance with time: Some ABI users demonstrated progress audiologically more than 8 years following activation. Additional reports, including a review of more than 60 ABI patients, have validated these findings, suggesting a significant improvement in audiologic test scores after ABI surgery with up to 55% open-set sentence recognition (City University of New York sentences) when ABI input and vision cues are combined.[28]

European experience with the Nucleus ABI has been similar to those outcomes appreciated in the United States. In one study, 27 patients with NF2 were tested under auditory-only, visual-only, and auditory-visual combined conditions.[27] Ninety-six percent of these patients achieved auditory sensation with device activation, with an average of 8 electrodes activated. Most users developed environmental sound awareness as well as recognition of speech stress and rhythm cues that enhanced lip reading. Few patients (7.4%) developed auditory-only, open-set speech recognition. Recent data and consensus opinion from an international, multicenter center group raise the possibility of achieving open-set recognition in some ABI users with NF2. In this study, 84 of the best performing patients who underwent surgery primarily via retrosigmoid craniotomy in the supine or semisitting position with tumor resection and ABI placement were reviewed. Patients with NF2 with poor performance were excluded to better identify factors that might correlate with improved performance. Twenty-six of these 84 best performing patients (31%) achieved open-set speech recognition (scores better than 30%).[29] Interestingly, 35.7% of patients operated on in the semisitting position achieved open-set speech recognition compared with 16.7% in patients positioned supine, suggesting this surgical position may facilitate improved ABI results. In the future, it will be essential to validate these findings with long-term follow-up of these patients to better determine the durability of the outcomes described.

In contrast to most ABI users with NF2, some non-NF2 ABI recipients seem to achieve open-set speech perception. Experience with these patients has been primarily gained through European studies, whereby non-NF2 patients have been implanted since the early 1990s. Vittorio Colletti and his colleagues[3,30] at the University of Verona have arguably the most extensive experience, reporting open-set, sound-only sentence recognition in 48 nontumor patients ranging from 10% to 100%, with an average performance of 59%. In contrast, 32 patients with NF2 from the same group had open-set, sound-only sentence recognition scores ranging from 5% to 31%, with a mean of 10%. In their data set, postlingually deafened adults, namely, those who had head trauma with damage to the cochlear nerve or developed cochlear ossification from meningitis or other conditions, had the best postoperative hearing outcomes,[3] with these patients showing significant improvement over the 10 years of follow-up.[3] In contrast, prelingually deafened patients with auditory neuropathy or anatomic malformations of the cochlea did not perform as well, although audiologic benefits are still realized. Consistent with these findings, 3 patients who had complete bilateral cochlear ossification from pneumococcal meningitis and underwent ABI surgery achieved mean open-set, sound and lip-reading sentence recognition scores of 82%.[31]

To better understand the differences between patients with NF2 and nontumor patients, Colletti and Shannon[2] compared cohorts of 10 patients with NF2 and nontumor patients, extensively testing these subjects to determine electrode placement, stimulation selectivity, modulation detection, and speech understanding. Although both groups had similar electrode placement with minimal interelectrode interference, patients with NF2 had significantly poorer modulation detection and speech comprehension than nontumor ABI patients. Although the reason for this difference remains unknown, it is possible that a subpopulation of neurons within the CN or pathways specific for modulation detection and speech recognition is disrupted in NF2 as part of the disease process or tumor resection. Although some have argued that traction or compression of the brainstem and auditory centers during surgery may result in anatomic or functional disruption of these anatomic regions, this hypothesis is undermined by the fact that larger tumor size does not correlate with poorer audiologic outcomes in patients with NF2. Thus, it is more likely that a secreted factor or a yet-to-be-determined molecular mechanism explains the discrepancies between patients with NF2 and nontumor patients that have now been consistently validated.

Dedicated studies of pediatric ABI outcomes remain sparse. Colletti and Zoccante[32] reviewed their experience with ABI surgery in 26 pediatric patients (14 months to 16 years old) with hearing loss caused by inner ear malformations/cochlear nerve aplasia, NF2, incomplete cochlear portioning defects, auditory neuropathy, meningitis-related ossification, and temporal bone fractures with nerve injury. Six of these children had undergone prior CI with no auditory benefit, and 14 had psychomotor delay. All patients underwent a retrosigmoid craniotomy approach with confirmed intraoperative and postoperative EABRs and were found to subsequently use their devices for 8 hours per day on average. Every child achieved environmental sound awareness and language development, including simple words and sentences. More substantial performance with bisyllabic word recognition and comprehension of simple commands was identified in 5 patients, and only one patient realized open-set word recognition. Category of auditory performance (CAP) testing revealed a substantial increase with ABI use; importantly, postimplant cognitive outcomes, such as visual-spatial attention, improved with gains in auditory performance. A recent long-term prospective analysis of 64 deaf children who were followed up to 12 years following ABI surgery revealed that all children showed improvements in auditory perception, with 7 children (11%) achieving the highest possible CAP score (able to converse on the telephone).[4] Twenty children (31.3%) realized open-set speech recognition (CAP score of 5), and an additional 30 (46.9%) achieved a CAP score of 4. These results suggest that with long-term ABI use, open-set auditory recognition may be achievable in many pediatric patients.

Additional pediatric ABI experience has been described by Levent Sennaroglu and colleagues[5] in Ankara, Turkey. In their report of 11 prelingually (30–56 months old) deafened children with severe inner ear malformations, they found that ABI surgery using a retrosigmoid approach had no adverse outcomes. Six children had sound recognition and discrimination, with environmental sound awareness within 3 months of ABI activation. There were improvements in MAIS scores for all patients, with 5 children able to discriminate LING 6 sounds and 2 children able to complete multisyllabic word recognition tests. Importantly, additional handicaps, such as attention deficit hyperactivity disorder, seem to limit audiologic progress, emphasizing the importance of a thorough multidisciplinary preoperative assessment.

Our own experience with pediatric ABI surgery in 4 pediatric patients ranging from 11 to 30 months old, including one patient who underwent revision surgery, is favorable (**Table 1**). Typical preoperative and postoperative radiographic, audiologic, and electrophysiologic parameters for a characteristic patient at our institution, a 16 month old with bilateral cochlear partitioning defects and bilateral cochlear nerve aplasia, are shown (**Fig. 9**). Duration of ABI use since activation with our series ranges from 3 months to 12 months, with 11 to 16 electrodes activated depending on the patient. Based on our experience, sound field thresholds of 20 to 30 dB are achievable, with auditory progress ranging from environmental sound awareness to vocalic play and detection of LING sounds.

Despite the promise of these early experiences and studies, not all reports are as favorable. A recent analysis of 12 pediatric patients at Medipol University in Turkey who underwent ABI surgery with the MED-EL ABI demonstrated reliable sound awareness in only 7 of the children, with the best performance consisting of closed-set word recognition and speaking simple words.[33] Clearly, further research from additional international centers is needed, including greater experience in North America, to better determine the critical factors leading to safe and effective pediatric ABI surgery and hearing outcomes.

One outstanding question is whether patients who have poor outcomes following CI might still be good candidates for ABI surgery. A review of 5 patients with poor audiologic outcomes following CI who subsequently underwent ABI surgery attempts to address this question. In this cohort, all 5 patients achieved audiologic benefits with ABI surgery, with one patient realizing open-set speech recognition in the sound-only condition.[30] More recent analyses from the same group describe 21 children with cochlear nerve deficiency who had initially undergone CI but failed to develop auditory perception and ultimately underwent ABI surgery. All 21 children benefited from ABI placement with an average preoperative CAP score of 0.52 that improved to 4.3 postoperatively.[34] Unfortunately, it remains unclear which factors portend favorable audiologic outcomes in ABI patients who initially have poor outcomes with CI. Certainly, future studies of this specific cohort are needed to better address this question and identify the patients that may truly benefit from ABI placement. In the meantime, improved imaging of the IAC to distinguish cochlear nerve hypoplasia from aplasia is sure to emerge as an important predictor of CI response and the need to proceed directly to ABI surgery.

Table 1
Initial audiologic outcomes following 5 pediatric ABI surgeries at a major US center (Massachusetts Eye and Ear-Harvard Medical School)

Patient ID	Age at Implantation	Duration of ABI Use Since Activation	Active Electrodes	Sound Field Thresholds (dB HL)	Report of Auditory Progress
S_01	2 y	4 mo	15	25–45	• Alerts to sound • More in tune with device • Parental report approximating *no* • Takes off device if told *no*
S_02	11 mo (Initial) 20 mo (Revision)	10 mo (Initial) 6 mo (Revision)	16	20–30	• Unhappy until has device on • Babbles • Responds to name • Detects Ling sounds • Identifies some environmental sounds and words with sign • Follows some practiced auditory play directions
S_03	15 mo	6 mo	11	25–30	• Vocalic babbling/ vocalizes with play • Understands simple phrases auditory only (14-mo level) • Spoken approximation of 3 words (10- to 12-mo level) • Understands 139 spoken words (14-mo level)
S_04	2 y	1 mo	13	60–75	• Alerts to environmental sounds • Requests TV volume on

Abbreviations: HL, hearing level; ID, identification.

FUTURE OF AUDITORY BRAINSTEM IMPLANT TECHNOLOGY

As described in previous sections, the ABI provides meaningful auditory benefits to patients with severe to profound hearing loss; however, outcomes are highly variable across similar cohorts of patients.[2,27,35] Further, many ABI users experience side effects, such as facial pain, involuntary motor movement, as well as dizziness, caused by activation of nonauditory neurons.[6] A possible explanation for the wide range of audiometric outcomes and side effects may be the nonspecific spread of electric current.[36–38] One approach to improve audiometric outcomes, such as speech perception, is by increasing the number of channels. The number of effective channels is diminished, however, by the longitudinal spread of electricity, resulting in channel crosstalk and activation of neuronal populations distant from the site of the electrode.[39–41]

There are several ongoing investigational pathways to improve the ABI in our laboratory at Massachusetts Eye and Ear: flexible electrode arrays and light-based neuronal stimulation. Several groups have begun to investigate flexible polymers for neuroprosthetics.[42] Electrode researchers have hypothesized that a new generation

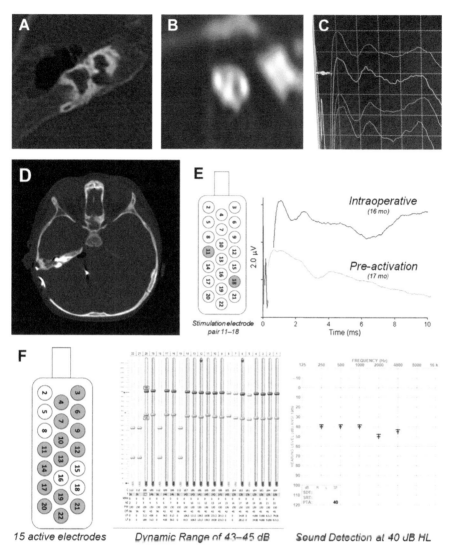

15 active electrodes   Dynamic Range of 43–45 dB   Sound Detection at 40 dB HL

Fig. 9. Radiologic and audiologic images from the case of a 16-month-old patient with bilateral cochlear partitioning defects and bilateral cochlear nerve aplasia who underwent a right-sided retrosigmoid craniotomy for ABI placement. (A) A preoperative axial CT demonstrates a right cochlear partitioning defect with a narrow basal turn. (B) Axial IAC MRI reformat showing cochlear aplasia on the right side. (C) Intraoperative EABRs confirming adequate device placement in the CN. (D) Postoperative axial CT demonstrating good positioning of the electrode. (E) Bipolar electrode stimulation (electrodes 11 and 18) with intraoperative and postoperative device activation. (F) Postoperative device programming with 15 active electrodes with a dynamic range of 43 to 45 dB and sound detection at 40 dB. HL, hearing level.

of polymers will provide a better neural interface and adapt to the curvature of neural tissue. In terms of the ABI, thin (<100 μm) and small (<200 μm diameter) electrodes integrated on flexible polyimide substrate may offer a better physical interface with the curvilinear surface of the CN and allow for a reduction of the stimulation currents thereby limiting the recruitment of neighboring nonauditory neurons.[43] Early studies have demonstrated the feasibility of manufacturing and placement of microelectrode arrays of flexible substrates in murine and rat models of the ABI.[43,44] Studies are ongoing to determine whether flexible arrays can provide improved spatial resolution compared with current electrode array designs.

The use of light-based neuronal stimulation also offers the promise to increase spatial resolution of current ABI arrays. In contrast to electricity, light offers a theoretic advantage as it can be focused and may allow for the selective activation of hundreds of independent channels. Over the past decade, researchers have explored the capacity for light to depolarize *unmodified* neurons in the auditory system via infrared neural stimulation (INS).[45,46] More recent studies, however, indicated that INS is an unlikely alternative to electrical stimulation at the level of the auditory brainstem. Efforts using INS in the central auditory system[47] and peripheral auditory system[48] demonstrated an optophonic artifact, and INS failed to elicit evoked responses in a deafened animal model, suggesting limited clinical utility.

An alternative and perhaps more promising approach is the use of light-sensitive proteins that can activate or silence cells by multiple colors of low-level visible light.[49,50] One such light-sensitive protein is derived from the opsin gene family. This family of genes has emerged as a primary tool for optogenetics, which can be defined as the combination of optics and genetics to control specific cellular events, such as action potentials, in neurons. Opsin genes are divided into 2 superfamilies: microbial-type opsins (type I) and animal-type opsins (type II). Type I opsin genes are found in prokaryotes, algae, and fungi and are the primary tool in neuroscience research. Type II opsin genes are present in higher eukaryotes. There are 4 major types of type I opsins: bacteriorhodopsin, proteorhodopsin, sensory rhodopsin, and channel rhodopsin (ChR). ChR and its variants are the most commonly used excitatory opsin. ChR is a light-gated transmembrane ion channel originally identified in the *Chlamydomonas reinhardtii*, a green unicellular algae from temperate freshwater environments. One variant, channel rhodopsin-2 (ChR2), opens to allow ions into the interior of the cell on stimulation by blue light[49,51] and is commonly used in neuroscience research (**Fig. 10**).

Several groups have investigated the use of opsins in both the central[52–55] and peripheral auditory systems.[25] Early studies demonstrated that adeno-associated viral vector-mediated delivery of ChR2 is possible in auditory neurons of the CN and that the auditory pathways can be activated by pulsed blue light.[52] More specifically, Darrow and colleagues[52] delivered blue light via an optical fiber placed near the surface of the infected CN. Optical stimulation evoked excitatory activity throughout the tonotopic axis of the central nucleus of the IC and the auditory cortex. The pattern and magnitude of the IC activity elicited by optical stimulation was comparable with a 50-dB sound pressure level acoustic click. These initial data suggested that optogenetic control of central auditory neurons is feasible; however, the channel kinetics of ChR2 may not be ideal to convey information at rates typical of many auditory signals.

To identify opsins with more favorable kinetic properties, Boyden and colleagues[56] screened a diversity of algal transcriptomes and identified a new channel rhodopsin called Chronos. In a recent study, the temporal resolution of light-evoked responses of ChR2 was compared with Chronos in a murine ABI model (**Fig. 11**).[54] Both ChR2 and Chronos evoked sustained responses to all stimuli, even at high pulse rates. In addition, optical stimulation evoked excitatory responses throughout the tonotopic axis of the IC. Synchrony of the light-evoked response to stimulus rates of 14 to 448 pulses per second was higher in Chronos compared with ChR2 mice ($P<.05$ at 56, 168, and 224 pulses per second) (**Fig. 12**). Results suggest that Chronos

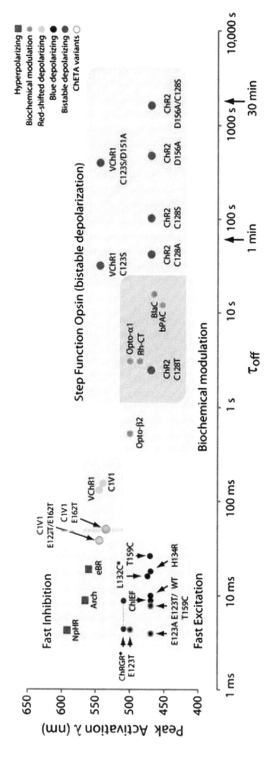

Fig. 10. Kinetic and spectral attributes of optogenetic tool variants. Arch, archaerhodopsin-3; ChIEF, channel rhodopsin-1/2 hybrid; ChRGR, channel rhodopsin-green receiver; eBR, Natronomonas halorhodopsin with addition of trafficking signal between bacteriorhodopsin (BR) and enhanced yellow fluorescent protein (EYFP); NpHR, halo-rhodopsin from Natronomonas pharaonis; WT, wildtype. (*Adapted from* Yizhar O, Fenno LE, Davidson TJ, et al. Optogenetics in neural systems. Neuron 2011;71(1):11; with permission.)

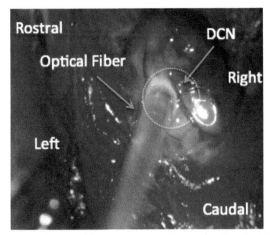

Fig. 11. Optogenetic stimulation of the murine CN. Placement of optical fiber on the surface of murine CN that has been directly transfected with Adeno-associated virus 2/8-Chronos. (*Adapted from* Hight AE, Kozin ED, Darrow K, et al. Superior temporal resolution of Chronos versus channel rhodopsin-2 in an optogenetic model of the auditory brainstem implant. Hear Res 2015;322:237; with permission.)

has the ability to drive the auditory system at higher stimulation rates compared with ChR2 and may be a more ideal auditory opsin for manipulation of auditory pathways.

In summary, there are new and exciting developments on the horizon for ABI technology. Both flexible arrays and light-based stimulation afford novel approaches for neuronal stimulation that may improve patient outcomes. Similar technology may be readily translated to CIs. Future studies will need to demonstrate that new neuronal stimulation paradigms exceed outcomes of current devices. Hybrid arrays, consisting of both established and new technology, may be an initial step to introduce recent technological advances to human auditory neuro-prosthetics.

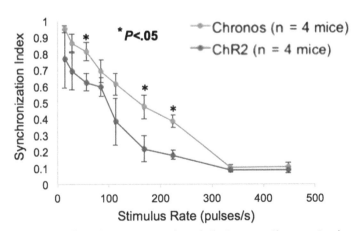

Fig. 12. Comparison of synchronization index of ChR2 versus Chronos. Synchrony of the light-evoked response to stimulus rates of 14 to 448 pulses per second was higher in Chronos compared with ChR2 mice. (*Adapted from* Hight AE, Kozin ED, Darrow K, et al. Superior temporal resolution of Chronos versus channel rhodopsin-2 in an optogenetic model of the auditory brainstem implant. Hear Res 2015;322:235–41; with permission.)

SUMMARY

Over the past several decades, there has been tremendous evolution in our understanding of auditory physiology and a deeper appreciation for the measures needed to improve hearing habilitation outcomes in deaf pediatric patients. Although CIs have become a mainstream option to improve hearing, this technology does not provide substantial benefits to individuals with profound hearing loss and small or absent inner ear anatomy. The ABI offers an alternative means of stimulating and activating neural pathways at the level of the auditory brainstem, thus bypassing deficits at the level of the cochlea and cochlear nerve. Additional advances will be needed to attain clinical audiologic outcomes in most ABI users comparable with modern multichannel CIs. Although some ABI patients achieve open-set speech recognition, most continue to have sound awareness that aids in lip reading.

Pediatric implant centers in the United States and abroad have begun using the ABI in children with severe anomalies of the cochlea or cochlear nerves. Expanding the utility and performance of ABI technology will only come with further experience and a careful analysis of long-term outcomes. Clinical and basic science ABI research, especially in the pediatric population, will be crucial for advancing the field.

ACKNOWLEDGMENTS

The authors would like to thank Elliott Kozin, MD and Aaron Remenschneider, MD, MPH at the Massachusetts Eye and Ear for their contributions to this article on pediatric ABI surgery.

SUPPLEMENTARY DATA

Supplementary data related to this article can be found online at http://dx.doi.org/10.1016/j.otc.2015.07.013.

REFERENCES

1. Young NM, Kim FM, Ryan ME, et al. Pediatric cochlear implantation of children with eighth nerve deficiency. Int J Pediatr Otorhinolaryngol 2012;76(10):1442–8.
2. Colletti V, Shannon RV. Open set speech perception with auditory brainstem implant? Laryngoscope 2005;115:1974–8.
3. Colletti V, Shannon R, Carner M, et al. Outcomes in nontumor adults fitted with the auditory brainstem implant: 10 years' experience. Otol Neurotol 2009;30:614–8.
4. Colletti L, Shannon RV, Colletti V. The development of auditory perception in children after auditory brainstem implantation. Audiol Neurootol 2014;19(6):386–94.
5. Sennaroglu L, Ziyal I, Atas A, et al. Preliminary results of auditory brainstem implantation in prelingually deaf children with inner ear malformations including severe stenosis of the cochlear aperture and aplasia of the cochlear nerve. Otol Neurotol 2009;30(6):708–15.
6. Colletti V, Shannon RV, Carner M, et al. Complications in auditory brainstem implant surgery in adults and children. Otol Neurotol 2010;31:558–64.
7. St. Clair EG, Golfinos JG, Roland JT Jr. Auditory brainstem implants. In: Waltzman SB, Roland JT Jr, editors. Cochlear implants. New York: Thieme Medical Publishers; 2006. p. 222–9.
8. Otto SR, Shannon RV, Wilkinson EP, et al. Audiologic outcomes with the penetrating electrode auditory brainstem implant. Otol Neurotol 2008;29(8):1147–54.

9. Samii A, Lenarz M, Majdani O, et al. Auditory midbrain implant: a combined approach for vestibular schwannoma surgery and device implantation. Otol Neurotol 2007;28:31–8.

10. Noij KS, Remenschneider AK, Kozin ED, et al. Direct parasagittal magnetic resonance imaging of the internal auditory canal to determine cochlear or auditory brainstem implant candidacy in children. Laryngoscope 2015. [Epub ahead of print].

11. Schwartz MS, Otto SR, Shannon RV, et al. Auditory brainstem implants. Neurotherapeutics 2008;5:128–36.

12. Plotkin SR, Stemmer-Rachamimov AO, Barker FG 2nd, et al. Hearing improvement after bevacizumab in patients with neurofibromatosis type 2. N Engl J Med 2009;361:358–67.

13. Sennaroglu L, Colletti V, Manrique M, et al. Auditory brainstem implantation in children and non-neurofibromatosis type 2 patients: a consensus statement. Otol Neurotol 2011;32:187–91.

14. Kim AH, Kileny PR, Arts HA, et al. Role of electrically evoked auditory brainstem response in cochlear implantation of children with inner ear malformations. Otol Neurotol 2008;29:626–34.

15. Kaplan AB, Kozin ED, Puram SV, et al. Auditory brainstem implant candidacy in the United States in children 0-17 years old. Int J Pediatr Otorhinolaryngol 2015; 79(3):310–5.

16. Sininger YS, Cone-Wesson B. Asymmetric cochlear processing mimics hemispheric specialization. Science 2004;305(5690):1581.

17. Puram SV, Tward AD, Jung DH, et al. Auditory brainstem implantation in a 16-month-old boy with cochlear hypoplasia. Otol Neurotol 2015;36(4):618–24.

18. Quester R, Schröder R. Topographic anatomy of the cochlear nuclear region at the floor of the fourth ventricle in humans. J Neurosurg 1999;91:466–76.

19. Friedland DR, Wackym PA. Evaluation of surgical approaches to endoscopic auditory brainstem implantation. Laryngoscope 1999;109(2 Pt 1):175–80.

20. Mass SC, Wiet RJ, Dinces E. Complications of the translabyrinthine approach for the removal of acoustic neuromas. Arch Otolaryngol Head Neck Surg 1999;125:801–4.

21. Charalampakis S, Koutsimpelas D, Gouveris H, et al. Post-operative complications after removal of sporadic vestibular schwannoma via retrosigmoid-suboccipital approach: current diagnosis and management. Eur Arch Otorhinolaryngol 2011; 268:653–60.

22. Arriaga M, Chen D. Facial function in hearing preservation acoustic neuroma surgery. Arch Otolaryngol Head Neck Surg 2001;127:543–6.

23. Otto SR, Brackmann DE, Hitselberger WE, et al. Multichannel auditory brainstem implant: update on performance in 61 patients. J Neurosurg 2002;96:1063–71.

24. Puram SV, Herrmann BS, Barker FG, et al. Retrosigmoid craniotomy for auditory brainstem implantation in adult patients with neurofibromatosis type 2. Journal of Neurologic Surgery – Part B (skull base), in press.

25. Herrmann BS, Brown MC, Eddington DK, et al. Auditory brainstem implant: electrophysiologic responses and subject perception. Ear Hear 2015;36(3):368–76.

26. Lenarz T, Moshrefi M, Matthies C, et al. Auditory brainstem implant: part I. Auditory performance and its evolution over time. Otol Neurotol 2001;22:823–33.

27. Nevison B, Laszig R, Sollmann WP, et al. Results from a European clinical investigation of the Nucleus multichannel auditory brainstem implant. Ear Hear 2002; 23:170–83.

28. Schwartz MS, Otto SR, Brackmann DE, et al. Use of a multichannel auditory brainstem implant for neurofibromatosis type 2. Stereotact Funct Neurosurg 2003;81:110–4.

29. Behr R, Colletti V, Matthies C, et al. New outcomes with auditory brainstem implants in NF2 patients. Otol Neurotol 2014;35:1844–51.
30. Colletti V. Auditory outcomes in tumor vs. nontumor patients fitted with auditory brainstem implants. Adv Otorhinolaryngol 2006;64:167–85.
31. Grayeli AB, Kalamarides M, Bouccara D, et al. Auditory brainstem implantation to rehabilitate profound hearing loss with totally ossified cochleae induced by pneumococcal meningitis. Audiol Neurootol 2007;12:27–30.
32. Colletti L, Zoccante L. Nonverbal cognitive abilities and auditory performance in children fitted with auditory brainstem implants: preliminary report. Laryngoscope 2008;118(8):1443–8.
33. Bayazit YA, Kosaner J, Cinar BC, et al. Methods and preliminary outcomes of pediatric auditory brainstem implantation. Ann Otol Rhinol Laryngol 2014;123(8): 529–36.
34. Colletti L, Wilkinson EP, Colletti V. Auditory brainstem implantation after unsuccessful cochlear implantation of children with clinical diagnosis of cochlear nerve deficiency. Ann Otol Rhinol Laryngol 2013;122(10):605–12.
35. Colletti L, Shannon R, Colletti V. Auditory brainstem implants for neurofibromatosis type 2. Curr Opin Otolaryngol Head Neck Surg 2012;20:353–7.
36. Eisen MD, Franck KH. Electrode interaction in pediatric cochlear implant subjects. J Assoc Res Otolaryngol 2005;6:160–70.
37. Nardo WD, Cantore I, Marchese MR, et al. Electric to acoustic pitch matching: a possible way to improve individual cochlear implant fitting. Eur Arch Otorhinolaryngol 2008;265:1321–8.
38. Venter P, Hanekom J. Is there a fundamental 300 Hz limit to pulse rate discrimination in cochlear implants? J Assoc Res Otolaryngol 2014;15(5):849–66.
39. Boëx C, de Balthasar C, Kós M-I, et al. Electrical field interactions in different cochlear implant systems. J Acoust Soc Am 2003;114:2049.
40. Karg S, Lackner C, Hemmert W. Temporal interaction in electrical hearing elucidates auditory nerve dynamics in humans. Hear Res 2013;299:10–8.
41. Qazi O, van Dijk B, Moonen M, et al. Understanding the effect of noise on electrical stimulation sequences in cochlear implants and its impact on speech intelligibility. Hear Res 2013;299:79–87.
42. Minev I, Musienko P, Hirsch A, et al. Electronic dura mater for long-term multimodal neural interfaces. Science 2015;347:159–63.
43. Guex A, Verma R, Hight A, et al. Electrical stimulation of the cochlear nucleus with a thin flexible polymer electrode array: designing the next generation auditory brainstem implant. In Association for Research in Otolaryngology MidWinter Meeting, San Diego, CA, February 22–26, 2014.
44. Guex A, Hight A, Vachicouras N, et al. Development and in vivo characterization of a novel microfabricated auditory brainstem implant array. In Association for Research in Otolaryngology MidWinter Meeting, Baltimore, MD, February 21–25, 2015.
45. Izzo A, Richter C, Jansen E, et al. Laser stimulation of the auditory nerve. Lasers Surg Med 2006;38:7450753.
46. Izzo A, Walsh J Jr, Ralph H, et al. Laser stimulation of auditory neurons: effect of shorter pulse duration and penetration depth. Biophys J 2008;94(8):3159–66.
47. Verma RU, Guex AA, Hancock KE, et al. Auditory responses to electric and infrared neural stimulation of the rat cochlear nucleus. Hear Res 2014;310: 69–75.
48. Thompson AC, Fallon JB, Wise AK, et al. Infrared neural stimulation fails to evoke neural activity in the deaf guinea pig cochlea. Hear Res 2015;324:46–53.

49. Boyden E, Zhang F, Bamberg E, et al. Multiple-color optical activation, silencing, and desynchronization of neural activity, with single-spike temporal resolution. PLoS One 2007;2:e299.

50. Warden M, Cardin J, Deisseroth K. Optical neural interfaces. Annu Rev Biomed Eng 2014;16:103–29.

51. Boyden E, Zhang F, Bamberg E, et al. Millisecond- timescale, genetically targeted optical control of neural activity. Nat Neurosci 2005;8:1263–8.

52. Darrow KN, Slama MC, Kozin ED, et al. Optogenetic stimulation of the cochlear nucleus using channel rhodopsin-2 evokes activity in the central auditory pathways. Brain Res 2015;1599:44–56.

53. Guo W, Hight AE, Chen JX, et al. Hearing the light: neural and perceptual encoding of optogenetic stimulation in the central auditory pathway. Sci Rep 2015;5: 10319.

54. Hight AE, Kozin ED, Darrow K, et al. Superior temporal resolution of Chronos versus channel rhodopsin-2 in an optogenetic model of the auditory brainstem implant. Hear Res 2015;322:235–41.

55. Kozin E, Darrow K, Hight A, et al. Direct visualization of the murine dorsal cochlear nucleus for optogenetic stimulation of the auditory pathway. J Vis Exp 2015;20:52426.

56. Klapoetke N, Murata Y, Kim S, et al. Independent optical excitation of distinct neural populations. Nat Methods 2014;11(3):338–46.

On the Distant Horizon— Medical Therapy for Sensorineural Hearing Loss

Kathleen M. Kelly, MD[a], Anil K. Lalwani, MD[b],*

KEYWORDS

- Hearing loss • Gene therapy • Spiral ganglion neuron • Hair cell

KEY POINTS

- The inner ear has several structural and functional characteristics that make it an appealing target for novel gene therapy, RNA-based therapy, and stem cell therapy for treatment of sensorineural hearing loss (SNHL).
- The most rapid advancements have been in gene therapy; for example, a recent phase 1/2 clinical trial uses adeno-associated virus (AAV)-mediated delivery of atonal homolog 1 (*Atoh1*) to promote hair cell regeneration.
- Further research will be aimed at optimizing gene therapy expression and timing of delivery, promoting appropriate connectivity between engineered and endogenous cells, and exploring alternative techniques, such as genomic editing.

INTRODUCTION

Hearing loss is the most common sensory deficit in developed societies.[1,2] According to the Centers for Disease Control, 2 to 3 children out of every 1000 births have hearing loss.[3] Hearing impairment in children, particularly of prelingual onset, has been shown to negatively affect educational achievement, future employment and earnings, and even life expectancy.[4,5]

SNHL, which refers to defects within the cochlea or auditory nerve itself, far outweighs conductive causes for permanent hearing loss in both children and adults. The causes of SNHL in children are heterogeneous, including both congenital and acquired causes. In neonates in particular, a genetic cause accounts for half of all cases of hearing loss. Of those with genetic causes, 30% can be considered syndromic (eg, Pendred, Usher, Waardenburg) and the other 70% nonsyndromic. The inheritance pattern of nonsyndromic SNHL follows this general distribution: 75% autosomal

[a] Department of Otolaryngology – Head and Neck Surgery, University of Texas Southwestern Medical Center, 5323 Harry Hinds Blvd, Dallas, TX 75390, USA; [b] Department of Otolaryngology – Head and Neck Surgery, Columbia University Medical Center, Harkness Pavilion, 180 Fort Washington Avenue, Floor 7, New York, NY 10032, USA
* Corresponding author.
E-mail address: akl2144@cumc.columbia.edu

Otolaryngol Clin N Am 48 (2015) 1149–1165
http://dx.doi.org/10.1016/j.otc.2015.07.012
0030-6665/15/$ – see front matter © 2015 Elsevier Inc. All rights reserved.

Abbreviations	
AAV	Adeno-associated virus
ABR	Auditory brainstem response
ASO	Antisense oligonucleotide
Atoh1	Atonal homolog 1
BDNF	Brain-derived neurotrophic factor
DFNA	Nonsyndromic deafness, autosomal dominant
DFNB	Nonsyndromic deafness, autosomal recessive
FGF	Fibroblast growth factor
GDNF	Glial cell line–derived neurotrophic factor
GJB2	Gap junction beta-2
HSV1	Herpes simplex virus 1
MYO7A	Myosin VIIA
NT-3	Neurotrophin 3
ONP	Oticlike neural progenitors
RNAi	RNA interference
SGN	Spiral ganglion neuron
SNHL	Sensorineural hearing loss
USH1C	Usher syndrome 1C

recessive, 20% autosomal dominant, 2%–5% X-linked, and less than 1% mitochondrial.[6] The mode of inheritance is important, as it guides the strategy of intervention, as explained in greater detail later.

The process of auditory transduction, in which mechanical sound waves are converted to electrical inputs, occurs at the level of the hair cell within the cochlea. The hair cell, located in the organ of Corti in mammals, contains specialized structures that project from the apical surface into the scala media and sense waves within the endolymph. The movement of these projections converts sound waves into electrical signals, which are subsequently carried via spiral ganglion neurons (SGNs) to the eighth cranial nerve. At any point along this pathway, a disruption in the conversion of mechanical signals to electrical signals propagated to the auditory nucleus results in SNHL. This article identifies potential mechanisms of intervention both at the level of the hair cell and the SGNs.

Approximately 16,000 hair cells are produced during early development in each cochlea, along with supporting cells and 30,000 to 40,000 afferent SGNs.[7] However, the fragile nature of hair cells makes them susceptible to damage and death because of genetic factors, exposure to noise, ototoxic drugs, and even early infection. Once damaged, these cells cannot be restored. However, since the discovery was made that avian species can spontaneously regenerate new hair cells after damage, translational research has been aimed at understanding this process so as to initiate a similar one in the human ear.[8]

Current treatment of SNHL cannot improve any cellular deficits; sound is either amplified with a hearing aid or the auditory nerve is stimulated with a cochlear implant. Both strategies use the remaining hair cells or auditory neurons. Yet, in recent years, new evidence suggests that future treatments may be able to improve SNHL at the cellular level through modification of hair cells or auditory neurons. These possible treatments follow 3 main approaches: (1) gene therapy to augment production of proteins that may protect or even regenerate hair cells, (2) RNA-based therapy to inhibit expression of detrimental proteins that promote hair cell damage, and (3) stem cell therapy to replace damaged or dead hair cells or auditory neurons. Although it is unlikely that any of these strategies will be a panacea for SNHL, they will add to the armamentarium of treatment options that can serve an individual patient.

GENE THERAPY FOR SENSORINEURAL HEARING LOSS

Conceptually speaking, gene therapy involves the transfer of a gene of interest to a target cell. This process can be accomplished through 2 main mechanisms: recombinant viruses and nonviral methods, which include liposomes and naked DNA. In the case of virally mediated gene therapy, the desired gene is packaged into a viral vector and the virus subsequently transfects the target cell and incorporates itself, including the desired gene, into the target cell's DNA. At this point, the target cell produces the protein of interest using its native translation machinery. Thus, long-term expression of a transgenic protein can be induced. Given the right promoter sequences, the target cell can be programmed to express the protein indefinitely or it can be situationally regulated. The alternative to gene therapy is direct administration of proteins, which are limited in their efficacy by their short half-lives and often require the use of continuous pumps.[9–13]

Several engineered replication-deficient viruses have been used for transfection of a variety of cell types in the nonprimate mammalian inner ear, including adenovirus,[14–16] lentivirus,[17] herpes simplex virus 1 (HSV1),[18,19] vaccinia virus,[18] and AAV.[20] Each of these vectors demonstrates a unique profile of strengths and weaknesses with regard to cell types transfected, efficiency of transfection, genetic carrying capacity, and potential side effects (**Table 1**; for review, see Ref.[21]). Adenovirus, a 36-kbp double-stranded DNA virus, has been found to be particularly suited for use in SNHL because of its large carrying capacity of up to 10 kbp, ease of production, and ability to efficiently transfect both hair cells and supporting cells[22] as well as neural and glial cells.[23] For these reasons, the first gene therapy clinical trial for SNHL used an adenoviral vector.[24]

The anatomy of the inner ear is unique and offers several advantages and disadvantages for the advancement of gene therapy treatment. The sensory organ is housed in bone and bathed in fluid, thereby protecting it and facilitating access. The presence of the blood-labyrinthine barrier is thought to prevent the dissemination of viral vector into the systemic circulation, thereby limiting potential side effects of the virus itself as well as reducing the risk of inappropriate gene insertion at distant sites. This protection also works the other way: the barrier prohibits interference by the immune system on exogenous cells or viral vectors.[25] Two injection sites are available for access depending on the strategy of interest: the round window provides access to the fluid surrounding the hair cell bodies, whereas a basal turn cochleostomy can be used for the hair cell bundles (**Fig. 1**).[26] Although both approaches showed expression of a green fluorescent protein reporter gene using an advanced-generation adenoviral vector in a guinea pig model, the basal turn cochleostomy group demonstrated high-frequency hearing loss, whereas the round window group preserved hearing.[27,28]

The small volume and small number of target cells that comprise the inner ear form the ideal scenario for gene therapy. The circumstances promote high concentrations of viral vector with few cells requiring transfection combined with a continuous flow of fluid throughout all segments of the inner ear. However, despite the continuity between chambers, studies have shown a transfection gradient after round window injection into the scala tympani, which occurs with multiple vector types, including AAV,[29] cationic liposome,[29,30] HSV1, and vaccinia virus vectors.[18] Because the volume is constrained, the injection of additional fluid into the cochlea may disrupt the tight junctions separating the endolymph and perilymph, resulting in loss of the endolymphatic potential through mixing of fluids, ultimately causing hair cell death.[31] Furthermore, future therapies targeting endolymphatic delivery of vectors will have to adapt to the high potassium content of the fluid, making the preparation substantially different from those intended for other delivery sites.[7]

Table 1
Characteristics of viral and nonviral mechanisms of gene therapy delivery

Mechanism of Delivery	Advantages	Disadvantages	Cellular Tropism
Viral			
Adenovirus	Easy to produce Large insert (7.5–10 kb) Cell division not required	Immunogenic Transient expression	Mesenchymal cells lining perilymphatic spaces Stria vascularis Fibrocytes of spiral ligament Supporting cells of OC Hair cells of OC and vestibule SGNs
Adeno-associated virus	No human disease Stable expression Cell division not required	Difficult to produce Small insert (4–5 kb) Variable transfection efficiency	Fibrocytes of SL Rm Supporting cells of OC SGNs Vestibular sensory hair cells and supporting cells
Herpes virus	Large insert (10–100 kb) Stable expression	Human disease Cytopathic	Mesenchymal cells lining perilymphatic spaces Fibrocytes of SL Rm Supporting cells of OC SGNs VGNs
Lentivirus (retrovirus)	Stable expression	Insertional mutagenesis Low transfection efficiency Cell division required	SGNs Glia
Nonviral			
Liposome	Easy to make Unlimited insert size Cell division not required Nonpathogenic Nonimmunogenic	Transient expression Low transfection	Fibrocytes of SL OHCs and SCs of OC Rm SGNs

Abbreviations: OC, organ of Corti; OHC, outer hair cell; Rm, Reissner membrane; SC, supporting cell; SGN, spiral ganglion neuron; SL, spiral ligament; VGN, vestibular ganglion neuron.

From Kesser BW, Lalwani AK. Gene therapy and stem cell transplantation: strategies for hearing restoration. In: Ryan AF, editor. Gene therapy of cochlear deafness: present concepts and future aspects. New York: Karger; 2009. p. 64–86; with permission.

There are 3 key ways in which gene therapy has been hypothesized to improve the function of the inner ear. In acquired hearing loss, gene therapy can be used to provide protective factors that promote SGN survival in the absence of healthy hair cells.[32–35] Similarly, it can be used to provide protective factors to prevent hair cell damage at the outset from chemical or noise-induced insult.[10,36,37] In these 2 examples, the results of gene therapy are supportive in nature, with the goal of preventing hearing loss. Gene therapy has also been used as a means of growth and replacement after hearing loss.

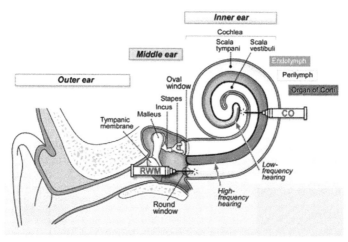

Fig. 1. Anatomy of the ear and the 2 prevailing injections sites for gene therapy administration. CO, cochleostomy; RWM, round window membrane. (*From* Holt JR, Vandenberghe LH. Gene therapy for deaf mice goes viral. Mol Ther 2012;20(10):1836–7; with permission.)

Some research groups are seeking to use gene therapy to promote hair cell rescue or regeneration to increase the population of remaining cells.[38–40] The same strategies have also been used in congenital hearing loss and include attempts to transform surrounding cells into expressing a hair cell–like phenotype.

Spiral Ganglion Neuron Survival

In the healthy ear, inner ear cells, including hair cells, secrete multiple neurotrophic factors. Both neurotrophin 3 (NT-3) and brain-derived neurotrophic factor (BDNF) have been associated with the maintenance of functional SGNs, which can be damaged through lack of adequate trophic support or through direct trauma to the afferent fibers or cell bodies.[41] Thus, hair cell loss negatively affects the survival of SGNs via the absence of these key trophic factors.[42,43] Although direct infusion of NT-3 and BDNF into the cochlea has been shown to improve SGN survival significantly,[44] the requirement of an osmotic mini pump is impractical for clinical use.[9] However, given that the hearing benefits of cochlear implants depend on functional SGNs and the auditory nerve, the question of how to provide sustained delivery of those trophic factors is of high importance. Gene therapy may prove to be a means to accomplish this goal.

Gene therapy has been successfully used to increase BDNF expression after hair cell loss using multiple viral vectors, including HSV[34] and AAV[33] in an aminoglycoside-deafening regimen and adenovirus after a deafening regimen in guinea pigs,[45] thereby increasing the versatility of this potential strategy. As several viral vectors have been compatible with this strategy, its versatility is a further potential benefit.

In addition, studies have demonstrated that glial cell line–derived neurotrophic factor (GDNF) can have protective effects for SGNs. Both direct application of GDNF to the cochlea in vitro as well as GDNF intratympanic infusion to the middle ear in vivo improved SGN survival in an ototoxic deafening model in guinea pigs.[46] Again, enhanced survival was seen after adenoviral-GDNF treatment in a similar guinea pig ototoxic model,[35] and interestingly, adenoviral-GDNF therapy combined with electrical stimulation was more effective at promoting SGN survival than either treatment alone.[47] These findings support the hypothesis that gene therapy may be best used as an adjunct to, instead of as a replacement for, other types of existing SNHL treatment.

Although most of these studies have tested trophic replacement in acquired SNHL models, BDNF supplementation has also been found to improve SGN survival in nonsyndromic SNHL. Mutations in the gene *POU4F3* in humans are responsible for DFNA15, a progressive nonsyndromic SNHL. Although the mutations are autosomal dominant, the phenotypic presentation varies greatly in age of onset and degree of hearing loss.[48–50] Unlike the human mutation, the *Pou4f3* mutation in mice is recessive and more uniform in phenotype, resulting in SGN loss at 2 to 6 weeks of age.[51,52] Fukui and colleagues[53] treated *Pou4f3* mutant mice with an adenoviral-BDNF vector. Treated mice were found to have significantly more viable SGNs than controls, and the surviving SGNs demonstrated substantial sprouting to the auditory epithelium.

Hair Cell Survival

The neurotrophic factors that have been shown to improve SGN survival, namely, NT-3,[54] BDNF,[54,55] and GDNF,[56,57] have also been shown to promote hair cell survival. In a gene therapy study with pharmacologic ototoxicity, an adenoviral-GDNF construct protected both vestibular and cochlear hair cells, which ultimately rescued hearing function.[40] In addition, damage caused by reactive oxygen species has been implicated as a mechanism of hair cell damage in acquired SNHL, including aminoglycoside- and noise-induced hearing loss.[58] Adenoviral vectors with catalase and Mn superoxide dismutase inserts curbed hearing loss when administered prophylactically in a model of aminoglycoside toxicity.[36]

Genetic Hearing Loss

Of particular interest in the pediatric population are gene therapy treatments for genetic hearing loss. As mentioned earlier, gene therapy can replace a defective allele with its wild-type counterpart and is a compelling strategy for treatment of patients with these types of diseases. Genetic causes for deafness are divided into 2 categories: (1) syndromic, in which deafness is associated with other deficits, and (2) nonsyndromic, in which deafness is the only deficit.

One of the well-studied syndromic causes of hearing loss is Usher syndrome, a disease characterized by congenital deafness, progressive vision loss, and vestibular dysfunction. The most common gene associated with profound congenital SNHL is Usher syndrome type 1B, in which mutations in myosin VIIA (*MYO7A*) cause the production of an atypical myosin in the sensory cells of the ears and eyes, resulting in retinitis pigmentosa and hearing loss. A phase 1/2 clinical trial initiated in 2013 is underway to test the effect of delivery of a corrected version of *MYO7A* on vision loss, based on the successful results of this approach in a mouse model.[59,60] Thus, in the future, it may be plausible to use a similar approach to treating the hearing loss caused by the same defective protein. In a related mouse model of Usher syndrome 1C (USH1C), Lentz and colleagues[61] were able to restore hearing and vestibular function using injections of antisense oligonucleotides (ASOs). The therapy reduced production of mutated harmonin in favor of translation of the wild-type protein. Further discussion of the strategy and mechanism are described in the RNA-based therapy section.

Nonsyndromic hearing loss is heterogeneous in inheritance with 32 autosomal dominant genes associated with 29 loci (DFNA1–DFNA67) and 60 autosomal recessive genes associated with 57 loci (DFNB1–DFNB103).[62] Mutations in the gap junction beta-2 (*GJB2*) gene, located at the DFNB1A locus, account for 20% to 50% of congenital recessive nonsyndromic SNHL, depending on the population. The *GJB2* gene encodes connexin-26, a protein found in the supporting cells of the inner ear whose aggregates form gap junctions.[63–65] These gap junctions are thought to facilitate potassium circulation between the hair cells and the stria vascularis during mechanosensory transduction.[66,67] Without proper potassium recirculation, the endolymph potential decays, and hearing loss ensues. Encouraging evidence from in vitro[68] and in vivo[69] studies shows that gene transfer of *GJB2* can restore expression of connexin-26 and even functional gap junctions. However, improvement in hearing has yet to be demonstrated in an animal model.

Hair Cell Regeneration and Supporting Cell Transformation

Although the aforementioned strategies seem more conducive to the treatment of congenital hearing loss, gene therapy also shows potential for the improvement of acquired hearing loss. Even in the pediatric population, SNHL can be attributed to infection (both viral and bacterial), acoustic trauma, or pharmacologic toxicity from aminoglycoside antibiotics, oncologic chemotherapy, or chelation therapy. These insults have the capacity to damage delicate hair cells, which, unlike those of avian species, do not spontaneously regenerate. However, recent research of these lower vertebrates capable of hair cell regeneration has led to strategies that may have the potential to promote the regeneration of hair cells themselves or to trigger differentiation of supporting cells to assume a hair cell–like phenotype.

For example, various groups have been able to generate hair cells by transfecting endogenous supporting cells with regulatory proteins that are normally found earlier in development. *Atoh1*, also referred to as Math1/Hath1 (mouse atonal homologue 1/human atonal homologue 1), is a basic helix-loop-helix transcription factor required for normal hair cell differentiation in the developing ear.[70,71] Initial in vitro studies by Zheng and Gao[72] induced overexpression of murine *Atoh1*, which resulted in ectopic hair cell production. Subsequently, the team used an adenoviral vector to overexpress human *Atoh1*, which generated increased numbers of hair cells both in a rat utricular macula model as well as after aminoglycoside injury.[73]

In in vivo studies, transfection of *Atoh1* into supporting cells has been shown to generate hair cells in a deafened guinea pig model, leading to lower thresholds on auditory brainstem responses (ABRs) than in deafened controls.[38] In an embryonic mouse model, a similar protocol showed generation of not only new hair cells from supporting cells but also new hair cells that could support mechanosensory function.[74] An adenoviral-packaged *Atoh1* delivery was found to increase hair cell numbers in the macular organs of an aminoglycoside-treated mouse model with resulting improvement in balance.[75] In more recent studies, increased expression of *Atoh1* has been shown to be protective of hair cells by means of induction of repair processes after noise-induced hearing loss.[76] The therapeutic window in which recovery can be maximized has yet to be determined and may likely require initiating therapy within a short time of injury.

The first clinical trial of gene therapy for hearing loss incorporates adenoviral delivery of *Atoh1* to the inner ear in adult patients to treat auditory and vestibular dysfunction. The clinical trial of the experimental drug CGF166, which is a collaboration between Novartis (Basel, Switzerland) and GenVec (Gaithersburg, Maryland), received approval of its Investigational New Drug application to the US Food and Drug Administration in 2014 and is currently in phase 1/2.[24] Although this clinical trial is approved only for adults older than 20 years who have noncongenital, severe to profound hearing loss, there is potential for the same treatment to be used in pediatric patients with acquired SNHL in the future.

RNA-BASED THERAPY FOR SENSORINEURAL HEARING LOSS

RNA-based therapies use viral vector technology similar to gene therapy and similarly result in the manipulation of the target cell's phenotype. One key difference lies in the outcome of the strategy: gene therapy inserts the genetic substrate necessary to produce a fully functional, missing protein, whereas RNA-based therapy disrupts the normal mRNA translation to purposefully prevent the formation of a deleterious protein. Two strategies have been developed to modulate protein expression at the RNA level: RNA interference (RNAi) and antisense technology. In the RNAi approach, short, complementary RNA sequences called microRNA or small interfering RNA bind to the mRNA sequence of the protein of choice. As double-stranded RNA is not capable of undergoing translation into a viable protein, the molecule triggers the formation of a nuclease complex for degradation called the RNA-induced silencing complex.[77] Antisense technology is similar in that it can turn a gene off by disrupting the translation of mRNA; however, the synthetic agent can be DNA, RNA, or a chemical analogue (**Fig. 2**).[78]

In a mouse model of Usher syndrome, the leading cause of combined congenital deafness and blindness,[79,80] Lentz and colleagues[61] restored hearing and vestibular function using a targeted ASO therapy. More specifically, the team modeled the recessive mutation in French-Acadian USH1C, which produces a cryptic splice site that results in a significantly truncated version of the protein harmonin.[81] Harmonin is an integral protein to the development and maintenance of stereocilia in hair cells.[82,83] Of 47 potential ASOs identified, 1 reduced cryptic splicing such that greater than 20% of harmonin production was wild type. Remarkably, after 1 intraperitoneal injection of ASO delivered neonatally, the mutant mice recovered normal vestibular function and some auditory function, as measured by ABRs as well as head-tossing and circling behavior. Improvement was sustained for several months, and postmortem investigation showed normal levels of harmonin and normal hair cell morphology.[61] Despite these impressive results, questions remain regarding the overall feasibility of this intervention in humans because of the administration of the ASO as well as the time line of treatment.

STEM CELL THERAPY FOR SENSORINEURAL HEARING LOSS

In recent decades, stem cell therapy has captured the attention of the scientific and medical communities with the hope that this technique could be used to replace deficient cell types within the human body, whether for treatment of diabetes, Parkinson disease, or hearing loss. Stem cells are self-renewing pluripotent cells whose development can be manipulated by use of various cytokines and growth factors. The basic strategy of stem cell therapy is to differentiate pluripotent stem cells into a missing cell type, such as hair cells or SGNs, or their progenitors, and then to transplant these new effector cells into the host. Three types of stem cells have been successfully differentiated into cell types that can be transplanted to improve SNHL: embryonic stem cells, adult inner ear stem cells, and neuronal stem cells.[84]

Transplant of these cells presents a unique problem given the accessibility and size of the structures involved as well as the complicated relationship between cell types. Injection approaches are similar to those used for gene therapy and include round window,[85] lateral semicircular canal,[86] posterior semicircular canal,[87] cochlear lateral wall,[86,88] internal auditory meatus,[89] and modiolus.[90] Of these approaches, only the cochlear lateral wall injection resulted in hearing loss.[86] Yet despite the success and variety of possibilities thus far, many questions regarding stem cell transplant remain. It is still unclear whether stem cells cause an immunologic response. Although the

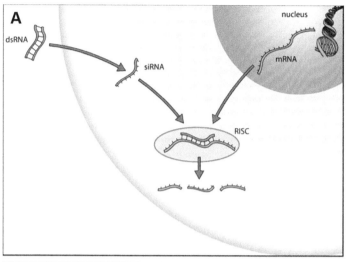

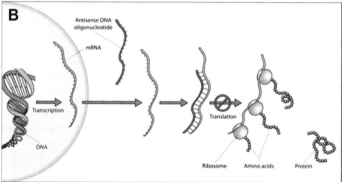

Fig. 2. (*A*) RNAi is a native process where small RNA molecules attach to mRNA sequences and activate an RNA-induced silencing complex (RISC), which results in the cleavage of the mRNA strand. (*B*) Antisense RNA or DNA (as in this schematic) is complementary to the target mRNA sequence and prevents normal translation by the ribosome from occurring. (*From* Robinson R. RNAi therapeutics: how likely, how soon? PLoS Biol 2004;2(1):E28.)

cochlea and brain are immunologically privileged sites and no inflammatory response has been noted in in vivo studies,[88,90,91] grafted stem cells have been found to aggregate at sites of injury.[92] This observation also calls to mind whether stem cells could provide a nidus for neoplasm development. The question remains as to whether these grafts have the potential to form adequate and appropriate connections.

Stem Cell Therapy for Generation of Hair Cells

In one of the first major studies to investigate stem cell therapy for use in hearing loss, Li and colleagues[92] determined that a stepwise differentiation protocol could be used to convert embryonic stem cells to inner ear progenitor and hair cells. Stepwise differentiation involves precisely executed cues that are present in normal development. The group isolated nestin-positive progenitor cells with markers present in the otic placode and otic vesicle. These cells were enriched with a 10-day treatment of epidermal growth factor/insulin-like growth factor 1, which was followed by treatment with basic fibroblast growth factor (FGF) in addition to the aforementioned factors. This process resulted in cells that expressed several marker genes attributable to those of the normal inner ear. The study also went on to show in vivo that these cells were capable of expressing hair cell markers and aggregating to form hair bundles in the cochlear or vestibular sensory epithelia.

Further research into stepwise differentiation by Oshima and colleagues[93] led to the successful generation of hair cell–like cells from otic progenitors derived from embryonic stem cells (**Fig. 3**). These hair cell–like cells formed hair bundle–like protrusions in vitro when cocultured with fibroblast-like cells derived from embryonic chicken utricles, which behaved in a manner similar to inner ear–supporting cells. Finally, on mechanical stimulation, the hair cell–like cells demonstrated responses consistent with normal immature hair cells.[94] Thus, although the resulting cells were mechanosensitive, additional developmental steps would need to be undertaken to reduce the response variability, increase the specificity of these cells, and improve the overall yield of the stepwise differentiation protocol.

Subsequent experiments by Koehler and colleagues[95] were able to further isolate cell types during stepwise differentiation in a 3-dimensional culture. Precise control over bone morphogenic peptide, transforming growth factor beta, and FGF led to a concerted developmental lineage from embryonic stem cell to nonneural, preplacodal,

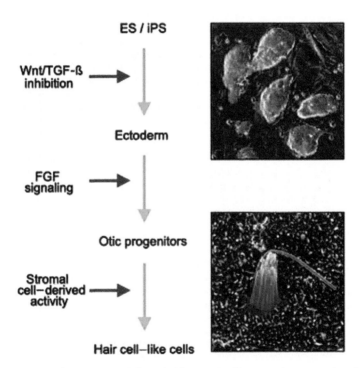

Fig. 3. Stepwise guidance protocol from Oshima and colleagues demonstrating the differentiation of embryonic stem cells (ES) and induced pluripotent stem cells (iPS) first into ectoderm, then into otic progenitors, and finally into epithelial clusters of hair cell–like cells with stereociliary bundles. FGF, fibroblast growth factor; TGF-β, transforming growth factor beta. (*From* Oshima K, Shin K, Diensthuber M, et al. Mechanosensitive hair cell-like cells from embryonic and induced pluripotent stem cells. Cell 2010;141(4):704–16.)

and finally otic placode–like epithelia. The otic placode–like epithelia were found to produce vesicles containing prosensory cells, which were structurally and functionally similar to vestibular end organs. These prosensory cells eventually formed hair cells with stereociliary bundles and kinocilium that were mechanosensitive and capable of forming viable synapses with sensory neurons that also originated from the otic placode. The protocol resulted in a more scalable process by which an inner ear organoid, that is, a collection of embryonic stem cell–derived hair cell–like cells, supporting cells, and sensory-like neurons, could be readily produced and used.[96]

Stem Cell Therapy for Generation of Auditory Neurons

Recent research has also led to the development of stem cell therapies for the generation of SGNs. This strategy could be useful in patients who have lost SGNs but have intact hair cells or those who have lost both and could use grafted SGNs to form sufficient connections with the auditory nucleus to become candidates for cochlear implant. Neuronal progenitors have been derived from cochlear stem cells,[84,97] neural stem cells of the lateral ventricle,[98] and embryonic stem cells.[99,100] In recent years, a series of steps have been elucidated to differentiate these stem cells into oticlike neural progenitors (ONPs), which behave with an SGN-like phenotype.[101,102]

In 2 pivotal studies, these ONPs were transplanted to investigate stem cell integration. In the first of the studies, Corrales and colleagues[103] deafened gerbils with ouabain, thus destroying hair cells while maintaining type I SGNs. After 10 weeks, ONPs were found to have created ectopic ganglia with projections to the organ of Corti as well as toward the brainstem. In a subsequent study with a similar model and protocol, Chen and colleagues[99] found that engrafted ONPs could survive, differentiate, and grow projections appropriately such that the animals showed improved auditory evoked responses. These improvements were detectable as early as 4 weeks postimplant, and at 10 weeks, improvement was almost 50%. Although these findings require replication, they provide an intriguing and exciting possibility for the future of stem cell–mediated generation of auditory neurons.

FUTURE DIRECTIONS

Many outstanding discoveries have been made regarding the genetic underpinnings of SNHL, with the potential to lead to novel therapies capable of helping individuals who have few to no other treatment alternatives. However, many questions regarding gene therapy, RNA-based therapy, and stem cell therapy remain.

With regard to gene therapy, further investigation is required to improve control over targeting and expression of genes of interest. Although there is evidence to suggest the selective gene transfer to supporting cells[104] and hair cells, there is minimal control over which cell types are transfected and what the resulting effect on that transfection might be for those cell types. In many instances, those effects may vary based on the stage of development of those cells. Thus, a greater understanding of the temporal requirements for each intervention is imperative to maximize therapeutic benefit.

A persistent concern surrounding gene therapy is the possibility of systemic side effects with viral vectors. Current clinical trials will help identify areas of potential risk. Another consideration may be to continue to explore nonviral means of cell delivery, such as electroporation. This technique in particular could be of interest in hearing loss because the electrode on a cochlear implant could be used to create a closed electric field capable of facilitating efficient gene delivery.[105]

A main concern regarding stem cell therapy is the ability to create as well as organize new cells to replace those lost in the deficient organ; this requires extensive organization within each cell type as well as integration between cell types. For example, not only would new hair cells need to assume biophysical properties depending on their location within the cochlea but they also need to interface properly with SGNs to closely replicate normal hearing. Similarly, new neurons would not only need to create appropriate connections based on the tonotopic structure of the cochlea but also need to project appropriately to the brainstem. The generation of replacement cells will not be able to achieve its full potential unless there is a greater understanding of how to support these integrative processes.

Another novel treatment strategy for hearing loss may be genomic editing. Although these approaches are still in their infancy, they have the potential to facilitate both the study of inner ear genes and repair mutations. RNA-guided DNA endonucleases based on clustered regulatory interspaced short palindromic repeats have been used in the mammalian inner ear in vivo.[106] What makes this technique so appealing, along with other genomic editing tools such as zinc-finger nucleases or transcriptional activator–like effector nucleases, is that it can be used to disrupt, modify, or add to existing genes. Genomic editing could prove useful for a large array of mutations, some of which may be difficult to target in other ways, such as single point mutations.

Restoration of hearing in the pediatric population is a complex problem with many potential solutions on the distant horizon. Given the importance of auditory learning in children, particularly for language development, advances in medical therapies would have a profound impact on the lives of these patients. As the number of treatment options increases, it is important to determine which ones are particularly suited to an individual's genotype and phenotype as well as the optimal delivery window for therapeutic efficacy. Although many questions still remain, these exciting new strategies have the capacity to redefine expected outcomes for those suffering from SNHL.

REFERENCES

1. Cruickshanks KJ, Wiley TL, Tweed TS, et al. Prevalence of hearing loss in older adults in Beaver dam, Wisconsin. The epidemiology of hearing loss study. Am J Epidemiol 1998;148(9):879–86.
2. Davis AC. The prevalence of hearing impairment and reported hearing disability among adults in Great Britain. Int J Epidemiol 1989;18(4):911–7.
3. Centers for Disease Control and Prevention (CDC). Identifying infants with hearing loss - United States, 1999-2007. MMWR Morb Mortal Wkly Rep 2003; 59(8):220–3.
4. Carvill S. Sensory impairments, intellectual disability and psychiatry. J Intellect Disabil Res 2001;45(Pt 6):467–83.
5. Mohr PE, Feldman JJ, Dunbar JL, et al. The societal costs of severe to profound hearing loss in the United States. Int J Technol Assess Health Care 2000;16(4): 1120–35.
6. Smith RJ, Bale JF Jr, White KR. Sensorineural hearing loss in children. Lancet 2005;365(9462):879–90.
7. Geleoc GS, Holt JR. Sound strategies for hearing restoration. Science 2014; 344(6184):1241062.
8. Ryals BM, Rubel EW. Hair cell regeneration after acoustic trauma in adult Coturnix quail. Science 1988;240(4860):1774–6.
9. Staecker H, Kopke R, Malgrange B, et al. NT-3 and/or BDNF therapy prevents loss of auditory neurons following loss of hair cells. Neuroreport 1996;7(4): 889–94.

10. Yagi M, Magal E, Sheng Z, et al. Hair cell protection from aminoglycoside ototoxicity by adenovirus-mediated overexpression of glial cell line-derived neurotrophic factor. Hum Gene Ther 1999;10(5):813–23.

11. Yamasoba T, Nuttall AL, Harris C, et al. Role of glutathione in protection against noise-induced hearing loss. Brain Res 1998;784(1–2):82–90.

12. Yamasoba T, Schacht J, Shoji F, et al. Attenuation of cochlear damage from noise trauma by an iron chelator, a free radical scavenger and glial cell line-derived neurotrophic factor in vivo. Brain Res 1999;815(2):317–25.

13. Ylikoski J, Pirvola U, Virkkala J, et al. Guinea pig auditory neurons are protected by glial cell line-derived growth factor from degeneration after noise trauma. Hear Res 1998;124(1–2):17–26.

14. Dazert S, Battaglia A, Ryan AF. Transfection of neonatal rat cochlear cells in vitro with an adenovirus vector. Int J Dev Neurosci 1997;15(4–5):595–600.

15. Holt JR, Johns DC, Wang S, et al. Functional expression of exogenous proteins in mammalian sensory hair cells infected with adenoviral vectors. J Neurophysiol 1999;81(4):1881–8.

16. Raphael Y, Frisancho JC, Roessler BJ. Adenoviral-mediated gene transfer into guinea pig cochlear cells in vivo. Neurosci Lett 1996;207(2):137–41.

17. Han JJ, Mhatre AN, Wareing M, et al. Transgene expression in the guinea pig cochlea mediated by a lentivirus-derived gene transfer vector. Hum Gene Ther 1999;10(11):1867–73.

18. Derby ML, Sena-Esteves M, Breakefield XO, et al. Gene transfer into the mammalian inner ear using HSV-1 and vaccinia virus vectors. Hear Res 1999;134(1–2):1–8.

19. Geschwind MD, Hartnick CJ, Liu W, et al. Defective HSV-1 vector expressing BDNF in auditory ganglia elicits neurite outgrowth: model for treatment of neuron loss following cochlear degeneration. Hum Gene Ther 1996;7(2):173–82.

20. Di Pasquale G, Rzadzinska A, Schneider ME, et al. A novel bovine virus efficiently transduces inner ear neuroepithelial cells. Mol Ther 2005;11(6):849–55.

21. Ryan AF. Gene therapy of cochlear deafness: present concepts and future aspects. Basel (Switzerland); New York: Karger; 2009.

22. Kesser BW, Hashisaki GT, Fletcher K, et al. An in vitro model system to study gene therapy in the human inner ear. Gene Ther 2007;14(15):1121–31.

23. Davidson BL, Allen ED, Kozarsky KF, et al. A model system for in vivo gene transfer into the central nervous system using an adenoviral vector. Nat Genet 1993;3(3):219–23.

24. GenVec I. CGF166-hearing loss. 2015. Available at: http://www.genvec.com/product-pipeline/cgf-166-hearing-loss. Accessed February 15, 2015.

25. Harris JP, Ryan AF. Fundamental immune mechanisms of the brain and inner ear. Otolaryngol Head Neck Surg 1995;112(6):639–53.

26. Rivera T, Sanz L, Camarero G, et al. Drug delivery to the inner ear: strategies and their therapeutic implications for sensorineural hearing loss. Curr Drug Deliv 2012;9(3):231–42.

27. Carvalho GJ, Lalwani AK. The effect of cochleostomy and intracochlear infusion on auditory brain stem response threshold in the guinea pig. Am J Otol 1999;20(1):87–90.

28. Praetorius M, Baker K, Weich CM, et al. Hearing preservation after inner ear gene therapy: the effect of vector and surgical approach. ORL J Otorhinolaryngol Relat Spec 2003;65(4):211–4.

29. Jero J, Mhatre AN, Tseng CJ, et al. Cochlear gene delivery through an intact round window membrane in mouse. Hum Gene Ther 2001;12(5):539–48.

30. Wareing M, Mhatre AN, Pettis R, et al. Cationic liposome mediated transgene expression in the guinea pig cochlea. Hear Res 1999;128(1–2):61–9.

31. Wangemann P. K+ cycling and the endocochlear potential. Hear Res 2002; 165(1–2):1–9.

32. Cooper LB, Chan DK, Roediger FC, et al. AAV-mediated delivery of the caspase inhibitor XIAP protects against cisplatin ototoxicity. Otol Neurotol 2006;27(4): 484–90.

33. Lalwani AK, Han JJ, Castelein CM, et al. In vitro and in vivo assessment of the ability of adeno-associated virus-brain-derived neurotrophic factor to enhance spiral ganglion cell survival following ototoxic insult. Laryngoscope 2002; 112(8 Pt 1):1325–34.

34. Staecker H, Gabaizadeh R, Federoff H, et al. Brain-derived neurotrophic factor gene therapy prevents spiral ganglion degeneration after hair cell loss. Otolaryngol Head Neck Surg 1998;119(1):7–13.

35. Yagi M, Kanzaki S, Kawamoto K, et al. Spiral ganglion neurons are protected from degeneration by GDNF gene therapy. J Assoc Res Otolaryngol 2000; 1(4):315–25.

36. Kawamoto K, Sha SH, Minoda R, et al. Antioxidant gene therapy can protect hearing and hair cells from ototoxicity. Mol Ther 2004;9(2):173–81.

37. Kawamoto K, Yagi M, Stover T, et al. Hearing and hair cells are protected by adenoviral gene therapy with TGF-beta1 and GDNF. Mol Ther 2003;7(4): 484–92.

38. Izumikawa M, Minoda R, Kawamoto K, et al. Auditory hair cell replacement and hearing improvement by Atoh1 gene therapy in deaf mammals. Nat Med 2005; 11(3):271–6.

39. Kawamoto K, Ishimoto S, Minoda R, et al. Math1 gene transfer generates new cochlear hair cells in mature guinea pigs in vivo. J Neurosci 2003;23(11): 4395–400.

40. Suzuki M, Yagi M, Brown JN, et al. Effect of transgenic GDNF expression on gentamicin-induced cochlear and vestibular toxicity. Gene Ther 2000;7(12): 1046–54.

41. Kujawa SG, Liberman MC. Adding insult to injury: cochlear nerve degeneration after "temporary" noise-induced hearing loss. J Neurosci 2009;29(45): 14077–85.

42. Ernfors P, Van De Water T, Loring J, et al. Complementary roles of BDNF and NT-3 in vestibular and auditory development. Neuron 1995;14(6):1153–64.

43. Morrison RS, Kinoshita Y, Johnson MD, et al. Neuronal survival and cell death signaling pathways. Adv Exp Med Biol 2002;513:41–86.

44. Miller JM, Chi DH, O'Keeffe LJ, et al. Neurotrophins can enhance spiral ganglion cell survival after inner hair cell loss. Int J Dev Neurosci 1997; 15(4–5):631–43.

45. Nakaizumi T, Kawamoto K, Minoda R, et al. Adenovirus-mediated expression of brain-derived neurotrophic factor protects spiral ganglion neurons from ototoxic damage. Audiol Neurootol 2004;9(3):135–43.

46. Kuang R, Hever G, Zajic G, et al. Glial cell line-derived neurotrophic factor. Potential for otoprotection. Ann N Y Acad Sci 1999;884:270–91.

47. Kanzaki S, Stover T, Kawamoto K, et al. Glial cell line-derived neurotrophic factor and chronic electrical stimulation prevent VIII cranial nerve degeneration following denervation. J Comp Neurol 2002;454(3):350–60.

48. Collin RW, Chellappa R, Pauw RJ, et al. Missense mutations in POU4F3 cause autosomal dominant hearing impairment DFNA15 and affect subcellular localization and DNA binding. Hum Mutat 2008;29(4):545–54.

49. Lee HK, Park HJ, Lee KY, et al. A novel frameshift mutation of POU4F3 gene associated with autosomal dominant non-syndromic hearing loss. Biochem Biophys Res Commun 2010;396(3):626–30.

50. Vahava O, Morell R, Lynch ED, et al. Mutation in transcription factor POU4F3 associated with inherited progressive hearing loss in humans. Science 1998; 279(5358):1950–4.

51. Erkman L, McEvilly RJ, Luo L, et al. Role of transcription factors Brn-3.1 and Brn-3.2 in auditory and visual system development. Nature 1996;381(6583): 603–6.

52. Keithley EM, Erkman L, Bennett T, et al. Effects of a hair cell transcription factor, Brn-3.1, gene deletion on homozygous and heterozygous mouse cochleas in adulthood and aging. Hear Res 1999;134(1–2):71–6.

53. Fukui H, Wong HT, Beyer LA, et al. BDNF gene therapy induces auditory nerve survival and fiber sprouting in deaf Pou4f3 mutant mice. Sci Rep 2012;2:838.

54. Shoji F, Miller AL, Mitchell A, et al. Differential protective effects of neurotrophins in the attenuation of noise-induced hair cell loss. Hear Res 2000;146(1–2):134–42.

55. Lopez I, Honrubia V, Lee SC, et al. The protective effect of brain-derived neurotrophic factor after gentamicin ototoxicity. Am J Otol 1999;20(3):317–24.

56. Keithley EM, Ma CL, Ryan AF, et al. GDNF protects the cochlea against noise damage. Neuroreport 1998;9(10):2183–7.

57. Shoji F, Yamasoba T, Magal E, et al. Glial cell line-derived neurotrophic factor has a dose dependent influence on noise-induced hearing loss in the guinea pig cochlea. Hear Res 2000;142(1–2):41–55.

58. Kopke R, Allen KA, Henderson D, et al. A radical demise. Toxins and trauma share common pathways in hair cell death. Ann N Y Acad Sci 1999;884:171–91.

59. Hashimoto T, Gibbs D, Lillo C, et al. Lentiviral gene replacement therapy of retinas in a mouse model for Usher syndrome type 1B. Gene Ther 2007;14(7): 584–94.

60. Lopes VS, Williams DS. Gene therapy for the retinal degeneration of Usher syndrome caused by mutations in MYO7A [review]. Cold Spring Harb Perspect Med 2015;5(6).

61. Lentz JJ, Jodelka FM, Hinrich AJ, et al. Rescue of hearing and vestibular function by antisense oligonucleotides in a mouse model of human deafness. Nat Med 2013;19(3):345–50.

62. Van Camp G, Smith RJ. Hereditary hearing loss: nonsyndromic genes. 2015. Available at: http://hereditaryhearingloss.org/main.aspx?c=.HHH&n=86307. Accessed July 13, 2015.

63. Dahl E, Manthey D, Chen Y, et al. Molecular cloning and functional expression of mouse connexin-30, a gap junction gene highly expressed in adult brain and skin. J Biol Chem 1996;271(30):17903–10.

64. del Castillo I, Villamar M, Moreno-Pelayo MA, et al. A deletion involving the connexin 30 gene in nonsyndromic hearing impairment. N Engl J Med 2002; 346(4):243–9.

65. Hand GM, Muller DJ, Nicholson BJ, et al. Isolation and characterization of gap junctions from tissue culture cells. J Mol Biol 2002;315(4):587–600.

66. Kikuchi T, Adams JC, Miyabe Y, et al. Potassium ion recycling pathway via gap junction systems in the mammalian cochlea and its interruption in hereditary nonsyndromic deafness. Med Electron Microsc 2000;33(2):51–6.

67. Rabionet R, Gasparini P, Estivill X. Molecular genetics of hearing impairment due to mutations in gap junction genes encoding beta connexins. Hum Mutat 2000;16(3):190–202.

68. Crispino G, Di Pasquale G, Scimemi P, et al. BAAV mediated GJB2 gene transfer restores gap junction coupling in cochlear organotypic cultures from deaf Cx26Sox10Cre mice. PLoS One 2011;6(8):e23279.

69. Yu Q, Wang Y, Chang Q, et al. Virally expressed connexin26 restores gap junction function in the cochlea of conditional Gjb2 knockout mice. Gene Ther 2014; 21(1):71–80.

70. Bermingham NA, Hassan BA, Price SD, et al. Math1: an essential gene for the generation of inner ear hair cells. Science 1999;284(5421):1837–41.

71. Rubel EW, Furrer SA, Stone JS. A brief history of hair cell regeneration research and speculations on the future. Hear Res 2013;297:42–51.

72. Zheng JL, Gao WQ. Overexpression of Math1 induces robust production of extra hair cells in postnatal rat inner ears. Nat Neurosci 2000;3(6):580–6.

73. Shou J, Zheng JL, Gao WQ. Robust generation of new hair cells in the mature mammalian inner ear by adenoviral expression of Hath1. Mol Cell Neurosci 2003;23(2):169–79.

74. Gubbels SP, Woessner DW, Mitchell JC, et al. Functional auditory hair cells produced in the mammalian cochlea by in utero gene transfer. Nature 2008; 455(7212):537–41.

75. Staecker H, Praetorius M, Baker K, et al. Vestibular hair cell regeneration and restoration of balance function induced by math1 gene transfer. Otol Neurotol 2007;28(2):223–31.

76. Yang SM, Chen W, Guo WW, et al. Regeneration of stereocilia of hair cells by forced Atoh1 expression in the adult mammalian cochlea. PLoS One 2012;7(9):e46355.

77. Hannon GJ. RNA interference. Nature 2002;418(6894):244–51.

78. Crooke ST. Progress in antisense technology. Annu Rev Med 2004;55:61–95.

79. Bermingham-McDonogh O, Reh TA. Regulated reprogramming in the regeneration of sensory receptor cells. Neuron 2011;71(3):389–405.

80. Bitner-Glindzicz M, Lindley KJ, Rutland P, et al. A recessive contiguous gene deletion causing infantile hyperinsulinism, enteropathy and deafness identifies the Usher type 1C gene. Nat Genet 2000;26(1):56–60.

81. Lentz JJ, Gordon WC, Farris HE, et al. Deafness and retinal degeneration in a novel USH1C knock-in mouse model. Dev Neurobiol 2010;70(4):253–67.

82. Michalski N, Michel V, Caberlotto E, et al. Harmonin-b, an actin-binding scaffold protein, is involved in the adaptation of mechanoelectrical transduction by sensory hair cells. Pflugers Arch 2009;459(1):115–30.

83. Verpy E, Leibovici M, Zwaenepoel I, et al. A defect in harmonin, a PDZ domain-containing protein expressed in the inner ear sensory hair cells, underlies Usher syndrome type 1C. Nat Genet 2000;26(1):51–5.

84. Chen W, Johnson SL, Marcotti W, et al. Human fetal auditory stem cells can be expanded in vitro and differentiate into functional auditory neurons and hair cell-like cells. Stem Cells 2009;27(5):1196–204.

85. Coleman B, Hardman J, Coco A, et al. Fate of embryonic stem cells transplanted into the deafened mammalian cochlea. Cell Transpl 2006;15(5):369–80.

86. Iguchi F, Nakagawa T, Tateya I, et al. Surgical techniques for cell transplantation into the mouse cochlea. Acta Otolaryngol Suppl 2004;551:43–7.

87. Sakamoto T, Nakagawa T, Endo T, et al. Fates of mouse embryonic stem cells transplanted into the inner ears of adult mice and embryonic chickens. Acta Otolaryngol Suppl 2004;551:48–52.

88. Tateya I, Nakagawa T, Iguchi F, et al. Fate of neural stem cells grafted into injured inner ears of mice. Neuroreport 2003;14(13):1677–81.

89. Sekiya T, Kojima K, Matsumoto M, et al. Cell transplantation to the auditory nerve and cochlear duct. Exp Neurol 2006;198(1):12–24.

90. Tamura T, Nakagawa T, Iguchi F, et al. Transplantation of neural stem cells into the modiolus of mouse cochleae injured by cisplatin. Acta Otolaryngol Suppl 2004;551:65–8.

91. Hu Z, Wei D, Johansson CB, et al. Survival and neural differentiation of adult neural stem cells transplanted into the mature inner ear. Exp Cell Res 2005; 302(1):40–7.

92. Li H, Roblin G, Liu H, et al. Generation of hair cells by stepwise differentiation of embryonic stem cells. Proc Natl Acad Sci U S A 2003;100(23):13495–500.

93. Oshima K, Shin K, Diensthuber M, et al. Mechanosensitive hair cell-like cells from embryonic and induced pluripotent stem cells. Cell 2010;141(4): 704–16.

94. Geleoc GS, Risner JR, Holt JR. Developmental acquisition of voltage-dependent conductances and sensory signaling in hair cells of the embryonic mouse inner ear. J Neurosci 2004;24(49):11148–59.

95. Koehler KR, Mikosz AM, Molosh AI, et al. Generation of inner ear sensory epithelia from pluripotent stem cells in 3D culture. Nature 2013;500(7461): 217–21.

96. Koehler KR, Hashino E. 3D mouse embryonic stem cell culture for generating inner ear organoids. Nat Protoc 2014;9(6):1229–44.

97. Shi F, Kempfle JS, Edge AS. Wnt-responsive Lgr5-expressing stem cells are hair cell progenitors in the cochlea. J Neurosci 2012;32(28):9639–48.

98. Wei D, Levic S, Nie L, et al. Cells of adult brain germinal zone have properties akin to hair cells and can be used to replace inner ear sensory cells after damage. Proc Natl Acad Sci U S A 2008;105(52):21000–5.

99. Chen W, Jongkamonwiwat N, Abbas L, et al. Restoration of auditory evoked responses by human ES-cell-derived otic progenitors. Nature 2012;490(7419): 278–82.

100. Shi F, Corrales CE, Liberman MC, et al. BMP4 induction of sensory neurons from human embryonic stem cells and reinnervation of sensory epithelium. Eur J Neurosci 2007;26(11):3016–23.

101. Kondo T, Sheets PL, Zopf DA, et al. Tlx3 exerts context-dependent transcriptional regulation and promotes neuronal differentiation from embryonic stem cells. Proc Natl Acad Sci U S A 2008;105(15):5780–5.

102. Reyes JH, O'Shea KS, Wys NL, et al. Glutamatergic neuronal differentiation of mouse embryonic stem cells after transient expression of neurogenin 1 and treatment with BDNF and GDNF: in vitro and in vivo studies. J Neurosci 2008; 28(48):12622–31.

103. Corrales CE, Pan L, Li H, et al. Engraftment and differentiation of embryonic stem cell-derived neural progenitor cells in the cochlear nerve trunk: growth of processes into the organ of Corti. J Neurobiol 2006;66(13):1489–500.

104. Sheffield AM, Gubbels SP, Hildebrand MS, et al. Viral vector tropism for supporting cells in the developing murine cochlea. Hear Res 2011;277(1–2):28–36.

105. Pinyon JL, Tadros SF, Froud KE, et al. Close-field electroporation gene delivery using the cochlear implant electrode array enhances the bionic ear. Sci Transl Med 2014;6(233):233ra254.

106. Zou B, Mittal R, Grati M, et al. The application of genome editing in studying hearing loss. Hear Res 2015;327:102–8.

Index

Note: Page numbers of article titles are in **boldface** type.

Otolaryngol Clin N Am 48 (2015) 1167–1174
http://dx.doi.org/10.1016/S0030-6665(15)00187-5
0030-6665/15/$ – see front matter © 2015 Elsevier Inc. All rights reserved.

United States Postal Service

Statement of Ownership, Management, and Circulation
(All Periodicals Publications Except Requester Publications)

1. Publication Title
Otolaryngologic Clinics of North America

2. Publication Number
4 6 6 - 5 5 5 0

3. Filing Date
9/18/15

4. Issue Frequency
Feb, Apr, Jun, Aug, Oct, Dec

5. Number of Issues Published Annually
6

6. Annual Subscription Price
$310.00

7. Complete Mailing Address of Known Office of Publication (Not printer) (Street, city, county, state, and ZIP+4®)
Elsevier Inc.
360 Park Avenue South
New York, NY 10010-1710

Contact Person
Stephen R. Bushing

Telephone (Include area code)
215-239-3688

8. Complete Mailing Address of Headquarters or General Business Office of Publisher (Not printer)
Elsevier Inc., 360 Park Avenue South, New York, NY 10010-1710

9. Full Names and Complete Mailing Addresses of Publisher, Editor, and Managing Editor (Do not leave blank)

Publisher (Name and complete mailing address)
Linda Belfus, Elsevier Inc., 1600 John F. Kennedy Blvd., Ste. 1800, Philadelphia, PA 19103-2899

Editor (Name and complete mailing address)
Jessica McCool, Elsevier Inc., 1600 John F. Kennedy Blvd., Ste. 1800, Philadelphia, PA 19103-2899

Managing Editor (Name and complete mailing address)
Adrianne Brigido, Elsevier Inc., 1600 John F. Kennedy Blvd., Ste. 1800, Philadelphia, PA 19103-2899

10. Owner (Do not leave blank. If the publication is owned by a corporation, give the name and address of the corporation immediately followed by the names and addresses of all stockholders owning or holding 1 percent or more of the total amount of stock. If not owned by a corporation, give the names and addresses of the individual owners. If owned by a partnership or other unincorporated firm, give its name and address as well as those of each individual owner. If the publication is published by a nonprofit organization, give its name and address.)

Full Name	Complete Mailing Address
Wholly owned subsidiary of	1500 John F. Kennedy Blvd., Ste. 1800
Reed/Elsevier, US holdings	Philadelphia, PA 19103-2899

11. Known Bondholders, Mortgagees, and Other Security Holders Owning or Holding 1 Percent or More of Total Amount of Bonds, Mortgages, or Other Securities. If none, check box ☐ None

Full Name	Complete Mailing Address
N/A	

12. Tax Status (For completion by nonprofit organizations authorized to mail at nonprofit rates) (Check one)
The purpose, function, and nonprofit status of this organization and the exempt status for federal income tax purposes:
☐ Has Not Changed During Preceding 12 Months
☐ Has Changed During Preceding 12 Months (Publisher must submit explanation of change with this statement)

13. Publication Title
Otolaryngologic Clinics of North America

14. Issue Date for Circulation Data Below
August 2015

PS Form 3526, July 2014 (Page 1 of 3 (Instructions Page 3)) PSN 7530-01-000-9931 **PRIVACY NOTICE:** See our Privacy policy in www.usps.com

---

15. Extent and Nature of Circulation

			Average No. Copies Each Issue During Preceding 12 Months	No. Copies of Single Issue Published Nearest to Filing Date
a. Total Number of Copies (Net press run)			1060	884
b. Legitimate Paid and/or Requested Distribution (By Mail and Outside the Mail)	(1)	Mailed Outside-County Paid/Requested Mail Subscriptions stated on PS Form 3541. (Include paid distribution above nominal rate, advertiser's proof copies and exchange copies)	504	340
	(2)	Mailed In-County Paid/Requested Mail Subscriptions stated on PS Form 3541. (Include paid distribution above nominal rate, advertiser's proof copies and exchange copies)		
	(3)	Paid Distribution Outside the Mails Including Sales Through Dealers And Carriers, Street Vendors, Counter Sales, and Other Paid Distribution Outside USPS®	245	302
	(4)	Paid Distribution by Other Classes of Mail Through the USPS (e.g. First-Class Mail®)		
c. Total Paid and/or Requested Circulation (Sum of 15b (1), (2), (3), and (4))		►	749	642
d. Free or Nominal Rate Distribution (By Mail and Outside the Mail)	(1)	Free or Nominal Rate Outside-County Copies included on PS Form 3541	28	26
	(2)	Free or Nominal Rate In-County Copies included on PS Form 3541		
	(3)	Free or Nominal Rate Copies mailed at Other classes Through the USPS (e.g. First-Class Mail®)		
	(4)	Free or Nominal Rate Distribution Outside the Mail (Carriers or Other means)		
e. Total Nonrequested Distribution (Sum of 15d (1), (2), (3) and (4))		►	28	26
f. Total Distribution (Sum of 15c and 15e)		►	777	668
g. Copies not Distributed (See instructions to publishers #4 (page 83))		►	283	216
h. Total (Sum of 15f and g)		►	1060	884
i. Percent Paid and/or Requested Circulation (15c divided by 15f times 100)		►	96.40%	96.11%

* If you are claiming electronic copies go to line 16 on page 3. If you are not claiming Electronic copies, skip to line 17 on page 3.

16. Electronic Copy Circulation	Average No. Copies Each Issue During Preceding 12 Months	No. Copies of Single Issue Published Nearest to Filing Date
a. Paid Electronic Copies		
b. Total paid Print Copies (Line 15c) + Paid Electronic copies (Line 16a)		
c. Total Print Distribution (Line 15f) + Paid Electronic Copies (Line 16a)		
d. Percent Paid (Both Print & Electronic copies) (16b divided by 16c X 100)		

☐ **I certify that 50% of all my distributed copies (electronic and print) are paid above a nominal price**

17. Publication of Statement of Ownership.
If the publication is a general publication, publication of this statement is required. Will be printed in the _December 2015_ issue of this publication.

18. Signature and Title of Editor, Publisher, Business Manager, or Owner

Stephen R. Bushing – Inventory Distribution Coordinator

Date September 18, 2015

I certify that all information furnished on this form is true and complete. I understand that anyone who furnishes false or misleading information on this form or who omits material or information requested on the form may be subject to criminal sanctions (including fines and imprisonment) and/or civil sanctions (including civil penalties).

PS Form 3526, July 2014 (Page 3 of 3)

Moving?

Make sure your subscription moves with you!

To notify us of your new address, find your **Clinics Account Number** (located on your mailing label above your name), and contact customer service at:

Email: journalscustomerservice-usa@elsevier.com

800-654-2452 (subscribers in the U.S. & Canada)
314-447-8871 (subscribers outside of the U.S. & Canada)

Fax number: 314-447-8029

Elsevier Health Sciences Division
Subscription Customer Service
3251 Riverport Lane
Maryland Heights, MO 63043

*To ensure uninterrupted delivery of your subscription, please notify us at least 4 weeks in advance of move.

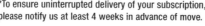

Printed and bound by CPI Group (UK) Ltd, Croydon, CR0 4YY

03/10/2024

01040497-0010